Running for the Average Joe

Fourth Edition

Bill Watts, NASM-CPT

Foreword by Marshall Ulrich

Edited by Kristen Bashaw

*Watts*Running

Please leave a review at
www.wattsrunning.com/reviews

Printed in the United States of America

The publisher makes every effort to use acid-free ∞, recycled paper ♻.

ISBN 978-0-9987261-0-6 Hard Cover $39.95 USD
ISBN 978-0-9987261-9-9 Paperback $29.95 USD
ISBN 978-0-692-63752-4 eBook $ 9.99 USD

4 6 8 10 9 7 5   Paperback, Hard Cover, eBook

WattsRunning Website   **WattsRunning Facebook Page**

AverageJoe Publishing

DEDICATION

This book is dedicated to my father, Gordon "Fuzz" Watts, whom I barely knew, but was, and always will be, my idol. As a friend to all, a coach, and a master motivator, he's the only one I knew that could persuade a penguin to fly.

To my mother Bonnie, who has always been there for me, and believed that I could do improbable, if not impossible things.

To my friend Keith Panzer, who somehow convinced me that I could run a marathon before I ran a single lap around the local track.

To ultra-runner Marshall Ulrich, for motivating me and thousands of other runners all around the world.

To the "average Joes" of the world, acknowledging their efforts, choices and commitments to living happier and healthier lives.

CONTENTS

FOREWORD

Running for the Average Joe

Another tall, thin, fit-looking guy walked up to me and I thought, "he looks like a runner," which wasn't unusual since I was at a marathon expo in Fort Collins, CO, selling my book *Running on Empty*, a memoir driven by the story of my record-setting run across America in 2008. But, as my wife reminds me, "Everyone has a story," and Bill Watts had come a long way, physically and psychologically, to look the part of a marathon runner at that race expo in 2011. Bill was humble and easy-going, despite the fact that he's an extremely intelligent and focused guy – qualities that have brought him success as an IT systems engineer (I can barely keep my computer running!), as well as a runner.

As we chatted, I shared some of my story: How I had started running back in 1979 as a way to manage the stress and resulting high blood pressure, from watching my first wife die of breast cancer. How I continued running, emotionally empty for almost 30 years, completing what I called the Triple Crown of Extreme Sports: over 125 running races averaging over 125 miles each; completing 12 expedition-length adventure races, including being one of only three people in the world to compete in all nine Eco Challenge races; and climbing the Seven Summits, including Mount Everest, all on first attempts (the mountain gods were kind to me!). Listening to Bill, I began to realize that he was a true student of the wonderful sport of running, as well as a runner extraordinaire in his own right. Despite decades of running, I realized I could learn stuff from this guy!

If I had met Bill back in 2001, I wouldn't have thought he looked like a runner at all, because he didn't. He weighed almost 200 pounds and suffered from high blood pressure and high cholesterol. Literally fearing for his life, he started running. Actually, he made a *lifestyle* change. He didn't want to be part of a fad, or simply look for a quick fix; he wanted to get in shape, and *stay* in shape... for a lifetime. He made the commitment, but when he looked for information about how running could help him keep his commitment, he found books for people that were already runners, not "average Joes" like him. He found books for people who could already run, say, "a tempo run at a 5:00-minute mile pace" – not someone like him who couldn't even run half a lap around a track! As the years went by, and Bill started competing in 5k and 10k races, then marathons and beyond, he continued to think about those running books – written for runners, and written only about running. He wished there was a book that covered all aspects of a lifestyle change, from psychology, to physiology, to nutrition; not just running and training plans. He wanted a book that would truly help others get in shape and stay in shape. To fill the void and help others, he started researching and writing *Running for the Average Joe*.

Having been a runner for over 37 years, I thought I knew a lot about running. But Bill has taken every aspect of running, physiologically and mentally, then dissected it, examined it, and related it to us in a useful way. He helped me to understand terminology that scientists and nutritionists use, that frankly, didn't make sense until Bill explained the how and why. The depth and breadth of the research is astounding – although I should have known to expect nothing less, knowing Bill's intelligence, focus, and attention to detail. This book is by far the best researched and most comprehensive yet written, by a very talented man who has the ability to explain complex topics in simple and always understandable language.

Average Joe is masterfully written, with personal stories from his own experience that will take you step by step through your own transformation. Packed with tips and suggestions, motivational quotes, mantras and challenges, this book will help you along through running *and* in life. You'll learn so much from this book, which I call the "A to Z Runner's Bible."

A labor of love fueled by years of running and research, Bill thoroughly addresses running in history, mind, body and soul. You'll find out how to take that initial first step (the most difficult) and how to maintain a style of living that we all deserve. You'll learn what equipment you need, how to build strength and conditioning through running and cross-training, how to handle injuries, and what to eat. Knowing that what you really need is *lifestyle change*, this book will take you on a journey with an emphasis on improving mental and physical health by setting and achieving your goals... and how to go beyond.

When Bill contacted me recently, asking me to write the foreword to his book, I thought back to our conversation at the marathon expo and remembered, "I could learn stuff from this guy." Little did I know how much I could learn! *Running for the Average Joe* is absolutely the most comprehensive running book – no, the most comprehensive book *on how to make a lifestyle change* – that I have ever read – and I've read more than a few! I invite and encourage you to delve into this book. But be careful, as you will get more than you bargained for. While it is a handbook chock full of information about running that you'll want to reference well into the future, *"Running for the Average Joe"* is really a book that can teach you how to enjoy a better life.

Marshall Ulrich

Extreme athlete and best-selling author of *Running on Empty, An Ultramarathoner's Story of Love, Loss, and a Record-Setting Run Across America*

Evergreen, Colorado, May 2016

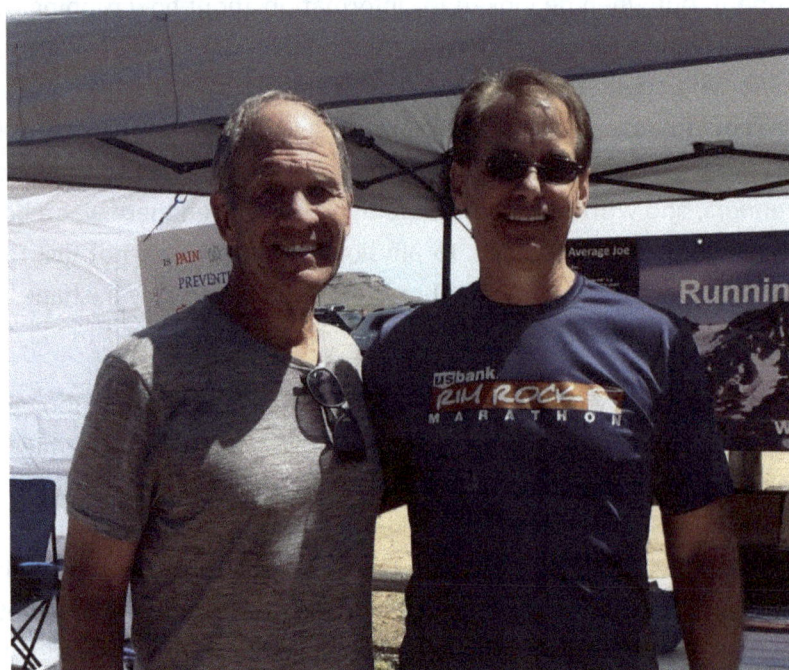

Ulrich and Watts at the 2018 Greenland 50k Ultra

PREFACE

While there are many good books about running, many of them seem to focus on the elite athletes, the gifted and talented runners of our time. This book was written for the rest of us, the "average Joes."

Running for the Average Joe

"Live to run, run to live..."

Prologue

For every story of running success, there seems to be one of failure. Running is difficult, especially when you're just beginning your running program. As with any success in life, you must begin with a *commitment* – and as many runners can attest, the most difficult step is the first one.

At some point in one's life, whether for health and fitness reasons or for less obvious ones, a decision is made to exercise or not to exercise; a decision is made to try a new diet plan or to avoid one altogether; a decision is made to monitor and manage your health, or to ignore it.

These decisions can be the by-product of an accumulation of events or they can be a "spur of the moment" choice. They can be based on personal decisions, peer pressure, advice from a doctor or a myriad of other reasons. Sometimes these choices are difficult and sometimes they make absolute sense, giving no reason to question them. For myself, after enjoying a relatively healthy childhood and adult life, I was suddenly confronted with what seemed to be a simple choice: life or death.

That may seem extreme and dramatic for many, but for me, it was as real as the air we breathe. Sure, I could have ignored the signs, but that's not the way I'm wired. By trade, I am a computer systems engineer and I MUST know how things work. The analogies I could conjure up in my technical thinking transitioned perfectly into what I thought about my health. I knew the data I saw in my charts were off kilter, but I also realized I had the choice to fix it.

So, I made the *commitment* – the leap of faith to better health – physically, mentally and emotionally. I made the *choice* for better health. To me, this choice was easy; however, I soon found out that the path itself was not so easy. I debated internally whether or not I could actually become healthy again, or if I even wanted to. After all, I was reaching the waning years of human health – why fight it?

Logically, there seemed to be only one choice, and that choice pushed me into a whole new realm of anatomical awareness and discovery. I soon found that this significant, solitary choice opened door after door of new opportunities, successes, and sometimes, failures.

January 2002

After being promoted to a supervisory role in my place of business, I found that in nine short months I was completely stressed, I couldn't sleep, and I felt like I couldn't eat, despite gaining over 30 pounds in such a short time.

My problems seemed miniscule, however, as our great country was still reeling from the attacks on the World Trade Center, the Pentagon, and Flight 93. The war in Afghanistan was intensifying and our soldiers were dying. My issues didn't compare to the constant rising costs of commodities and a host of other international, cultural, financial and world-health problems.

I knew I couldn't do much about the attacks on American soil; I couldn't fix Wall Street and all its schemes and uncertainty, and I definitely couldn't cure the world's diseases. Nonetheless, I knew that I could try to alter my rapidly deteriorating health. It was something that I made a *choice* to do and I fully *committed* to that choice.

Back in 2002, my LDL (bad) cholesterol had climbed to 212 and should have been below 100. My blood pressure was 154 over 110 when I woke up in the morning and my heart rate was around 90 beats per minute. I was barely able to walk the four flights of stairs at my job without feeling dizzy. And I was just 44 years old.

Every health indicator and blood level I had seemed to be threatening and uncontrolled. I was weighing in at more than 200 pounds, on a frame that was meant to hold significantly less. People said that I looked great as I was able to hide my weight with the clothes I wore, but I certainly didn't feel great. On the inside was a growing beast that was taking over my body – and my life....

As most people do with diet plans, they like to start with a "New Year's Resolution." And why not? It's a great time to put the holidays behind you and your best foot forward, no matter what your goal is. I decided to set my resolution, but unlike others who had failed before me, I was determined to be steadfast and successful.

On January 1st of 2002, I hit the scale at 199.5 pounds, up some thirty-two pounds from just a few months earlier. That was the last time I weighed myself and am certain I was closer to 210 pounds. In retrospect, I should have seen the signs. I didn't think twice when I gained eight pounds in September of 2001, acknowledging the fact that summer was coming to a close and my activities were slowing down. In October, and without fully realizing it, I gained another eight or nine pounds. Then came November and December and all of the holiday festivities. Surprisingly, I gained another ten pounds. How quickly it crept up on me. By disregarding my health and habits, whether deliberate or not, I suddenly added on more weight than I had realized. How could this happen? How could this happen to *me*?

At that point, it didn't matter. It happened, and I was solely responsible for it. Luckily, my co-worker, Keith, got me interested in running. Keith is a great friend and mentor, and he encouraged me (and sometimes tricked me) into things I never thought conceivable. Keith had well over 100 marathons under his belt and he was experienced at all of the popular race distances. He urged me to take a few laps around the track to get things going. That shouldn't be a problem – or so I thought. I immediately went to the local track and attempted to run my first lap. I was only able to jog half way around without gasping for air and having the sensation that I would black out with the very next step.

I went home that night dejected but not defeated. I vowed to go back the next night, and the next, and the night after that. During the first couple of weeks of that exceptionally cold winter, I lost a few pounds, but I really thought they would come off more quickly. Still, I was determined, so I began researching some popular diet plans.

Eventually, I tried the Atkins Diet, the South Beach Diet, vegetarian and vegan diets, and my own "custom" diet plans – such as not eating at all during the day – only to gorge myself later in the evening. For obvious reasons, my custom diet did not work. I finally established a diet plan that I DO NOT, and WOULD NOT recommend to anyone. It could not have been healthy and it undoubtedly didn't satisfy me. But it was effective, at first anyway. For breakfast, I drank a can of Ensure®, Boost® or SlimFast® as I was convinced I'd get my minimum daily requirements from these vitamin-loaded beverages. Mid-morning, I ate an apple, orange, or banana. For lunch, I popped up a 3.5-ounce bag of unsalted, unbuttered popcorn. I'm convinced that there were few health benefits, if any, but it made me feel "full" until dinner time, when I would devour a regular meal.

In early February, I lost about seven pounds and was able to jog two complete laps around the track. By the middle of February, another eight pounds were shed and I was able to run one mile without stopping!

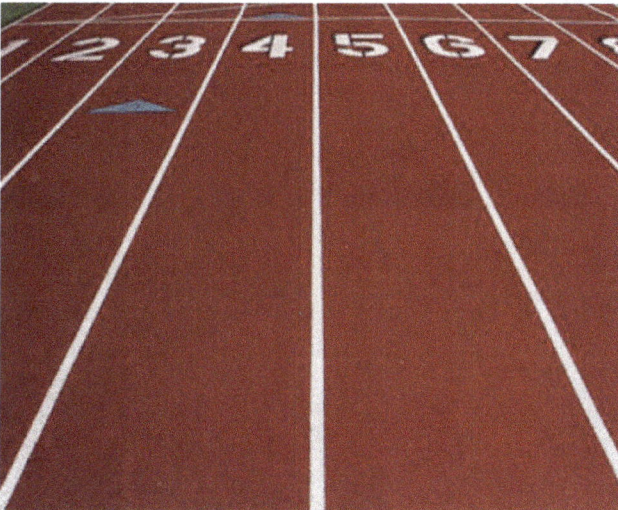

The month of March arrived and I plummeted another ten pounds. My running had increased to three or four miles at the track, but now I had a new problem. The diet plan I was on hadn't changed, and while I was losing a significant amount of weight, I was also losing valuable strength. Ultimately, I decided to trade the mid-morning fruit and popcorn for a lunchtime veggie sandwich from the local Subway® restaurant. My weight soon stabilized and I noticed a physical change in my appearance for the first time in nearly a year.

I was becoming leaner but more importantly, I was beginning to *feel* better. I soon discovered that my blood pressure was "down" to 146 over 90 – not great by common health standards but certainly a substantial drop from six months earlier. I scheduled a physical with my doctor and the results were positive and conclusive.

Remarkably, my LDL (bad) cholesterol had plunged from 212 to 95. My resting heart rate was at a comfortable 65 beats per minute, previously at 90 beats per minute. Today, as I write this after several years of a life-changing commitment, my normal blood pressure registers 110 over 63 with a resting heart rate of 46. My LDL cholesterol averages around 84.

So convinced that I was becoming stronger, lighter and healthier, I continued to run, and ultimately entered the BolderBOULDER 10k race. At the time, I wasn't sure if I could even run 6.2 miles, but the pre-registration into the race forced my motivation. Keith also told me I could go the distance; therefore, it must be true. The race was scheduled for Memorial Day, as it always is, and come Hell or high water, I was going to run it.

I vaguely remember that first race in May of 2002, with all of the hype, race day tensions and confusion that can accompany a first-time runner. I finished at a pace that I was satisfied with, but more importantly, I showed up at the start line having lost 31 pounds in just five months.

From there, my obsession for running had taken a firm hold on me. Since then, I've competed in some 350 races, with more than 100 marathons, 60 half marathons and all of the distances between 5k and 50-mile ultramarathons. I estimate that I've run about 6,700 race miles and 73,000 training miles since 2002. According to my calculations, I've burned more than ten million calories and climbed more than six million feet of elevation gain while going through about one hundred and thirty pairs of shoes. The numbers may seem staggering, but to me, I'm still an "average Joe." I believe that anyone without debilitating handicaps or injuries can do this too.

That's how I got into running, but enough about me. What motivates you? Are you willing to make the *choices* and *commitments*? If so, let's get out the door and put one foot in front of the other.

My Story

Throughout this book, I'll include "My Story" snippets. Watch for these sections, and I'll share my own personal experiences and perspectives with you.

Tip

Watch for my tips and suggestions throughout this book. These tidbits of advice may help you as they have helped me!

Motivation

Quotes and mantras, from professional athletes, politicians and "average Joes," to get you going and keep you going!

Challenge!

I'll create a "challenge" at the end of most chapters that will help you by allowing you to experience what you read in this book. All of the "challenges" will help you with your end goal – enjoying a happy and healthy lifestyle.

Chapter 1 - Getting Started

The question always beckons: Who *should* run and who *should not* run? There are no facts in my response to these questions, only feelings and beliefs. So here is my non-scientific belief: I feel that anyone who has enough coordination, balance, pain tolerance and determination can run. This includes people who have had chronic problems, whether real or perceived, and people who have handicaps such as blindness and partial loss of limb(s). Most of all, it includes normal, able-bodied people who may not have taken the opportunity to run. People like you and me: *"Average Joes."*

So how does one get started running? You may have many reasons to get started, or it may be that you simply want to try it. The health benefits are numerous, well documented and proven. In most cases, running will improve your overall health, decrease your health risks and possibly add years to your life. Of course, you should always consult your doctor and submit to a full physical evaluation before you start your training.

You may be new to the sport, or you may be returning after an absence from the sport. Either way, it can lead to a happier and healthier lifestyle.

The Coach in Me

My father was a math teacher and high school football coach, amassing a phenomenal record of high performers, both in the classroom and on the gridiron. Apparently, I inherited that "gene" with a desire to share the knowledge I've obtained over the years.

I am a Certified Personal Trainer, receiving my accreditation from the National Academy of Sports Medicine (NASM-CPT). In this book however, I'll refer to myself as simply an "average Joe." I am a person who realizes that all of us have some personal or physical constraints, but from a mental perspective, I also believe in ultra-runner Marshall Ulrich's statement: "The only limitations are in your mind." (I'll tell you more about Marshall and other running legends later in Chapter Four.) Suffice to say, I think I have enough personal training and real life "average Joe" experience to get you out the door and down the road.

Get Started Today!

Some people will never enter a race. Some will run around the local track, and some will run multistage events across all seven continents. It all comes down to your choices and the benefits and thrills you get from your running, jogging or walking. It doesn't matter how far or how fast you go. What matters is that you *enjoy* your experiences. Running has few boundaries – you can run indoors or outdoors. You can run just about any time of the day or night, and with the right gear, any time of the year.

I'd like to share my experiences as the "average Joe" and hope that you adopt and adapt some of my philosophies and visions.

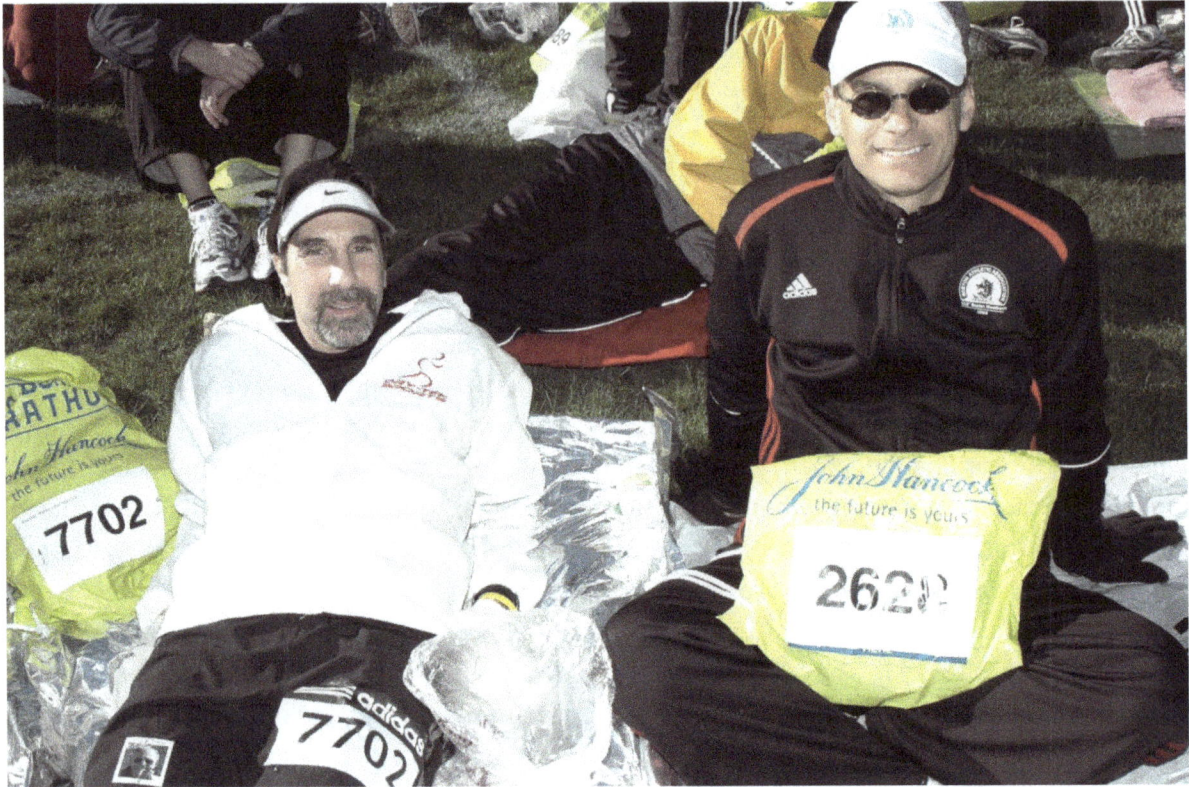

Relaxing with Keith Panzer (#7702), friend and mentor before the start of the 2010 Boston Marathon

Motivation

"I find that the harder I work, the more luck I seem to have." – *Thomas Jefferson*

Challenge!

In the prologue, I described myself as a person who was struggling with increasing weight and declining health. When I finally accepted these facts, I immediately challenged myself to take a realistic view of my entire well-being.

How do you perceive yourself? Are you as fit as you want to be? Do you need to make minor adjustments or wholesale changes to your life? Whatever your answer is, look in the mirror and *challenge* yourself to a happier and healthier lifestyle. Turn the page to the next chapter and let's begin this journey together, shall we?

Chapter 2 – History of Running

It is generally assumed that Homo sapiens developed the ability to run long distances about 200,000 years ago in an attempt to hunt for animals and to provide food and clothing for themselves. Early man was so adept in this skill, that he was able to out-distance or simply "wear out" his prey. Even though man is not the fastest mammal, he certainly has the most endurance. It's said that a man can outrun a horse in a 25-mile foot race and one of the primary reasons is the human's ability to cool the body by sweating and dispersing the heat. No other mammal has such an efficient cooling system as ours, thus cannot endure a sustained cadence as long as we can.

Although hunting was the primary reason for early man's adaptation to running, he most likely had to use running for a means of escape as well. As man developed, his running became more efficient and eventually he used his running for sport and competition.

Many incorrectly assume that the Greeks may have started competitive running and sports with the Olympic Games, but early history shows us that it actually dates back to the Tailteann Games in Ireland nearly 4,000 years ago.

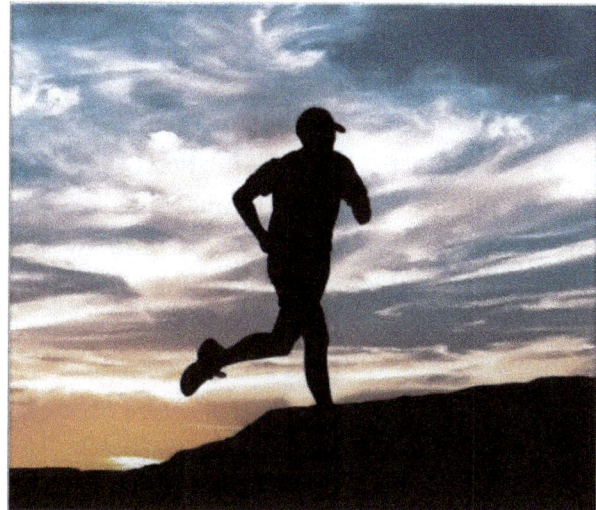

The Tailteann Games took place during the last two weeks of each July, at the end of the harvest season. The games included three functions: honoring the dead, proclaiming laws, and the games and festivities. They would sing songs in memory of the dead for several days, followed by laying down new laws and truces to the people. When these functions were complete, they would begin the physical and mental games that included running, chariot races, horse riding competition, archery, swimming, hand to hand combat, and sword fighting. Other less physical competitions included story-telling, singing and dancing, along with fine arts competitions for the local craftsmen and women of the time.

Motivation

"Out on the roads, there is fitness and self-discovery and the persons we were destined to be."
– George Sheehan

Early Olympic Games

Nearly 1,000 years later, in 776 BC, the Greeks held the first "Olympic Games." This was a series of athletic games and competitions to honor the Greek god Zeus and took place every *Olympiad*, or every four years. Even during times of war and political unrest, an "Olympic Truce" was put in place to allow safe passage for the athletes and contestants to travel from their home or region, to the Olympic host location. This truce was quite remarkable for its time. The roots of the Olympic Games originated in Olympia, Greece, and featured annual foot races in a competition to give the title of "priestess for Hera, the Greek goddess" – to the "chosen" females. By the fifth and fourth centuries, however, the competition was limited only to male competitors.

Back in 776 BC, the only running competition held was the *stadion* race, a foot race roughly 190 meters long. The word *stadium* is derived from this foot race. These games continued until AD 394, when the games were abolished by emperor Theodosius I, as part of his tactics to force Christianity and remove all pagan events throughout the Roman Empire. Despite his best efforts, archeological records indicate that "the games went on."

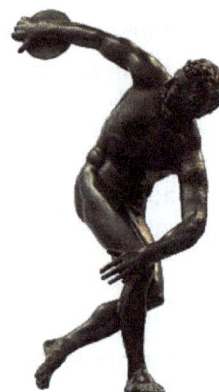

Pheidippides, *pronounced: "fahy-**dip**-i-deez"*

No running book would be complete without the inclusion of Pheidippides, the ancient Greek hemerodrome (rough translation "day-runner"). This folk hero lived between 530 BC and 490 BC and is said to have been labeled as a "long running courier" or "day long runner." The story tells us that Pheidippides was sent to Sparta to ask for military assistance when the Persians came ashore in Marathon, Greece.

According to lore, he ran nearly 150 miles (240 kilometers) in just two days. He then ran an additional 25 miles from the Marathon battlefield to Athens, Greece, with news of the battle. "We have won," he announced, only to collapse and die from his laborious effort. Since 1983 there has been an annual footrace from Athens to Sparta, known as the Spartathlon. This race commemorates Pheidippides's historical run of over 240 kilometers of Greek countryside.

Later on, when you're training for your first marathon, you'll know the history of Pheidippides and how the name "Marathon" originated!

There have been several variations of the official length of the Marathon. In the beginning, it was approximately 25 miles (40 km), the approximate distance run by Pheidippides and his enormous effort to deliver the big victory news.

Today's marathon distance has changed a number of times, from approximately 25 miles to exactly 26.2 miles (42.195 kilometers). This change was constituted at the request of Alexandra, the reigning Queen of England. Once the race organizers set the course, the Queen insisted that the race should begin at Windsor Castle and finish at the royal entrance of White City Stadium. Ultimately, the race organizers extended the course to yet another entrance to the stadium, effectively increasing the course mileage to 26 miles and 385 yards.

Olympic Marathon Distances

Year	Distance km	Distance Miles
1896	40	24.85
1900	40.26	25.02
1904	40	24.85
1906	41.86	26.01
1908	42.195	26.22
1912	40.2	24.98
1920	42.75	26.56
1924-today	42.195	26.22

In the month of May, 1921, after numerous marathon distance changes, the International Amateur Athletic Federation (IAAF) finally ratified the distance and it's still in use today.

Modern Olympic Games

After nearly 1,500 years of absence, the modern Olympic Games were reborn in Athens, Greece, in 1896. The return of the Olympic Games attracted 241 participants from 14 nations. The competing nations were Australia, Austria, Bulgaria, Chile, Denmark, France, Germany, Great Britain, Greece, Hungary, Ireland, Italy, Sweden, Switzerland, and the United States.

With all of the high stakes and hype in the 1896 Olympics, Greece wanted to win the Marathon race desperately. And win, they did! Spyridon Louis, born in Marousi, Greece in 1873, ran the 40 kilometers in 2 hours, 58 minutes and 50 seconds at the age of 24. Apparently, *during the race*, Louis stopped at a local pub for a glass of wine, and was asked if he was pulling out of the race. With confidence, he finished his drink and announced that he would overtake the other two runners in front of him. Race leader Albin Lermusiaux of France collapsed, and shortly after he went down, Australian Edwin Flack collapsed with just 4 kilometers to go, giving Louis the eventual win.

France, Great Britain, Germany and Greece had the greatest number of participants; the United States took home the most first-place medals of any nation with 11, followed by Greece and Germany. The United States had top 3 finishes in 20 different events, while Greece placed in 46 different events. Germany was a distant third place in the medal count with 13. The only running events in the 1896 Olympics were the 100 meter, 110 meter hurdles, 400 meter, 800 meter and 1,500 meter runs, along with the marathon. At that time, there were no 5 or 10 kilometer races and no women were entered in the 1896 Olympics.

Motivation

"Gold medals aren't really made of gold. They're made of sweat, determination, and a hard-to-find alloy called guts." – *Dan Gable*

As the Olympics and the sport of running evolved, so did the performance and caliber of the competitors. In Chapter Four, we'll look at some of these legendary athletes and how they've impacted the sport of competitive running. Later, we'll apply their techniques and philosophies to the "average Joes.".

Perhaps the greatest marathoner to date is the unrivaled Eliud Kipchoge, winner of the 2016 and 2020 Summer Olympic games (held in 2021). At the time of this writing, he also held the marathon world record, with a time of 2:01:39 during the 2018 Berlin Marathon. In addition to his official world record in Berlin, Kipchoge also ran the first sub-two-hour "unofficial" marathon on October 12, 2019. This was done on a closed course in Vienna, and does not count as an official marathon record because there was no other competition and he utilized rotating pacers during the historic run. He completed the 26.2 mile course in just 1 hour, 59 minutes and 40 seconds.

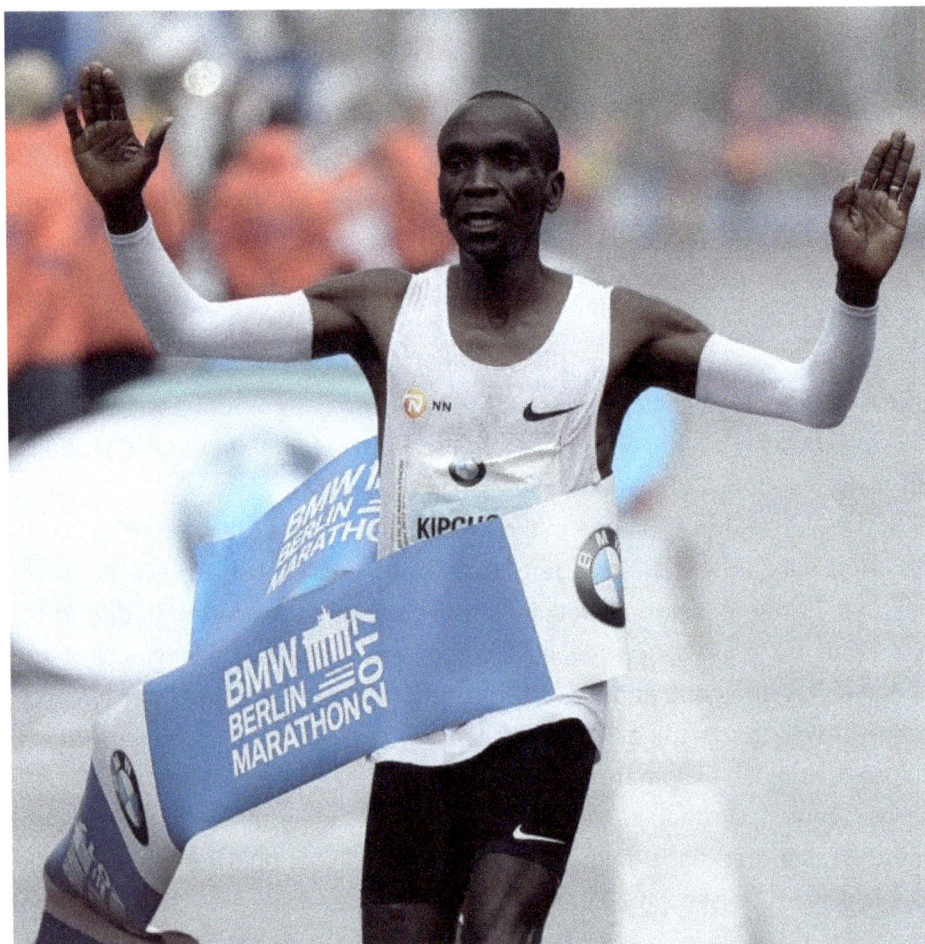

Eliud Kipchoge nears the finish of the 2018 Berlin Olympics marathon

Motivation

"Win if you can, lose if you must, but never quit!" – *Cameron Trammell*

Chapter 3 – What is Running?

Run [ruhn] - verb (used without object), ran, run, running.

- to go quickly by moving the legs more rapidly than at a walk and in such a manner that for an instant in each step both feet are off the ground
- to move with haste; act quickly
- to depart quickly; take to flight; flee or escape
- to have recourse for aid, support, comfort, etc.
- to make a quick trip or informal visit for a short stay at a place
- to go around, rove, or ramble without restraint (often followed by about)

By its simplest definition, *running* is the act of motion that allows humans to move rapidly on foot, in which at regular points of the running cycle, both feet are off the ground. *Walking* is the act of having at least one foot on the ground, with fairly straight legs and propelling yourself in a generally forward motion.

There are four phases of the running cycle: *foot strike, midstance, propulsion* and *swing*. Why are these phases important? In this chapter, you will see how these phases can affect your performance and efficiency, as well as the health of your feet, legs and back.

Foot Strike

The foot strike is defined as the point at which the foot makes contact with the ground. Runners commonly strike the ground in one of three ways: forefoot – which is a toe-to-heel landing, where the ball of the foot lands first; midfoot – where the heel and ball of the foot land simultaneously; heel strike – which occurs in a heel-to-toe progression when the heel of the foot lands first, then the plantar flexes to the ball of the foot. Many researchers classify the different foot strikes by the initial center of pressure to the foot. Forefoot strikers contact the ground with the front one third of their foot. Midfoot strikers contact with the middle of their foot, while heel strikers contact the ground with the rear third of their foot. The foot strike can vary between walking and running, and running with shoes or without shoes. The foot strike cycle could also be known as the *absorption* cycle, during which time the hip joint is undergoing extension from being in maximal flexion and the knee joint should be flexed. The ankle should be aligned slightly ahead of the body. The absorption cycle is a key to running efficiently, as we'll discover later in this book.

Midstance

Midstance occurs when the foot has landed on the ground and all of your body weight is supported on one leg. It is at this stage of the running cycle where the most common running-related injuries occur, such as Iliotibial band syndrome, runner's knee, stress fractures, shin splints, Achilles tendinitis, and plantar fasciitis. This is because the body is exposed to more weight for a longer period of time than at any other part of the cycle. During this phase, the body absorbs more than 2-1/2 times its body weight.

Multiply that figure by an optimal cadence of 1,400 foot strikes per mile and you suddenly find out how important this phase of the running cycle becomes. Strong muscles are very important during this phase to provide stability to the joints and tendons. Later in this book, we'll work on exercises that can help strengthen and improve your stability. At this point, your foot begins to roll inwards (pronation) and your arch flattens out. Pronation is a natural occurrence, and is a requirement to properly absorb the ground forces and into an efficient running position. During midstance, the focus is in knee flexion directly underneath the trunk, pelvis and hips.

Propulsion (toe-off) phase

The big toe is used to lift or propel you forward. As you move forward, your arch heightens and provides stability to push off with your toe. This is the time when your heel first rises off the ground, just after the midstance phase ends, and just before the swing phase begins. This phase is quite different than the two previous phases in that during the foot strike and the midstance phases, your body is actually absorbing energy. During the propulsion phase, your body is expelling that same energy to make an upwards and forward motion to begin the swing phase. A runner can reap the most benefits during this cycle by fully extending the hips. By extending and flexing the hips more, we can tap into and maximize the potential energy stored during the foot strike and midstance phases. To improve hip flexors and range of motion, focus on exercises such as stretches, deep lunges and cross-training with cycling.

Swing Phase

In the beginning of this phase, the trailing foot begins to swing forward and it ends when the same foot touches the ground in front of you. Since the act of running never includes both feet on the ground at the same time, one leg is always in this phase, while the opposite leg is in either the propulsion or foot strike phase. The distance covered by the swing phase is what many people refer to as your *stride.*

Upper Body Function

The upper body functions provide balance and momentum for the leg movement. The movement of each leg is paired with the opposite arm, which gives counterbalance to the running motion. The elbows should be bent at approximately 90 degrees, and fists should be relaxed. The torso should rotate slightly, serving mostly for balance. A strong core is invaluable for efficient running.

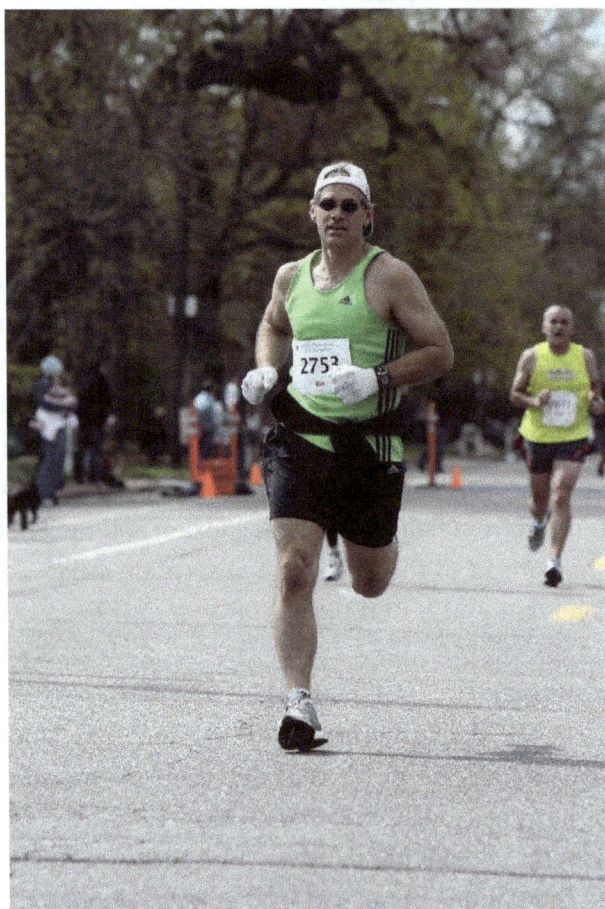

Upper body rotation aids in running efficiency

Foot Strike Types

As previously mentioned, there are three basic foot strike types: forefoot, midfoot and heel strike. Each one of these types can depend on running shoes, your body type and weight, and your running technique.

By nature, those who run on forefront and midfoot striking will be more efficient runners. These types absorb more shock with their knees, and spend less time in contacting the ground. Heel strikers tend to spend more time contacting the ground, and are less efficient in the propulsion phase.

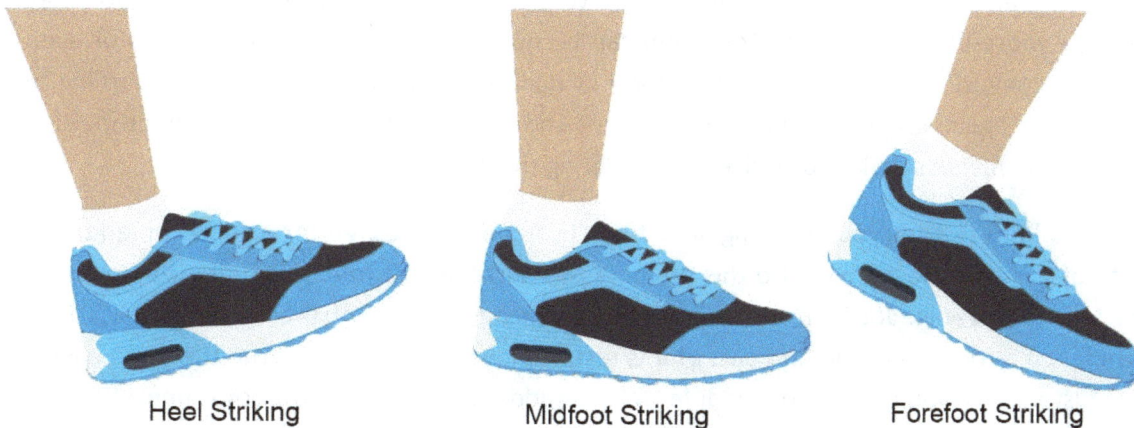

Heel Striking	Midfoot Striking	Forefoot Striking

Distance runners in particular, can lose their form during a race. They may start out with a fore or midfoot strike, but as the race wears on, their bodies fatigue and they end up landing more on their heels. Maintaining good form and core strength is essential during a long race.

Even though heel-striking is the most common, it is possible for runners to change how they strike. Shoes with a lower heel can change the geometry of how and when your foot strikes the ground. A lower heel may allow you to strike the ground at midfoot but it should be noted that forcing this can cause a change in your natural biomechanics and you may injure yourself. On the other hand, those of us who have successfully changed our foot strike from a heel strike may have *fewer* pains because we are now running more efficiently.

Tip

What type of *foot strike* do you have? When you run, do you strike with your forefoot or your heel? There are several reasons that you might consider a change of your strike type. The first reason may be to increase your running efficiency and the second may be to reduce pain. Be sure to read "My Story" in **Chapter 7 – Dealing with Injuries**.

Research* indicates that about 90 percent of all "average Joe" (middle-of-the-pack) runners

....continued

The International Journal of Sports Physiology and Performance – May 2013

Tip…. Continued

are "heel strikers" and it doesn't matter if they have a fast pace or not. Research also shows that it isn't gender specific. Furthermore, most elite runners are fore- or midfoot strikers, which is why they are generally more efficient at running. So, the question remains: Can you change your running style to become a better runner? Unfortunately, this answer is not straightforward. There are many variables to this question, and many parts of the equation are based on pain tolerance and body mechanics. When you change your running style, you may become more efficient, but the transition can be quite painful. It may take months or even years to convert from a heel-strike to a fore- or midfoot strike. For some, it's like learning to run all over again, using different muscle groups and changing the way you launch (propulsion phase) and absorb shock (foot-strike phase) during the run cycle.

Here's a little test for you. Wearing your favorite running shoes, go for a short run and take note of your foot strike type. Do this on a grassy course, a soft trail or a rubberized outdoor track. As an "average Joe" runner, you may quickly recognize that you are indeed a heel striker. When you're done with the first part of this test, remove your shoes and run the same course and distance. If you're like most people, you've suddenly become a forefoot runner! Put the shoes back on, and you'll more than likely return to your heel striking ways.

If we analyze this, does it mean that our "natural" running style uses a forefoot strike? Are the heels of our shoes so high that we're forced to strike the ground with our heels first? Would a flat-soled shoe be healthier and make us more efficient? There is currently a great debate regarding overall foot health and strengthening, and much of it is driven by the increasing number of barefoot runners. This debate will most likely continue for years to come because barefoot running has been shown to strengthen the fascia (connective tissue on the bottom of the feet), and may allow runners to run greater lengths using a fore or midfoot strike.

It should be noted however, that making the transition may or may not be the best thing for you. You may successfully change to a fore- or midfoot striker only to find out that you've not become a more efficient runner, or worse yet, you are now slower than you were before. You may now have more frequent injuries and suffer more pain. Really, it comes down to biomechanics and adaptability.

Motivation

"Excellence is the gradual result of always striving to do better." — *Pat Riley*

My Story

Several years after I started running, I was able to make the transition to become a mid-foot striker and eventually, a more efficient runner. This was not an easy transition but was necessitated by an injury to my foot. I quickly found out how bad habits and fatigue could change my running style back to a heel striker. This was especially noticeable on long training runs or marathons. As my body fatigued, my core muscles weakened, my leg strength diminished, and my style actually reverted during my run.

If you are going to be successful to the conversion from heel to fore- or midfoot striking, you must constantly monitor your stride length, stride rate and how you're striking the ground at all times. As noted in the next section, your stride rate can really help you with your running style. Always keep the turnover rate over 180 – it not only helps you with your race times, but it helps you focus on your running style. (See **Stride Rate** in the upcoming pages.)

Pronation

Pronation is the natural side-to-side movement of the foot when you walk or run. With a normal gait, the foot begins to roll inwards slightly and then it should start to roll outward during the propulsion (toe-off) phase. For some people, however, the ankle rolls too far downward and inward with each step, a condition known as overpronation. This can lead to pain, injury and premature shoe wear, but can usually be corrected with the proper shoes or insoles, or the use of orthotics.

There are three main types of pronation in the human gait; neutral pronation, overpronation, and underpronation, which is commonly known as supination. Both supination and overpronation can occur when standing or walking, but they're usually more pronounced and the effects amplified while running. People with high arches tend to supinate.

Neutral Pronation

Pronation is a very natural occurrence in normal body movement, however, overpronation and underpronation can lead to injury and long lasting foot, ankle and leg alignment problems. Rather than overpronating or supinating, healthy foot movement signifies neutral pronation.

In healthy movement, more of the forefoot is used when pushing off compared to unhealthy movement. In neutral pronation the weight is distributed fairly evenly among all of the toes with an emphasis on the big and second toes, which are better tailored to handle load. People with normal or medium arches tend to be neutral pronators.

Motivation

"Continuous effort – not strength or intelligence – is the key to unlocking our potential." – Liane Cardes

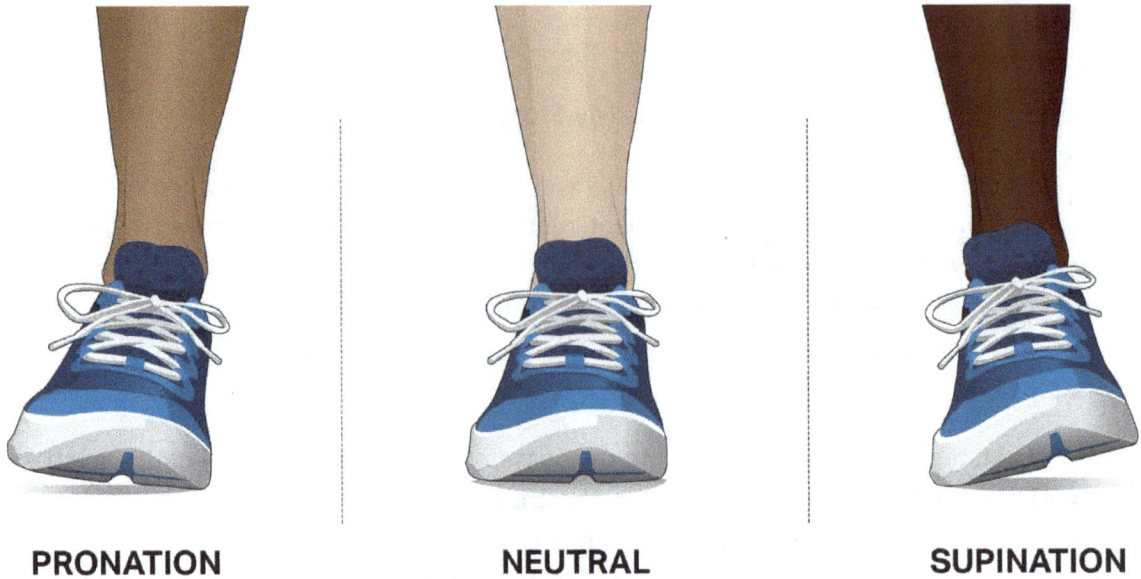

PRONATION   **NEUTRAL**   **SUPINATION**

(All views showing a right leg and foot)

Overpronation

  Overpronators tend to propel themselves nearly entirely from the big and second toes. Because of this, the load is not spread evenly throughout the forefoot and stabilization of the foot and ankle become an issue that can affect inequalities of balance and strength throughout the rest of the body.

  These anomalies cause unnatural angles to develop between the ankle and foot which can cause the foot and toes to splay out abnormally. Additionally, it's not uncommon for people with neutral pronation to have varying degrees of angulation, but not to the extent of over pronators. Weight is usually distributed evenly with normal pronation. Determining whether you are an overpronator is vital to selecting the right running shoes. Overpronators should buy motion control shoes to help correct their pronation issues and reduce the risk of injury. People with low arches or flat feet tend to overpronate.

Causes

  Causes for overpronation usually center on angles of the lower leg bones – the tibia and fibula, leg length discrepancy and arch height. Muscle tightness or weakness in the foot, ankle and lower legs, can also contribute to angulation problems that result in overpronation.

  Your shoe type can have a profound effect on how much you pronate or supinate. This is why it is very important to have the correct shoe type when running. We'll get into that in greater detail in **Chapter 11 – Equipment and Safety.** In that chapter, we'll look at common shoe wear patterns that can help you determine if you pronate normally, and we'll look at shoe types that can help with arch anomalies.

Motivation

"I'm all about breaking mental boundaries, and training for a marathon falls right into the Jedi mind-training I need." – *Liane Cardes*

Running Technique - Running form and posture for distance runners

Correct Running Form   **Incorrect Running Form**

Looking straight ahead   Head looking down
Shoulders relaxed   Shoulders high and tight
Upright torso   Leaning too far forward
Hands held in unclenched fist   Arms held too tight
Arms relaxed, swinging at sides   Hips turned out
Hips pointing straight ahead   Stride too long
Legs beneath body, knees slightly bent   Landing on heel
Landing between forefoot and midfoot

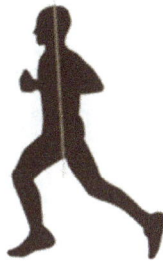

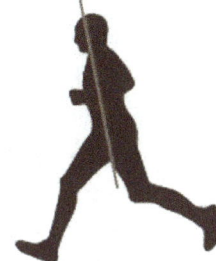

To run efficiently, you should have a slightly forward lean. This places the center of mass on the front portion of the foot and keeps the heel from striking the ground harshly. It's also very important to maintain a relaxed frame and strengthen your core muscles during training. This helps you to avoid injuries and allows you to run more efficiently. Make sure you don't clench your fists, scrunch your shoulders or keep your head and neck too stiff while running. Keep a shorter stride – the longer the stride, the more energy you consume.

Stride Length

Stride length is most likely more important in short and medium distance running than it is in long distance running. Stride length is directly related to the Swing Phase of the running cycle and depends on increased hip flexion to be possible.

Stride Rate

Elite runners, running experts, sports doctors and physiologists have all agreed in recent years, that a stride rate (cadence, turnover or footfall) is optimum when it is between 180 and 200 steps per minute. This optimum rate of turnover is consistent across all running distances, whether it is a sprint or a long distance race. The principal difference between sprinters and distance runners is the *length* of the stride, not the *rate* of the stride.

Obviously, the easiest way to measure your stride rate is to wear a foot pod that measures the number of steps by one of your feet. The foot pod can send the information electronically to a GPS enabled watch or a smart device and can very accurately measure your running cadence.

You can also count your stride rate by counting the number of times your left foot hits the ground within 60 seconds. Simply multiply the foot strikes by two to calculate your stride rate.   For instance, if your left foot hits the ground 85 times, you have a stride rate, or cadence, of 170. (85 x 2 = 170)   If your left foot hits the ground 94 times per minute, you have a stride rate of 182. (94 x 2 = 182)

Motivation

"Motivation is what gets you started. Habit is what keeps you going." – Jim Ryun

Tip

Ideally, for "Average Joe" runners, I suggest that you try to have a stride rate of 180 (90 steps per foot, per minute.)

Finally, you should always try to adjust your stride and rate when running hills. During your hill running, regardless if it's up or down the hill, you should *shorten* your stride by taking smaller steps and *increase* your stride rate.

Combining Stride Length with Stride Rate

With any race, try to optimize your stride rate, and once you have accomplished your target rate, you can try increasing your stride length. For distance runners especially, stride rate is much more important than stride length.

Limits of Speed

Foot speed is normally described as the maximum speed at which a human being can run. The fastest human foot speed on record is 44.72 km/h (12.42 m/s, 27.79 mph), observed during a 100-meter sprint by Usain Bolt in 2009.

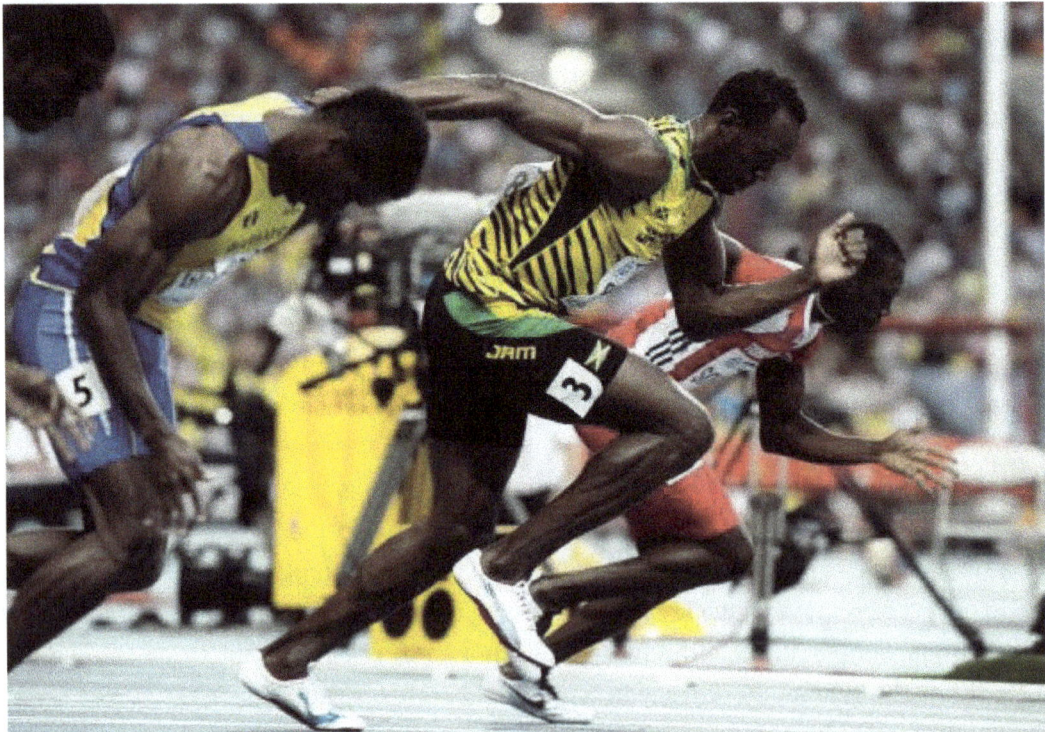

Usain Bolt set the foot speed record in Berlin in 2009

Motivation

"The starting point of all achievements is desire." – *Napoleon Hill*

While good running form can help your overall speed, it's been proven that most above-average runners move their legs approximately the same speed. The difference however, is in the amount of energy that they exert from their muscles. Top athletes exert as much as four times their body weight on their legs than do average runners. This is because they possess more muscle mass than the casual runner and have more strength to rebound from the downforce. This results in faster maximum speed. Although there seems to be many variables to reach the maximum foot speed, one of the key components is the type of muscle fiber the athlete has. All athletes have a combination of fast-twitch and slow-twitch muscles. Most humans have an equal amount of both muscle types, but elite sprinters may have up to 80% of the fast-twitch muscles compared to distance runners that may only have 20% of the fast-twitch muscle type. These variations in muscle type are typically due to genetic design; however, some sports physiologists suggest that training can actually produce changes in muscle types.

Running Events

As previously mentioned, running events and competition have been around for thousands of years, from the Tailteann Games of 4,000 years ago, the early Olympic nearly 2,800 years ago, the modern Olympics of 1896, the running boom of the 1970s, and all the way up to today.

Running dominates nearly all modern sports, or is at least part of the training effort for them. Even swimmers and skiers engage in running to strengthen and enhance their specific sports activities. There are a number of variations and classes of running, divided into groups and sub-groups. For instance, road racing defines one of the classes of running types, and can be further subdivided into varying distances, from 5k to marathon distance events. Each of these variations can require different training methods and tactics, as well as different types of competitors.

The aforementioned running boom of the 1970s was triggered by an upsurge of American competitor wins in the marathon by the likes of Amby Burfoot, Bill Rodgers, Alberto Salazar and Frank Shorter, just to name a few. Additionally, new statements from the Surgeon General's office regarding smoking and other health-related issues prompted people to take a look at their overall health and ways to become healthier. Running was an attractive option to those who wanted to improve their health and at-risk concerns. It's estimated that over 25 million Americans were engaged in some form of jogging or running at a competitive level, which at that time, accounted for nearly 10 percent of the US population. In 2015 alone, more than 10 million people participated in road racing from 5k to marathon distance events. Of those participants, nearly 57% were women, compared to 25% in the 1990s.

In this section, we'll take a look at some of the more popular types of running competitions, which include road racing, track racing, trail running and cross-country events.

Track Running

Track events are held on oval quarter mile or 400-meter distance running tracks with athletes competing in sprints, relays and hurdling categories. Modern tracks with a soft rubber substrate are ideal for new and experienced runners alike. They offer great traction with a soft underfoot to help prevent injuries.

> **Motivation**
>
> **"Nothing will work unless you do."** – *Maya Angelou*

Road Running

Road running is quite different than track running, in that it is usually run on common roads with varying distances ranging from 5 kilometers to longer distances such as half marathons, marathons and ultramarathons, and they may involve large numbers of competitive as well as non-competitive runners and wheelchair participants.

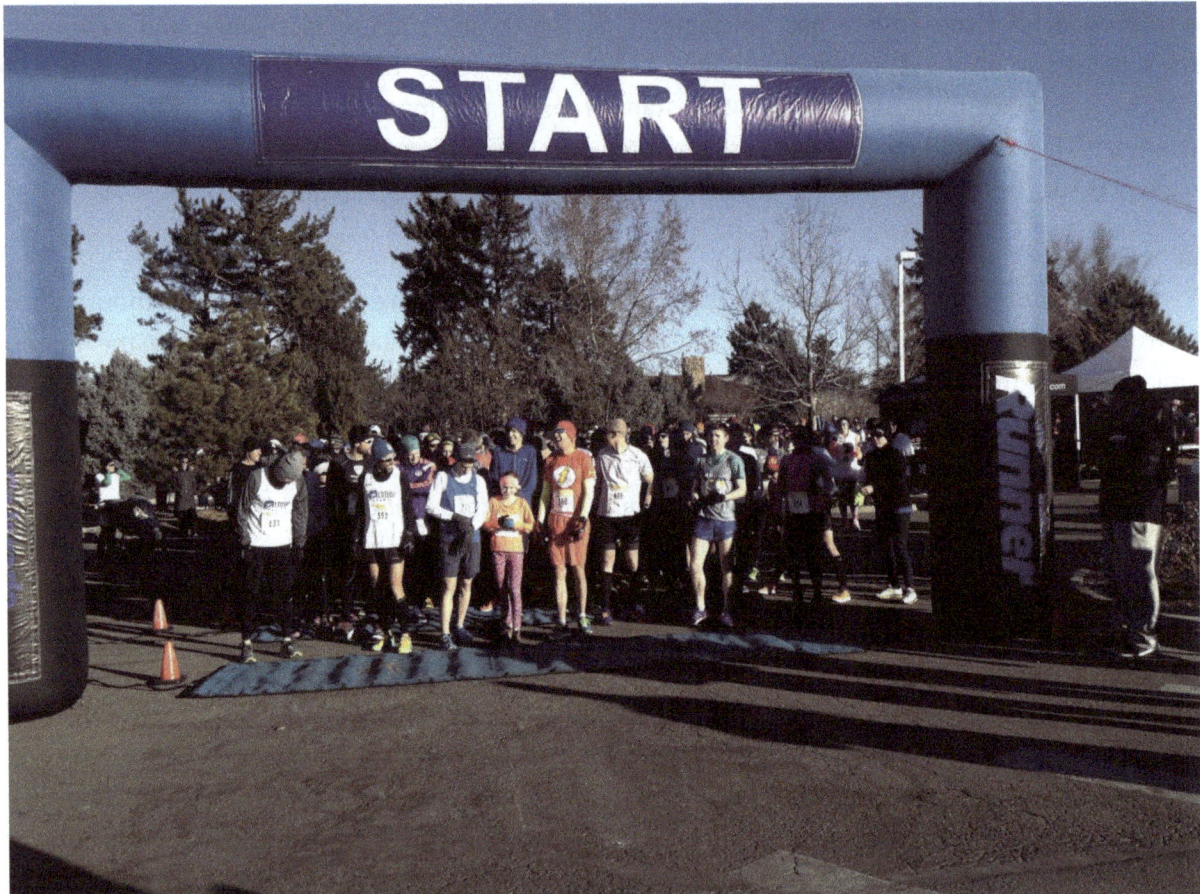

Cross Country Running

Cross country runners compete on an open course that consists of rough terrain that can even include grassy, muddy, wet or hilly conditions. Many of today's competitive runners have their roots originating in cross country running, primarily because it is very popular in high school and collegiate athletic programs.

Trail Running

Trail running races have also grown in popularity, combining the length of the road race courses with the terrain of the cross country running.

Motivation

"I've missed more than 9,000 shots in my career. I've lost almost 300 games. 26 times, I've been trusted to take the game winning shot and missed. I've failed over and over and over again in my life. And that is why I succeed." – *Michael Jordan*

Sprints

Sprints are usually considered short running events from 100 to 400 meters (or 440 yards) in length, and sometimes use several athletes in a relay situation. Sprinting was part of the original events in the Ancient Olympic Games with the only event – the "Stadion" race, which was a sprint from one end of the stadium to the other. Today, there are three sprinting events in the World Championships and modern Olympic games: the 100 meters, 200 meters, and 400 meters. These events originated in races of imperial distance measurements and were later changed to metric equivalents; the 100 meter evolved from the 100-yard dash; the 200 meter from the 1/8 mile; and the 400 meter that succeeded the 440-yard dash or quarter-mile race. Human physiologists tell us that a sprinter's top speed can only be maintained for thirty seconds or so, as lactate builds up and leg muscles begin to be deprived of oxygen.

Middle Distance

Events that are considered to be middle distance are races longer than the sprint distance but rarely longer than 3,000 meters. The 800 meter, 1,500 meter, and the one mile run are all considered to be middle distances, and the 3,000 meter teeters between middle and long distance races, depending on which running camp you believe. The 880 yard run (half mile) was the predecessor to the 800-meter distance and has its competitive roots in the United Kingdom around 1830.   ·

The 1,500-meter race also originated in Europe in the early 1900's as the result of running three laps around a 500-meter track.

Long Distance

Examples of long distance running events include the 3,200 meter, the 5,000 meter and 10,000 meter races. 20,000 and 25,000 meter races are also becoming more popular. Other long distances which are more familiar include the 13.1 mile half marathon and the 26.2 mile marathon.

Ultra distances

Ultramarathons are considered to be anything longer than the standard marathon and include popular distances such as 50k, 50 mile, 100k and 100 mile races. Finally, multiday or multi-stage races are growing in popularity, in which participants will run predetermined distances for several or many consecutive days. If that's not enough, timed endurance runs are also available, in which contestants compete against the clock and see how many miles they can run in a given time, such as 24 or 72 hour races.

Running Trends

Since the running boom began in the 1970s, record numbers of participants have been involved in road racing. It's interesting to note the gender trends over the past 40 years.

In 1990, males dominated with all race distances by a whopping 75% to 25%, a 3 to 1 ratio, but in just five years (1995), those percentages had shifted to 68% of men and 32% women. Then in 2005, male entries were down to 52%. By 2010, females had taken over the majority of entries with 53% to 47% for men. This trend has continued through 2019, with an average of 57% of all registered runners being women. These statistics are based on all race distances from one mile to marathon distance.

Women's race registrations still dominate nearly all distances, from 5k's to half marathons, but when it comes to the marathon, men still claim more finishes with about 59% to 41% for women.

Despite the COVID-19 pandemic of 2020 through 2022, 55 percent of runners on tracking apps scored personal records in the 5, 10k, half marathon and marathon distances.

Long Distance running statistics since 2004 for United States finishers:

Year	Marathon Finishers	Half-marathon Finishers
2004	386,000	612,000
2005	396,000	658,000
2006	410,000	724,000
2007	412,000	796,000
2008	425,000	900,000
2009	467,000	1,113,000
2010	507,000	1,385,000
2011	518,000	1,610,000
2012	487,000	1,850,000
2013	541,000	1,960,000
2014	550,637	2,046,600
2015	509,000	1,986,600
2016	618,411	1,900,000
2017	722,855	1,940,200
2018	984,616	1,916,400
2019	1,098,248	1,979,321
2020	1,121,016	2,143,789
2021	1,118,546	1,968,711

The top five marathons with the most amount of annual entries are New York City (51,267), Chicago (40,523), Boston (26,640), Los Angeles (20,608) and Honolulu (around 20,117) – approximations based on 2021 figures. During the pandemic, more people became physically active to help deal with the stressors of COVID-19. Coincidentally, even more running records were broken during this time (2020 to 2022).

5k (Road)	12:49	Berihu Aregawi	Dec 21, 2021
5k (Track)	12:35	Joshua Cheptegei	Aug 14, 2020
10k (Road)	26:24	Rhonex Kipruto	Jan 12, 2020
10k (Track)	26:11	Joshua Cheptegei	Oct 7, 2020
Half Marathon	57:31	Jacob Kiplimo	Nov 21, 2021
50k (Road)	2:42:07	Ketema Negasa	May 23, 2021

Motivation

"There are no shortcuts to any place worth going…" – *Beverly Sills*

Chapter 4 – Running Legends

The great debate has continued for years: whether or not man was meant to run. In this chapter, we'll look at some of the gifted and talented individuals who, without a doubt, were meant to run. Some excelled in short races and some are able to go incredible distances. Despite their obvious differences, one thing they all had in common: DETERMINATION! These runners are NOT your "average Joes," but can inspire anyone who follows the running culture and communities.

Short Distance Runners

While it is difficult to pick a favorite from past and present runners, one rises above the rest because of his relentless conquest of the "four-minute mile."

Born in Harrow, England, March 23rd, 1929, **Roger Bannister** posed the first serious attempt to break the four minute mile. Bannister made the effort several times in the late 1940s and early 1950s. Many experts and prognosticators said that it was impossible for a human to run that fast and that it could not, and would not, ever be done.

Bannister's running career started at the young age of 17. In 1947, he ran the mile in 4:24.6, despite having trained for only three weeks. He was listed as one of Britain's Olympic "hopefuls" for the 1948 Olympics. Bannister eventually declined the invitation, instead focusing on the 1952 Games in Helsinki. Over the next few years, Bannister flirted with the record on several attempts. In 1948, he ran one mile in 4:11, followed by a 4:14.2, just six weeks later. His record attempt in 1950 dropped to a "slow" 4:13, but he ran an unbelievable final lap in just 57.5 seconds. This gave him more motivation to renew his hope in breaking the barrier. On December 30th of 1950, he ran a 4:09.9 pace, followed by two races in 1951 of 4:08.3 and 4:07.8. In his quest, Bannister ran a 4:03.6 on May 2nd, 1953.

While he was attempting to break the records, others realized that it might be possible after all. American Wes Santee ran a 4:02.4, and Australian John Landy ran a blistering 4:02.0. In early 1954, Landy tried three more attempts – once at 4:02.4, and 4:02.6 twice.

All the while, Bannister was watching these attempts unfold, and on May 6th, 1954, at a meet at Iffley Road Track in Oxford, he toed the start line. The race went off as scheduled at 6:00PM, and Chris Brasher and Bannister went immediately to the lead. Brasher, wearing jersey number 44, led both the first lap in 58 seconds and the half-mile in 1:58, with Bannister (#41) tucked in behind, and Chris Chataway (#42) a stride behind Bannister. Chataway moved to the front after the second lap and maintained the pace with a 3:01 split at the bell. Chataway continued to lead around the front turn until Bannister began his finishing kick with about 275 yards to go (just over a half-lap), running the last lap in just under 59 seconds. The stadium announcer for the race was Norris McWhirter, who went on to co-publish and co-edit the *Guinness Book of Records*. He excited the crowd by delaying the announcement of the time Bannister ran as long as possible:

"Ladies and gentlemen, here is the result of event nine, the one mile: first, number forty-one, R. G. Bannister, Amateur Athletic Association and formerly of Exeter and Merton Colleges, Oxford, with a time which is a new meeting and track record, and which—subject to ratification—will be a new English Native, British National, All-Comers, European, British Empire and World Record. The time was three..."

The roar of the crowd drowned out the rest of the announcement. Bannister's time was three minutes, 59.4 seconds. As it turned out, the four-minute mile proved to be more of a mental barrier than a physical one, as many more athletes broke the four-minute mile record within months of Bannister's "impossible" feat.

Bannister later went on to medical school where he became a neurologist and Master at Pembroke College, Oxford, before retiring in 1993. Bannister was diagnosed with Parkinson's disease in 2011 and passed away on March 3rd, 2018.

In the last 50 years, the mile record has been lowered by almost 17 seconds. Running a mile in four minutes translates to a speed of 15 miles per hour.

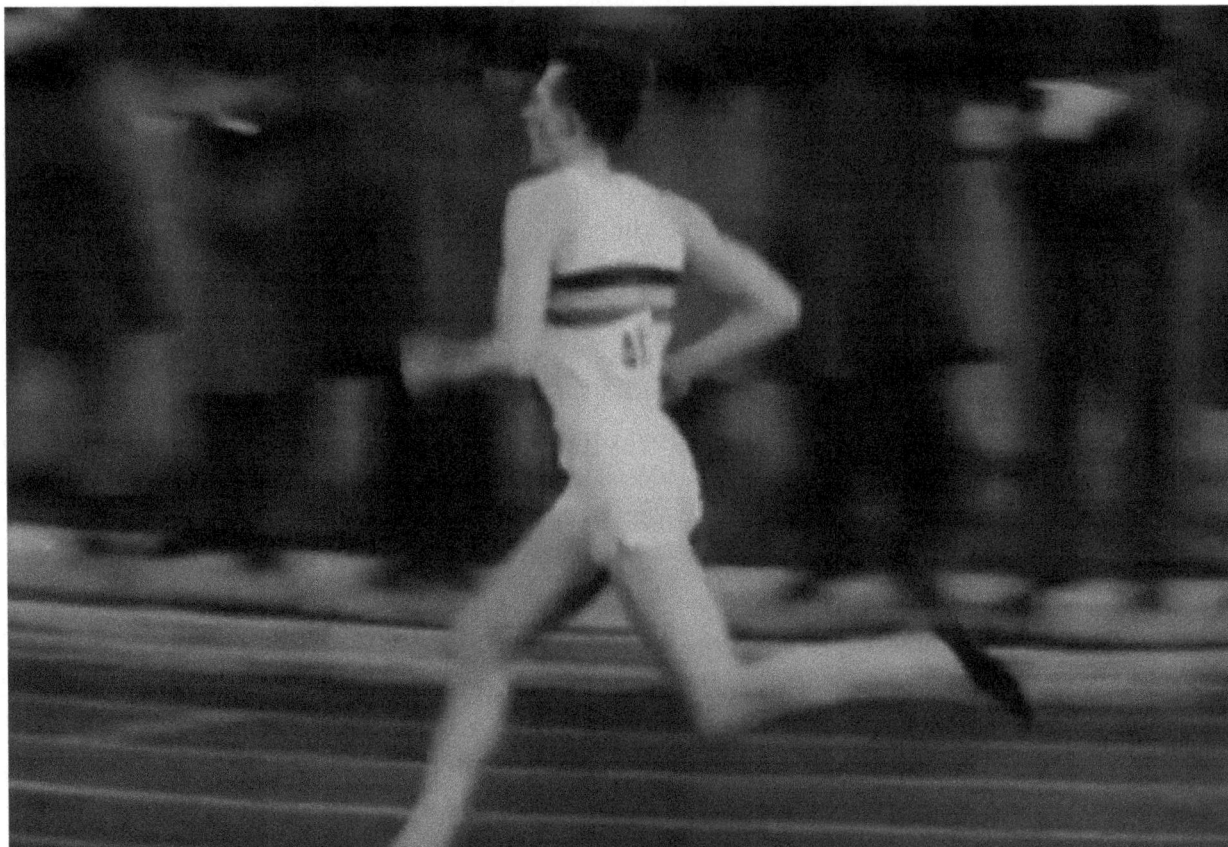

Roger Bannister on his way to breaking the 4-minute mile barrier in 1954

In 1964, Jim Ryun became the first high school athlete to break the four-minute mile with a time of 3:59.0. As a senior in 1965, Ryun once again broke the record with a time of 3:55.3. This record stayed intact until Alan Webb ran a 3:53.43 mile in 2001. As of this writing, the world record for the mile was 3:43.13, set by Hicham El Guerrouj, of Morocco. He set the world record in 1999 in Rome, Italy. The fastest mile set by a woman is 4:12.56, recorded in 1996 by Russian Svetlana Masterkova.

While these athletes are anything but "average Joes," their stories tell us that records are meant to be broken, and hard work can pay dividends to those who choose to commit to their goals. It all starts with belief in yourself and setting achievable goals.

Middle Distance Runners

No one believed in themselves more than the late, great, **Steve Prefontaine**. "Pre," as most call him, was an outstanding collegiate athlete for the University of Oregon in the 1970s. He was the epitome of a committed runner, leaving nothing behind whenever he raced. Prefontaine was an American middle distance runner and competed in the 1972 Olympics in Munich, Germany. At one time, he held the American record in seven different events from the 2,000 meter to the 10,000 meter distances.

Prefontaine joined the Marshfield High School cross country team in 1965, coached by Walt McClure, Jr. In his collegiate years, he ran under the leadership of Bill Bowerman, at the University of Oregon. He was recruited by most of the top track programs in the United States, but ultimately settled on Oregon. Prefontaine was defeated in the mile race only a few times during his college career but won four 5,000 meter titles, three times in a row. In college, he never lost a 5,000 or 10,000-meter race.

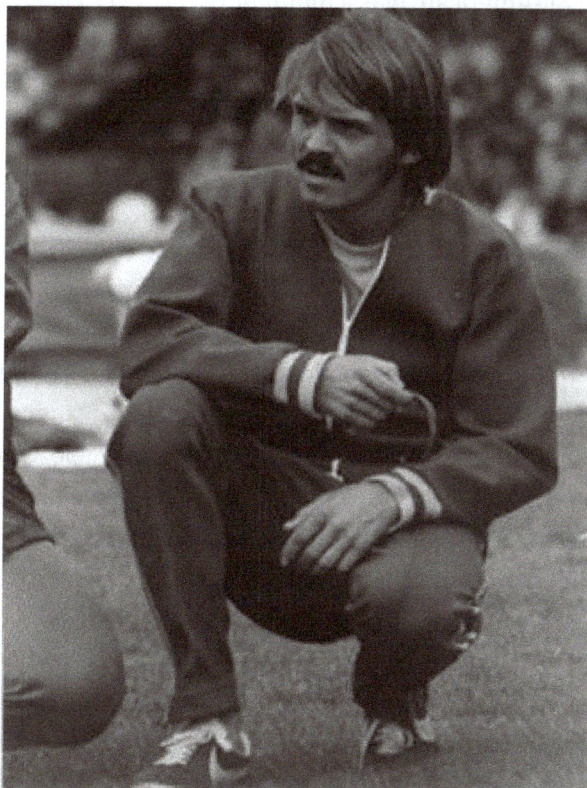

Steve Prefontaine

He was most known for his aggressive running style, giving everything he had from the beginning to the end of the race. He was once quoted as saying: "No one will ever win a 5,000 meter by running an easy two miles. Not against me." He would later state, "I am going to work so that it's a pure guts race. In the end, if it is, I'm the only one that can win it."

Prefontaine died in a car accident in May of 1975 at the age of 24.

Motivation

"I don't have any more skill or talent than the next guy – I only have more will power." – *Bill Watts*

Long Distance Runners

While Bannister and Prefontaine set the standards for the short and medium distance runners, a new group of long distance runners was beginning to emerge, along with a new running culture. In the 1970s, long distance American runners Frank Shorter and Bill Rodgers, joined forces with short and medium distance runners (Bannister and Prefontaine) to kick-start the boom of running in America. It's said that over 25 million people were active runners during this time.

The media escalated this new culture, and many great running books were authored by the likes of Dr. George Sheehan, Amby Burfoot, Ken Cooper, Hal Higdon, Joe Henderson, and Jim Fixx.

Running theorists began to develop their own running plans, schedules and techniques. These included marathoner **Jeff Galloway** and ultra-runner and columnist **Bart Yasso**. Each has made key contributions to running technique and theory, especially for the "average Joe" runner.

Galloway, a collegiate All-American, was a member of the 1972 Olympic team in the 10,000 meter run. He was also a marathon alternate for the Munich games. While proficient in the longer distances, he was also very good at the short distances, with times of 4:12 in the mile, 9:06 in the two mile, and 14:10 in three miles. In 1973, he set the American 10-mile record with a time of 47 minutes, 49 seconds. He was one of the first advocates of "more rest and fewer miles," combined with one long run per week, a program that to this day has proven very successful.

Later, his training methods prescribed a "run/walk" progression for beginners or less talented runners. His theory proved successful for many first time marathoners and those who felt they couldn't run an entire marathon. The technique he used was to get the runners to run for the first seven or eight minutes, followed by a one-minute walk. He maintained that if the runners did this for every mile, beginning at the first mile, they would be able to complete the 26.2 distance. This was especially helpful for first timers of the marathon distance. The walk breaks at each mile allow the body to re-oxygenate the blood cells, possibly reducing lactate. The breaks also help avoid constant pounding of the joints and muscles, offering quicker recovery and response time. To this day, Jeff is still an avid runner and continues to promote the run/walk training method. Many runners claim success with his training program and as an "average Joe," I urge you to try this training method. If you're just starting out, this method will also work for shorter distances.

Bart Yasso, a great runner in his own right, also came up with a training method, actually, more of a formula, to estimate marathon times. His theory has also been proven time after time. In the "Yasso 800" strategy, he states that if you can run 800 meters in 4 minutes, you can complete a marathon in 4 hours. If you run it in 3 minutes, he estimates that you have the potential to run a marathon in 3 hours. This method doesn't take the effort out of the running; you still have to work hard. It does however, eliminate the math and "thinking" while you run, so you can focus on the perceived effort.

Motivation

"To uncover your true potential, you must first find your own limits and then you have to have the courage to blow past them." – *Picabo Street*

My Story

I put the "Yasso 800" theory to the test in 2009 when I ran the St. George Marathon in Utah. I trained hard, running long segments of the Colorado Trail, weekend after weekend. The hill work and altitude had a dramatic effect on my strength and conditioning. Prior to this difficult training, I struggled to run a 3:30 marathon. Up to that point, I hadn't yet tested my speed for 800 meters, but I decided to give it a try. After about 20 track sessions, my time for the 800 meters gradually decreased from 3 minutes, 44 seconds, to 3 minutes and 2 seconds. In October of that year, I ran my first sub-three-hour marathon, with a time of 2:59:01. That was a banner year for me, and I set several personal records at different race lengths, but the big takeaway was that the Yasso 800s really do work. As I aged, my times slowed dramatically, but the Yasso 800 theory still works. As an "average Joe," I fully endorse this training method.

With regards to the marathon, my favorite distance, it should be noted that America has had a number of world class marathoners. In the 70s and 80s, we had stars like Frank Shorter, Bill Rodgers, Alberto Salazar, Dick Beardsley, Greg Meyer, Amby Burfoot, and Joan Benoit-Samuelson. In recent years, we've had the privilege of watching Meb Keflezighi, Ryan Hall, Dathan Ritzenhein, Khalid Khannouchi, Deena Kastor, Kara Goucher, Shalene Flanagan and Des Linden. All of these world class athletes have contributed to the marathon's popularity. Ryan Hall holds the American Men's marathon record at 2:04:58 (Boston 2011), but Meb Keflezighi has proven to be the better big race finisher with wins in both the New York Marathon in 2009 and the Boston Marathon in 2014. Keflezighi also finished 2nd in the 2004 Olympics and 4th in the 2012 Games. Deena Kastor held the American woman's marathon record of 2:19:36 for 16 years, until Kiera D'Amato broke it at the 2022 Houston Marathon, registering a blistering time of 2:19:12. Kastor has maintained other American records in the 8k, 12k, 15k, 10-mile, and 20-km distances. She also won the bronze medal in the marathon at the 2004 Olympics. The women's half-marathon American record was shattered by Sarah Hall at the 2022 Houston Half Marathon.

Ultra-Distance Runners

Next, we'll focus on the Ultrarunners. This is a completely different breed of runner defined by living on the edge and going to great lengths to find the most difficult races, in the harshest of places. Unlike track runners and road racers, these folks rarely seek acknowledgement from their hard work; they may get a mug, a coaster, or a belt buckle, but for the most part, Ultrarunners don't seek notoriety, nor do they receive it.

As mentioned in Chapter Three, an *ultramarathon* is defined as any race longer than the standard marathon of 26.2 miles. The most popular "ultra" events are the 50k (31 miles), the 50 mile, the double marathon (52.4 miles), the 100k (62 miles) and the 100 mile. Even longer are the extreme ultras, such as the Badwater competition held annually in Death Valley, California. This race is labeled as the "World's Toughest Footrace" – 135 miles across the hottest place on Earth in July, when the average daytime temperature is 117 degrees with highs as much as 130 degrees. With a starting location of 282 feet below sea level, it finishes at the portal of Mount Whitney at 8,360 feet above sea level.

Who runs Ultramarathons?

Marshall Ulrich (b. 4 July 1951) epitomizes the term "ultramarathon runner," with more than 130 ultramarathons averaging over 125 miles. Labeled as the "Endurance King" by *Outside* magazine, this extreme athlete has climbed the highest mountains on every continent, each on his first attempt, and has competed in multiple "adventure" races in the harshest environments.

By far, Marshall's most famous ultramarathon experiences lie in Death Valley, California, where he has finished the "Badwater" footrace more than 20 times and won the race a record four times. While most of the runners stop at the Mt. Whitney portal at 8,360', Marshall always continues on to the summit at 14,505', the highest point in the lower 48 states. (See page 32 for more information on Badwater.) Ulrich still holds the record for the lowest (-282') to highest (14,505') crossing of Death Valley in 33 hours and 54 minutes.

Ulrich has crossed Death Valley a record 29 times, including circumventing the entire park in a little over 16 days. Running with his friend, Dave Heckman, they completed the first-ever trip around the perimeter of the park in July of 2012, covering 425 miles in the blistering heat. He also covered the course four times (out and back twice), and ran the first-ever solo run – completely unsupported by a crew, pulling a cart that was loaded with more than 220 pounds of water and supplies. (See photo on page 29.)

In 2008, at the age of 57, he attempted to break the 3,063 mile trans-America crossing record. The trek began in San Francisco and finished in New York City. Even though he didn't break Frank Giannino's 28-year-old record, he was able to complete the journey in just 52.5 days, shattering the Masters (40+ age) and Grand Masters (50+ age) records. Along the way, he authored a bare-the-soul book called *"Running on Empty,"* a masterful writing that tells of the trials and tribulations of his run across America. If you'd like to get inside the head of an elite ultramarathon runner, I encourage you to read the book, along with the other books that he's co-authored and contributed to.

Ulrich is one of only two people in the world to have competed in all nine Eco Challenge adventure races, and has competed in 17 expedition-length adventure races with 12 ranked finishes. Other records include the 258-mile *Run Across Ohio* (64 hours, 09 minutes), and three wins of the 310-mile *Run Across Colorado*. He was the first person to complete the *Death Valley Cup* finishing the *Badwater Ultra* AND the *Furnace Creek 508* in the same year. Ulrich is one of only two athletes to ever complete the *Leadville Trail 100* run and the *Pikes Peak Marathon* combination on the same weekend, and the only person to complete *The Leadville Triple Crown* – Leadville 100-mile bike, 100 mile run, and 100-mile kayak on consecutive weekends. He was the first person to compete in all six American 100-mile trail races in one year, and has five *Western State 100* finishes in less than 24 hours. He's competed in an astonishing thirteen *Leadville 100* trail races, accumulating four top-10 finishes and has won the coveted silver buckle seven times by finishing in less than 24 hours. He placed 6th in the *Iditafoot 100-mile* race in Alaska.

> **Motivation**
>
> **"The only limitations are in your mind."** *– Marshall Ulrich*

Outside of the United States, he's competed in the *Marathon Des Sables* (Africa), the *4 Deserts Races* (finishing 28th in the Sahara desert in Egypt, and was on the 3rd place team in the Gobi desert in China. His personal bests include running 202 miles in 48 hours, 142 miles in 24 hours, 100 miles in 15 hours, 28 minutes, and 50 miles in six hours and 19 minutes.

As previously cited, his skills go well beyond the running trails - and places where there simply are no trails. Marshall has demonstrated phenomenal athleticism in all nine Eco Challenge Adventure races that brings together the most extreme athletes from all over the world.

His mountaineering adventures include climbs to the highest summits on all seven continents, including Mount Everest, Aconcagua, Denali, Kilimanjaro, Elbrus, Vinson, Kosciusko, Blanc, the Mexican Volcanoes of Orizaba, Ixta and Toluca, as well as other technical peaks in Ecuador, Italy, France and Switzerland.

In 2020, Ulrich released a new book dubbed "Both Feet on the Ground: Reflections from the Outside" – a fantastic book about disconnecting from technology and reconnecting with nature, urging you to spend more time unplugged, eat food whose origins you understand, and push yourself to try something bold and personally compelling.

Ulrich has raised over $850,000.00 for various charities, including the Religious Teachers Fillipini. Ulrich is an experienced public speaker who delivers his speeches to business-oriented, motivational, technical, and entertaining presentations, and caters to businesses, universities, sports teams, and professional conferences. Marshall resides with his wife Heather, in Colorado.

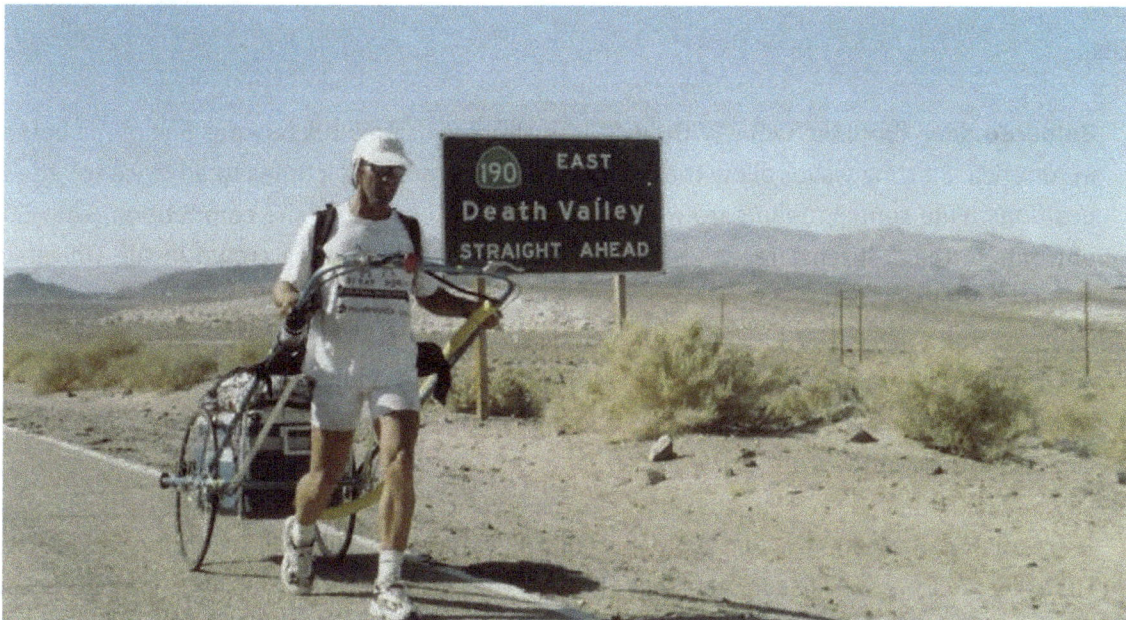

Ulrich with his 220-pound elephant, on his solo run across Death Valley

Motivation

"Always make a total effort, even when the odds are against you." – *Arnold Palmer*

Now that we've discussed what running is, and the various distances that are available, let's examine some of the more popular races in the United States. The "Best" races are based on course reviews and popular sentiment.

Best Middle Distance Races

Best 5ks

Susan Komen Race for the Cure (various locations) – What could be better than saving lives and running? Susan G. Komen Race for the Cure 5k events are held all over the country to fund research and create awareness for breast cancer.

Boston 5k (Boston, MA) – This race takes place during the Patriots Day weekend, along with the Boston Marathon, and brings in runners from all over the world. The race offers nearly $40,000.00 in prize money. If you stay until the following Monday, you can watch (or run) the Boston Marathon.

Anthem Fitness Classic 5k (Louisville, KY) – Held in March, this relatively new 5k race has become a favorite for middle distance runners across the US. There are normally around 6,000 people entered in this race!

Best 10ks

BolderBoulder (Boulder, CO) – With "wall-to-wall" crowds, this 10k ranks as one of the best races in America. Starting waves allow those with the fastest qualifying times to advance to the front positions. Elite running teams from all over the world enter into the competition, with 60,000 entrants in the "Citizens" race. The finish concludes with a roaring crowd in the University of Colorado football stadium.

AJC Peachtree Road Race (Atlanta, GA) – This race is held on Independence Day each year and has developed into one of the premier road races in the country. Starting waves allow qualifying runners to start at the front of the pack.

Statesman Cap 10,000 (Austin, TX) – A beautiful course in a beautiful city. This race ranks as a runner's favorite, not just for the race, but for the location itself. This race usually has about 25,000 registrants.

Best Long Distance Races

Best Half Marathons

Surf City USA Half Marathon (Huntington Beach, CA) – Run nearly six miles along the Pacific Ocean with 15,000 of your best friends. Enjoy southern California at its finest and get an awesome surfboard finisher's medal.

Canyonlands Half Marathon (Moab, UT) – See the Southwest and run on one of the finest half marathon courses in the nation. Held in March, this race is a great early season trainer and tune-up for Boston runners.

Slacker Half Marathon (Georgetown, CO) – Do you like running at altitude? Do you like downhill running? If you said yes to these questions, you will love this race. Starting at Loveland ski resort at nearly 11,000 feet, this course drops nearly 3,000 feet and finishes in Georgetown, CO. A half marathon relay team and a 4 mile course are also available.

Best US Marathons

Walt Disney Marathon (Orlando, FL) this is a perfect family destination for marathon runners and their families. Run through all four theme parks! This one is held in January each year when temperatures and humidity levels are down.

Boston Marathon (Boston, MA) – "Average Joe's" are capable of running the oldest Marathon in the US. In most cases, you must meet a qualifying time, but if you work hard enough, this race can be the biggest accomplishment in your running achievements.

New York City Marathon (New York, NY) – If you want to experience a big city marathon, this is for you. The weather can be unpredictable in November, but it's too good to pass up. Put this on your bucket list.

Big Sur Marathon (Pfeiffer Big Sur State Park to Carmel, CA) – If you don't want to experience a big city marathon, this is for you. Watch the migrating whales along the Pacific Ocean. See the giant redwoods near the start line, and finish in beautiful Carmel. This is one of the finest racing getaways you can find.

Best Long Distance Relays – Besides the urban and rural races, there are a number of fine multi-person relays that are great for the adventurous runners.

Wild West Relay (Fort Collins to Steamboat Springs, CO) – Get your ass over the pass! This is Colorado's longest-running relay for 12 member and four to six member ultramarathon teams covering over 200 miles.

Hood to Coast (Mount Hood to Seaside, OR) – Another legendary relay, this one features 12-member running teams that run 197 miles, from Mt. Hood's Timberline Lodge (6,000' above sea level) to the Pacific Ocean in Seaside, OR. This is a must for any serious endurance relay event runner.

Reach the Beach Relay (Cannon Mountain to Hampton Beach, NH) Another 200-mile race, this relay features some of the most spectacular scenery in the eastern United States. The net elevation loss is around 2,050 feet – but that's after you've climbed over 13,000 feet and dropped 11,000 feet. This relay is set up for 12 member teams.

Best Ultramarathons

Badwater Ultramarathon

Starting in the mid-1970s, Badwater is one of the most notorious of the modern ultramarathon races. Dubbed as the "World's Toughest Footrace," the Badwater ultramarathon proceeds through Death Valley, California. The original course started at 282 feet below sea level and finished at the summit of Mount Whitney. The course has been altered several times, sometimes with safety reasons in mind, and sometimes because of Mother Nature. This difficult 135-mile course winds through Death Valley, the hottest known place in the United States and takes place in July which is the hottest month. Starting in the Badwater Basin, it finishes at the portal of Mount Whitney, the highest mountain in the 48 contiguous states. During the race, runners gain over 13,000 feet of elevation, crossing two mountain ranges. Due to environmental and safety concerns, the 2014 course was modified for a "safety assessment" by the National Park Service. This revised course gained over 17,000 feet of elevation gain over three mountain passes, 4,000 feet more than previous years. The course was changed back to the previous route in 2015.

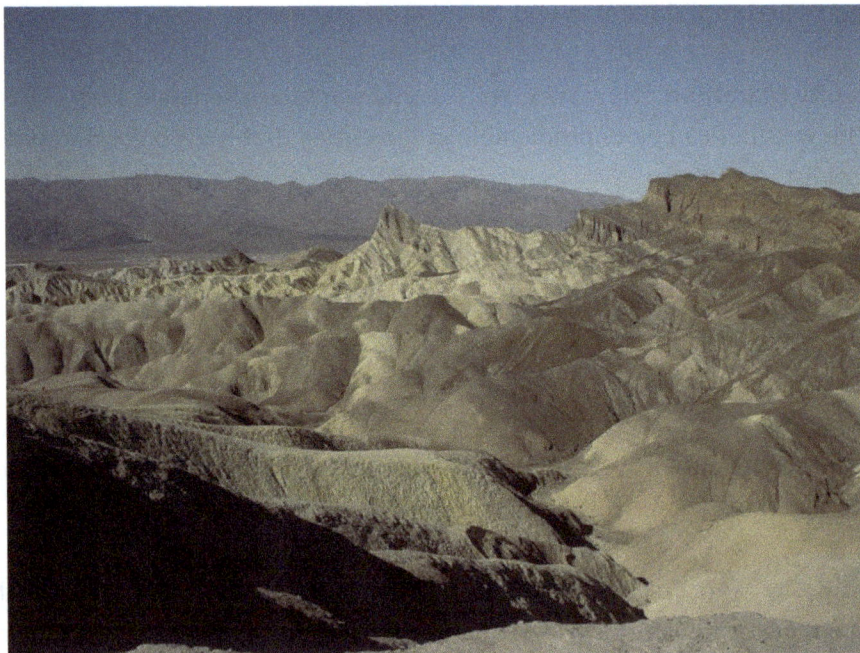

Death Valley

Western States 100

The Western States 100-Mile Endurance Run actually began as a horse trail ride, but after Gordy Ansleigh's horse pulled up lame at mile 29 in 1973, he decided to attempt the course on foot the following year. In his first attempt, Ansleigh proved that a runner could complete this difficult course in one day, covering the 100 miles in just 23 hours and forty-two minutes. It's now considered the world's oldest and most prestigious ultramarathon trail race. The race begins in Squaw Valley, California, not far from the site of the 1960 Winter Olympics, and finishes in Auburn, California nearly 102 miles later. The race is held in June of each year, when weather conditions can dip well below freezing in the upper Alpine regions, to more than 100 degrees in the dry, dusty valleys below.

Runners climb nearly 18,100 feet and descend 22,970 feet before they reach the finish line at Placer High School in Auburn. During the race, runners might experience snow several feet deep as they cross Emigrant Pass and the Granite Chief Wilderness and may encounter several rushing water river crossings of the Middle Fork of the American River. The race usually begins at 5:00AM and for many, continues into the night and next day. Runners who complete the course in less than 24 hours receive a silver commemorative belt buckle, while those who complete it in less than 30 hours receive a bronze buckle.

Hardrock 100

This ultramarathon race begins and ends near Silverton, Colorado, and is considered one of the most difficult of the 100 milers. The loop includes 33,992 feet of ascent and descent, the most of almost any ultramarathon in the world. The cut-off time for this race is 48 hours, with average times of 41 hours. Much of the course is run above tree line, which is near 11,000 feet. A lottery system allows only 140 runners each year.

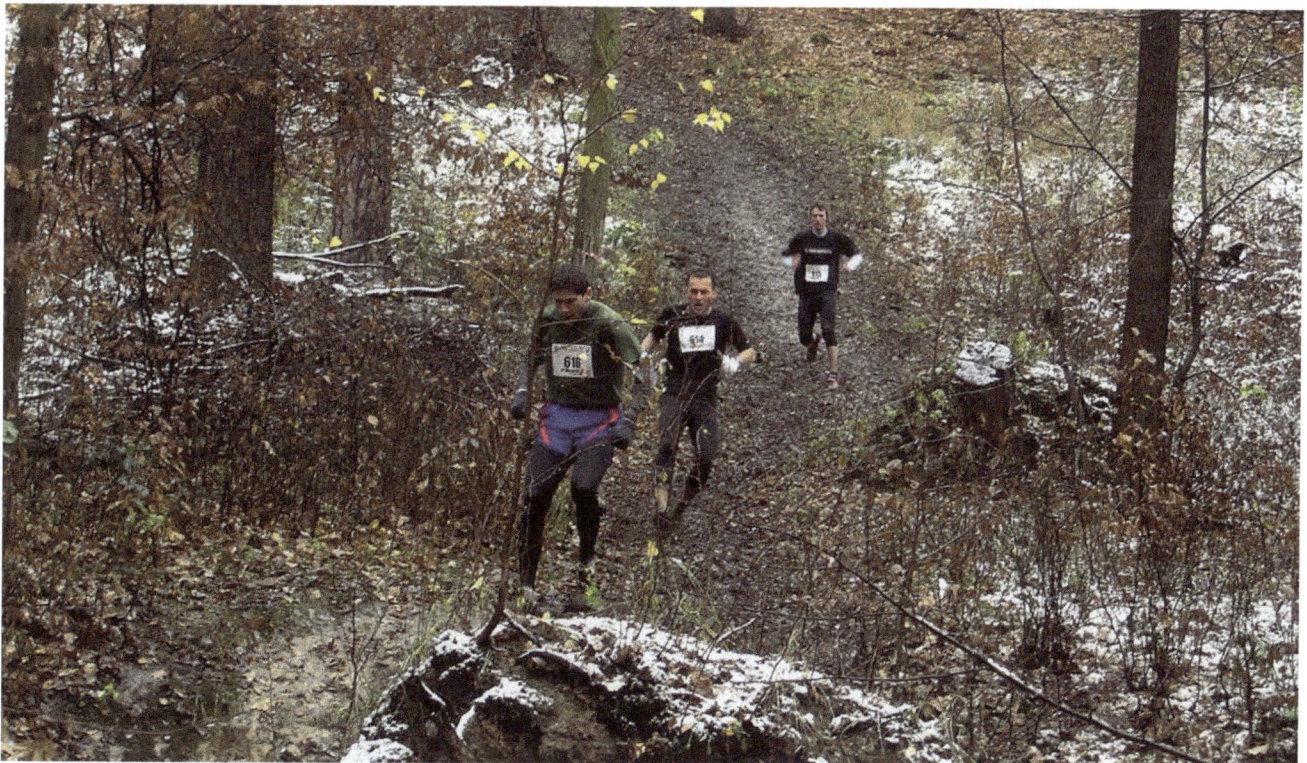

Trail Running

Motivation

"You must expect great things of yourself before you can do them." – Michael Jordan

My Story

I was fortunate enough to run the Death Valley Trail Marathon in 2005. It starts at 3,460 feet above sea level, in Beatty, Nevada, and climbs to 5,250 feet over the Grapevine Mountains. The course then drops into the desert, with a finish near Furnace Creek at 242 feet above sea level. This was not the "Badwater" ultramarathon; it was a standard 26.2-mile marathon and held in February. The temperature was about 38 degrees at the start of the race, but quickly climbed into the low 90s by the time I finished. The marathon winds through Titus Canyon and the colors that Mother Nature has painted on the canyon walls are truly breathtaking. Despite the drop of nearly 5,000 feet during the last 14 miles, this ranks as one of my favorite marathons.

Tip

Running in the desert is a different experience. The air is much drier there, as low as 2% or 3% humidity, and your sweat will dry almost instantly. You need to make sure you stay hydrated by drinking plenty of water and electrolyte fluid (Gatorade or equivalent). During my marathon in Death Valley, I lost nearly 8 pounds in just a few hours. Be prepared!

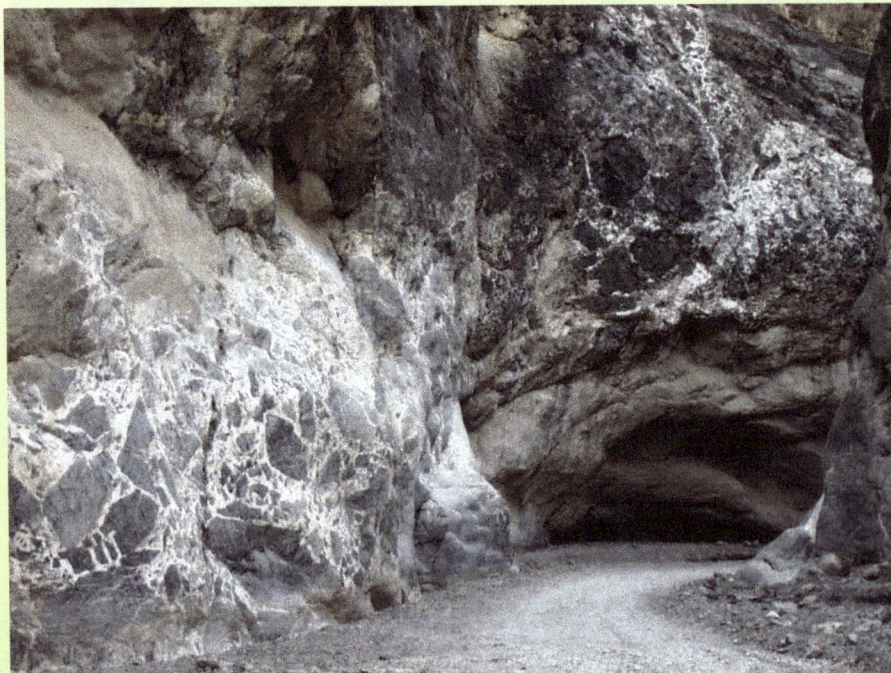

The beautiful scenery of Titus Canyon

My Story

Running an ultramarathon is never an *easy* task, but it can be *fun!* In June of 2010, I had my first experience with an "ultra" – the Angel Island 50 kilometer in the San Francisco Bay. Adjacent to Alcatraz Island, it offered a fantastic view of the Bay area. Circumventing the island six times and climbing nearly 5,000 feet of elevation, this ranked as my favorite ultramarathon. I ran a very pedestrian pace that took nearly six hours, but I loved every step of the 31-mile race!

Sadly, this race is no longer held.

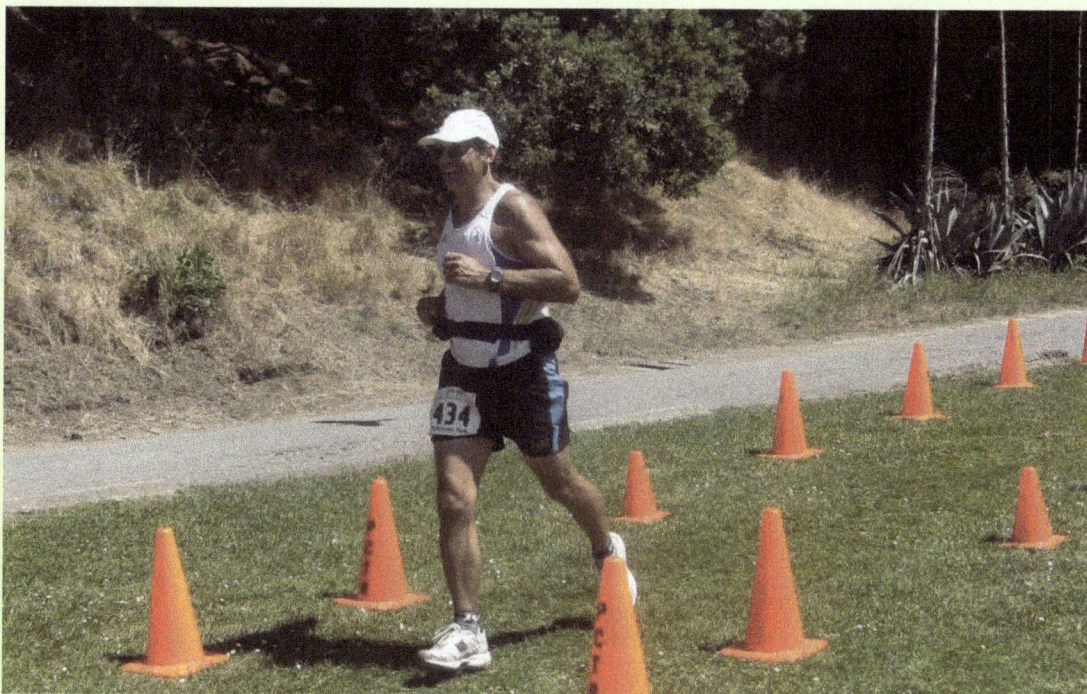

Finishing up the Angel Island 50k

Motivation

"Pain is temporary. It may last a minute, or an hour, or a day, or a year, but eventually it will subside and something else will take its place. If I quit, however, it lasts forever."
– Lance Armstrong

Are Ultramarathons for "average Joes"?

So, why do I include all of these ultramarathon stories in a book that is meant for "average Joes?" At some point, you may feel compelled to challenge yourself to an ultramarathon. Would you try one? Should you try one? That is entirely up to you as a runner and a competitor, or someone who just likes to set and achieve challenging goals.

Before I got caught up in running, I could never even imagine running a half or full marathon, let alone an ultramarathon. As I progressed through the different running variations, I finally found the courage to sign up for one and was glad I did, as my "ultra" experiences were some of my fondest running memories!

Again, I truly believe that any able-bodied person, with enough initiative and drive, can compete in an ultramarathon. Go for it!

Additional Resources and Inspiration

Recommended reading for middle distance running:

- *Galloway's 5k and 10k Running* by Jeff Galloway
- *The Competitive Runner's Handbook: The Bestselling Guide to Running 5Ks through Marathons* by Shelly-Lynn Florence Glover, Bob Glover
- *5k and 10k Training: Customizable Effort-Based Programs for Better Workouts and Faster Racing* by Brian Clarke

Recommended reading for long distance running:

- *Advanced Marathoning* by Pete Pfitzinger
- *Half Marathon* by Jeff Galloway
- *Marathon: The Ultimate Training Guide: Advice, Plans, and Programs for Half and Full Marathons* by Hal Higdon

Recommended reading for ultramarathons:

- *To the Edge* by Kirk Johnson
- *Running on Empty* by Marshall Ulrich
- *Ultramarathon Man: Confessions of an All-Night Runner* by Dean Karnazes
- *Running Beyond Limits: The Adventures of an Ultramarathon Runner* by Andrew Murray
- *Eat and Run - My Unlikely Journey to Ultramarathon Greatness (Scott Jurek)* by Steve Friedman

Recommended video documentaries for ultramarathons:

- *Desert Runners* produced by Dean Karnazes
- *Running America* produced by NEHST
- *Running the Sahara* produced by NEHST
- *The Distance of Truth* produced by Roger Hendrix and associate producer Chris Kostman

Motivation
"With self-discipline, all things are possible." – *Theodore Roosevelt*

Recommended reading for additional inspiration at any distance:

- *The Long Run* by Matt Long and Charles Butler
- *My Life on the Run* by Bart Yasso
- *PRE: The Story of America's Greatest Running Legend – Steve Prefontaine* by Tom Jordan
- *Bowerman and the Running Men of Oregon* by Kenny Moore
- *Finding Ultra* by Rich Roll
- *The Race Before Us: A Journey of Running and Faith* by Bruce H. Matson
- *Devoted — The Story of a Father's Love For His Son* by Dick Hoyt and Dan Yaeger.

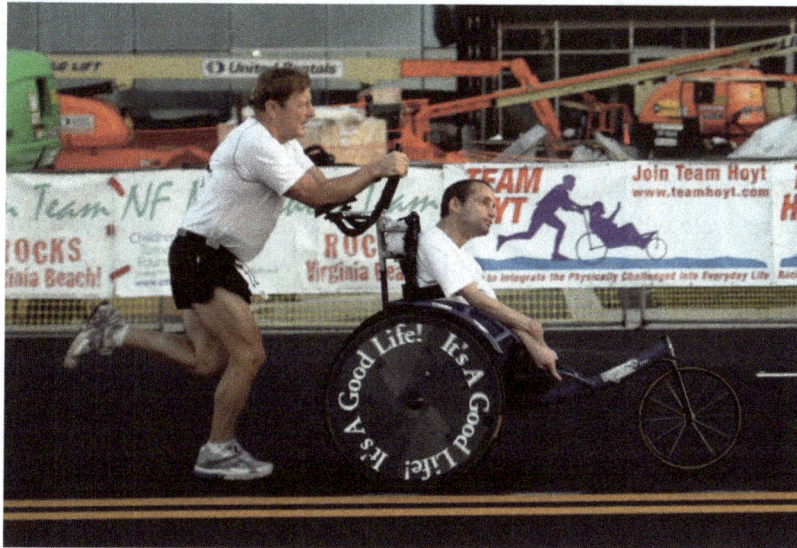

Dick Hoyt and his son Rick   *(Courtesy: www.teamhoyt.com)*

If you're looking for inspiration, look no further than Dick and Rick Hoyt. This father and son duo competed in more than 1,100 races in the span of 38 years, including more than 70 marathons – 32 of which were Boston Marathons. In the spring of 1977, Rick, stricken with cerebral palsy, told his father that he wanted to participate in a 5-mile benefit run for a Lacrosse player who had been paralyzed in an accident. Far from being a long-distance runner, Dick agreed to push Rick in his wheelchair and they finished all 5 miles, coming in next to last. That night, Rick told his father, "Dad, when I'm running, it feels like I'm not handicapped." According to Team Hoyt, the 2014 running of the Boston Marathon was their last marathon together, but went on to compete in 15 to 20 shorter distance races and triathlons each year after that. Unfortunately, Dick died of congestive heart failure March 17, 2021.

Challenge!

This chapter introduced us to several running legends.

Challenge: *Run inspired! I've found that you don't need to be THE best – you need to be YOUR best. Find a reason to run. Run with heart; run with passion.*

Chapter 5 – Running Psychology

My Story

I woke up one day, not wanting to get out of bed and not really caring if I ran that day or not. And then I did it again the next day and the following four days before I realized that after only six months, I was already burned out. Why did my passion for running disappear so quickly? My body certainly wasn't screaming in agony; as a matter of fact, this was the best I'd felt in years. My problem was that I was *mentally* depleted from running. My life felt out of balance and I realized that I needed to find other ways to keep my running interest intact. Over the years, this has happened many times, and I realize now that it's just another "cycle" in my running regimen. I've seen other people go through the same phases – buildup, over-training, injury or burnout. These phases seem to cycle with alarming regularity, and one is almost always a precursor to the next cycle. You start out with enthusiasm and eagerness, which can lead to over-training, and eventually, physical injuries or mental burnout. This chapter can help you deal with this predictable and avoidable issue.

So far, we've looked at *who* can run, *what* running is, *where* we can run, *when* we do it, and *how* running started. What we haven't examined is *why? Why* do we accept failure and pain, and see it as growth? *Why* do we *pay* to run? *Why* do some of us feel the need to compete? *Why* can we talk ourselves out of an important training session? Ask five different people, and you will most likely get five different answers. What would seem like the easiest question – *Why?* – is probably the most difficult one to answer. The one thing we all have in common is that we're all different, and as individuals, we seek different reasons to run. As I mentioned in the prologue, some will do it for health reasons and some will do it for pleasure. Others will run simply because they can.

In this chapter, we'll look at the psychology of running to see if we can solve the mystery of *why*. It's easy to understand the questions of *who, what, where, when* and *how* because these questions don't require the human brain to help us *reason* with them.

Motivation

"Make sure your worst enemy doesn't live between your own ears." – *Laird Hamilton*

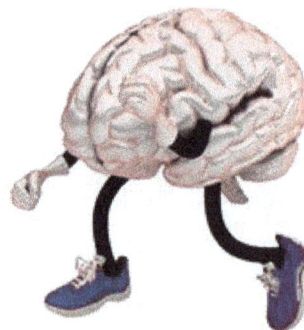

Mind Over Gray Matter

The human brain is the most complex organ of any animal, with 85 to 100 billion nerve cells – it is simply mind-boggling to try and understand the amount of instructions the human brain can comprehend and execute in just a few milliseconds. It controls bodily functions and issues instructions to the many subsystems of the body, such as muscle movement and coordination. It allows us to balance on one leg, for example, or touch our nose with one finger, with our eyes closed. It tells us when we're hungry or thirsty, or feeling pain. The brain sends commands to the legs to set them in motion to walk or run, frontwards or backwards. It allows us to leap and jump. But, none of these attributes answers the question of *why.* The only logical reason that may answer the question of *why,* is because, as humans, we have the ability to *think.* Unfortunately, this same function can fool us or play mind games (literally) with us. As humans, we can *accept* various conditions and pain tolerance, or *adapt* to them, whether they're real or not. But because we can think, we can also *doubt, perceive* and *criticize* our own efforts. Our mind can be our best friend or our worst enemy when it comes to running.

The Little Engine That Could….

Back in 1930, a children's book was published by Pratt & Munk. It was a story about a little train that was asked to haul a heavy load over a mountain, something that was normally reserved for the larger, more powerful locomotives. The Little Engine repeatedly said, "I think I can, I think I can…" as he struggled to carry the payload up the mountain. When he finally reached the top and started his descent, he proclaimed, "I thought I could, I thought I could!" This story reminds us to stay optimistic, and remain hopeful in the midst of adversity. This same concept applies not only to running, but to all aspects of life. Imagine where we would be if we didn't have any goals. Imagine how often we'd fail if we weren't able to convince ourselves with positive thinking. This is where psychology comes into play.

Psychological Influence

The Denver Broncos American football club plays in Denver, Colorado at an altitude of one mile above sea level. There are several signs in the stadium that remind the visiting team: "Elevation: 5,280 Feet above Sea Level." These gentle reminders are also part of sport psychology – they can be positive for the Broncos, but negative for the opposition. This type of psychological message or ***mantra*** can be either a detriment or benefit, depending on the way it's interpreted. It's very important to always have a positive mantra, one that you can believe in to achieve your goals. Following are a few examples of how psychology can work for you or against you.

Are there psychological influences or limitations within these words or phrases?

- Red: Simply wearing red clothing has been found to give a significant advantage in sports competitions which may be because psychology links red color with health, anger, and dominance.
- When you run with a training partner or against competition, do you unknowingly run faster? Statistics prove that you do!
- Can the change of one word in a sentence make an impact on how you feel or perform? If someone says, "You *should* have done better" or "you *could* have done better," which phrase has a negative connotation to it?

- You're at mile 23 of a marathon, and a spectator says, "One more mile to go!" Do you take it as encouragement, or does it frustrate you knowing that you really have three miles to go?
- How well do you adapt when the weather changes right before your planned run?

If you look around, you'll see psychological barriers in words, colors, trends, records and even people moods! To understand better, let's look at the medical definition of psychology, what its effects are, and how you can adapt to these effects.

Sport Psychology combines the knowledge from several inter-related fields that include kinesiology (the study of the mechanics of body movements), psychology (the study of behavior, behavioral disorders and mental illness), and physiology (the study of functions, activities and processes of living organisms and their components). Sport psychology is the study of how psychological factors influence performance and how exercise affects psychological elements. Sport psychology is used by doctors, coaches, athletes and parents for communications, rehabilitation, mental persuasion, team building and career transitions.

Originally, sport psychology was used by physical educators seeking to explain the various phenomena associated with sport and physical activity. Most of the early studies were done in Germany, with scientists measuring the physical abilities and aptitude in sports. Sport psychology started in Russia around 1925, followed by formal sport psychology departments that were established around 1930.

Later, the Cold War period spurred an escalation of significant growth, primarily because of the military competition between the United States and the Soviet Union, but also in an attempt to increase the medal counts for the Olympics. America thought that they could no longer compete with their Soviet rivals, so they invested more time, money and resources that would help the athletes from a psychological standpoint.

In its short history, sport psychology has lacked consistent accreditation because no one seems to be able to decide if a psychologist possesses enough knowledge of a particular sport, or if someone within the sport has enough knowledge to understand psychology. To be effective, a good sport psychologist would need to know both.

The Olympic games of 1984 brought about an insurgence of sport psychologists as the various teams began to hire them as full time, paid employees. By 1995, the United States had over 20 sport psychologists working with their athletes. Today, nearly all professional and collegiate teams and many high school teams utilize sport psychologists at some level. Sport psychologists are sometimes used for addiction intervention and excessive anger and aggression management, as well as other non-sports related issues.

Effective sport psychology consists of teaching the athletes, coaches, parents and fitness professionals, the psychological characteristics of their particular sport to maximize performance and enjoyment.

Motivation

"Obstacles don't have to stop you. If you run into a wall, don't turn around and give up. Figure out how to climb it, go through it, or work around it." – *Michael Jordan*

Generally speaking, the two types of sport psychologists come from either educational or clinical backgrounds. Some of the professional athletes or teams have one of each, and they work together to provide the best psychological solutions. The primary goal of an educational psychologist is to emphasize the understanding of the sport, provide confidence and teach goal setting, self-talk and energy management.

Medical sport psychologists understand more about the kinesiology, biomechanics and medicine to help maintain top performance in the athlete. A good sport psychologist will focus on a number of functions and variations of those functions, which may include, coping skills, conflict resolution, motivation, recovery from injury, and team and athlete performance. They may even need to possess more specialized training for topics such as career transition, team building and Post Traumatic Stress Disorder (PTSD) for veterans or anyone else who has experienced a life-changing event.

One of the common areas of study includes how personality and performance interact with each other. Topics such as *mental toughness, confidence* and *motivation* are usually focal points for most sport psychologists. The knowledge gained from these studies is then passed to coaches, fitness instructors, and medical staff for youth and professional sports alike. This knowledge is used to improve athletic performance at all levels by creating positive relationships between the coach and the athlete.

Sport psychologists are usually asked to track and interpret trends, tendencies, beliefs, rumors and issues at the individual and team levels. This allows *team cohesion* – the ability for a team to work together for a common goal. It also allows them to find out which member or members of the team are the true leaders.

Goal setting is crucial to the success of running, as it often is in life. Goals are defined as *measureable, specific,* difficult but *attainable, time-based and documented.* These can be a combination of short-term and long-term time frames. As an "average Joe," you must be motivated enough to create and accomplish your own goals.

- **Measurable** – You can measure your goal in a number of ways – How long does it take you to run your race? How much have you achieved since your previous goal? How much distance has been covered, etc.?
- **Specific** – you must know exactly what the end result should be. Do you want to run a 5k or a 50k? Without specificity, you cannot achieve your goal.
- **Attainable** – All races can be difficult but most are attainable. Will power and motivation are a must. Believe in yourself!
- **Time-based** – What is your timeline for achieving your goal? Once again, specify your goal, and if you don't make it on the first pass, reschedule it. Whether your goal moves or not, make sure you keep it!
- **Documented** – Keep running logs of your training, races and accomplishments.

We'll take a deeper dive in **Chapter 15 - Setting Goals**.

Motivation

"You don't have to be *the* best – you have to be *your* best." *– Bill Watts*

Another important aspect of sport psychology includes arousal regulation for those who get too anxious in the days or hours before a race or activity. This includes, but is not limited to, progressive muscle relaxation, meditation and breathing exercises. All of these can help the athlete perform better on race day. A pre-performance routine can also greatly reduce stress and provide time for physical benefits such as stretching, ingesting proper nutrition, and warming up.

It also helps to use *imagery* and *self-talk (mantras)* to help prepare the mind for your work ahead. Imagery allows you to use multiple senses to create or adapt to existing images in your mind. You may want to drive the race course before the race and then play it back in your memory before you run. This can help you build a strategy that will help you succeed on race day. Imagine where the turns are, where the hills are, and where you might be able to perform your best. Professional skier Lindsey Vonn uses this technique before her races to develop and enhance an image of the course in her mind.

In order to maintain a positive attitude, you might already possess enough mental discipline to overcome the frequent negativity that you may encounter. If you don't already have this mental toughness, or if you lose it during your training or in a race, you can still convince yourself to have a positive outlook and to keep going, even when your body wants to call it quits.

To create a mantra, keep it simple and keep it focused. Make it short and memorable so that you can repeat it over and over, especially when you're struggling. Here are some examples of some from our running heroes:

- **"I can run faster."** — *Haile Gebrselassie, distance runner, marathoner and Olympian*
- **"Negative split every run."** — *Sean Wade, Olympic marathoner*
- **"Think strong, be strong, finish strong."** — *Renee Metivier Baillie, long-distance runner*
- **"This is what you came for."** — *Scott Jurek, ultramarathon runner*
- **"Run the mile you are in."** — *David Willey, marathoner and editor of Runner's World*
- **"The only one who can beat me is me."** — *Michael Johnson, Olympic sprinter*
- **"As we run, we become."** — *Amby Burfoot, marathoner*
- **"All I have to do is manage this moment."** — *Stu Mittleman, ultra-distance runner and coach*
- **"I don't stop when I'm tired. I stop when I'm done.** — *Unknown*
- **"Today is my day."** — *Unknown*
- **"I'm a runner. This is what I do."** — *Unknown*
- **"I can dig deeper. I'm almost there."** — *Unknown*

My Story

Music can also help conquer psychological barriers, particularly in longer distances. When I ran the Angel Island 50k in 2010, I was really struggling at mile 27. With four miles to go, and facing another arduous climb of nearly 800 feet, I finally "plugged in" to my iPod. Before then, I had only occasionally listened to music during a race. This time, it proved its worth, and I cruised to a finish that I was satisfied with.

Motivation

"Most people never run far enough on their first wind to find they've got a second." – *William James*

How to Beat the Running Blues

Runners usually go through many cycles as they progress through their training. Once I made the commitment to start my running program, I was very motivated and excited. But I questioned my sanity after my first night of training and questioned it again in the following days, as my shin splints developed, my quads ached, and my lungs seared. I stayed with it and endured the startup discomforts, and found that I was really beginning to take pleasure in my running. By enjoying it so much, I unknowingly began to over-train, which fostered a real injury within the first two weeks. Again, I had to enter a new cycle: the "I'm not quite ready for prime time" cycle. Once I began to feel better, I decreased my training frequency and found that running three or four days per week was plenty, and made me feel "fit." I sustained this cycle for several months, entered a couple races, and found that I actually *liked* running.

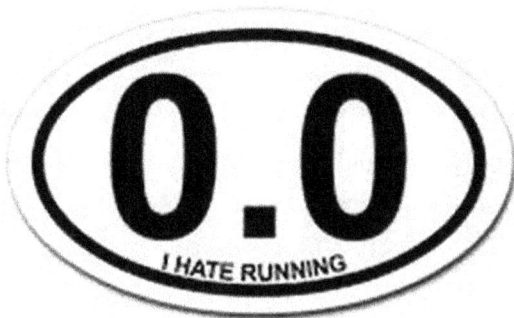

I bring this topic up because I think it happens to nearly every runner, and it hits some harder than others. More than likely, you'll go through these same cycles and you too will see this as "normal" once you've gone through them a couple of times. Beware that the longer you stay in the "burnout" stage, the more difficult it is to return to your running program!

So, what *do* you do when your motivation drops off? Here are a few things you can do to prevent the burnout stage.

- **Cross-Train!** I've found that one of the best ways to beat over-training, injury and burnout is to engage in cross-training. Adding variety to your program will help fend off the temptation to stop your training. Be sure to read **Chapter 14 – Cross-Training** to get ideas on how to stay stronger and avoid burnout.

- **Pick a Mantra!** Picking a short phrase that you play over and over in your head while running can help you stay focused and centered. It can be your inner motivation when you need it most. Finding a mantra isn't hard; it can pop into your head as you're listening to your iPod, chatting with training partners, or flipping through a running magazine. Pick one that fits your running style, mood or personality, such as: "This too shall pass" or "Work builds strength" or "Never give up." Create one, just as "The Little Train That Could" did to get through difficult times.

- **Get Off (or on) the Treadmill!** The treadmill can work for you or against you, depending on your situation. For many runners, a treadmill can be the only place to run during a recovery period or inclement weather. If you're injured, a treadmill can help you get back on pace, offering a static, but softer surface to run on. It allows you to run at a slower pace and keeps you from reinjuring yourself. And when you absolutely can't get outside, it makes a great alternate venue. Many of us refer to this as the *dreadmill* and will find just about any way to stay away from it, although we're sometimes forced to use it when there is no other choice.

- **Treat Yourself!** Make a deal with yourself – If you get out and run on a day when you don't feel like it, reward yourself with a special treat – a movie, a dinner out, or a massage.

- **Change Your Goals!** If you find yourself getting bored with the same routine over and over, try a different goal. Instead of signing up for a 5k, challenge yourself with a 5 *mile* race. Or, if you don't have time to run your usual 60 minutes, go for 30 instead. Don't develop an "all or nothing" attitude. Take what you can get, when you can get it.

- **Run With Friends!** Many runners shy away from the running crowd because they like to run at their own pace. Some of us feel intimidated by our faster friends, but we don't need to. Running with friends can be a real boost to your running program. If you run at a different pace than your friends, it's quite all right. Simply make a plan to meet afterwards and stay focused on *your* pace. And if you're the faster runner, be sure to encourage the others!

- **Keep It Fun!** That's really what it's all about. Don't make running another stressor in your life. Maybe your mantra could be "No run, no fun," instead of "no pain, no gain."

- **Change Your Route!** Running the same route over and over is a really good way to initiate burnout. Mix up your route – the distance, the terrain, even the time of day.

- **Log It!** Document your run and keep track of what you ate the night before, the weather conditions, and what your mood was that day. Did you get enough sleep last night? We'll take a closer examination of runner's logs in **Chapter 13 – Training Basics.**

- **Remember Why You First Started Running!** Finally, remember what brought you to the start line in the first place. Stay focused on your *choice* and *commitment* to running, for better health and happiness!

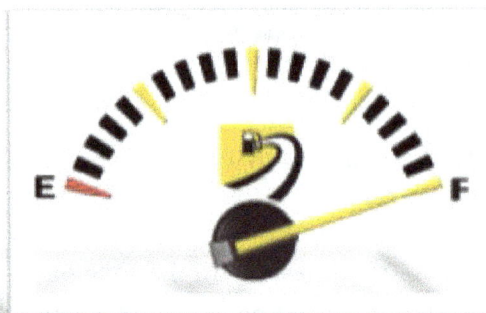

Motivation

"When you wake up in the morning, you have two choices: go back to sleep and dream, or wake up and chase those dreams." – *Unknown*

Challenge!

BEFORE you become mentally or physically depleted, create a list of different scenarios that could affect your running plans and find ways to enhance and revitalize your training program when you're struggling. Make sure you have a running plan! Talk to experienced runners and read magazines, books and online blogs for valuable tips and information. Your challenge: *Make entries in your running log of how you feel, physically, mentally and emotionally, so you don't repeat the same mistakes.*

Chapter 6 – Running Physiology

My Story

In 2009, I had my best year as a runner. I ran the St. George Marathon in less than three hours. The conditions were perfect for running – a nice downhill course, with a tailwind and cool temperatures. I went back in 2010 and suffered greatly in the marathon with a time of just over four hours. It was extremely hot, near or over 90 degrees on the course, and it certainly didn't help that I trained minimally and ineffectively. In 2010, my training (or lack thereof) was not nearly what it should have been. I had forgotten how hard I worked to run my sub-3-hour marathon, and took it for granted the following year. The St. George Marathon starts just before dawn, and most of us at the start line that day could tell that it was going to be a hot one. By 8:30 a.m., temperatures were already in the 80s. By the time I finished four hours after the start, it was already 93 degrees. Much like the 2007 Chicago marathon, where temperatures soared into the high 80s, finishers at St. George were collapsing near or at the finish line. The biggest difference between the 2010 St. George Marathon and the 2007 Chicago Marathon was the humidity, however, which contributed to two deaths and many heat stroke victims in Illinois.

The year 2011 was a totally different experience, however. I did, in fact, come prepared for the distance and the heat. Even though it was slightly cooler in 2011, I experienced **postural hypotension,** a condition that is frequently mistaken for heat exhaustion. I didn't have a fast race in 2011, but it was a very enjoyable run – until I stopped at an aid station. Each time I stopped, I started to feel faint. When I finally crossed the finish line, I collapsed in the exit corral. I couldn't even sit up, for fear of blacking out. I thought it was heatstroke at the time, but we took my blood pressure and found that it was an extremely low 86 over 38. Postural hypotension in effect, is a sudden loss of blood pressure. Since then, I've seen various runners on numerous occasions collapse near, or at the finish line of different races, even in cool or cold conditions. I had a first-hand experience with this anomaly and I caution all long distance runners and finish line volunteers to be aware of it.

This is just one of many running-related problems that can confront any runner at any time. Take time to understand the issues presented in this chapter, and prepare for the possibility of encountering them.

What is Physiology?

This chapter will focus on *physiology*, the study of how our cells, muscles and organs function together. There are many functional key components that are important to healthy running, and I will show them in a ***bold*** font. Physiology is a sub-science of biology and can be further divided into subsets of physiology, including plant, animal, cellular, viral, microbial, bacterial, and many others. In this chapter, we'll concentrate primarily on human and cellular physiology, the two that are most relevant to running.

The brain consumes up to twenty percent of the energy used by the human body, more than any other organ. Brain *metabolism* normally relies upon blood *glucose* as an energy source, but during times of low glucose such as fasting, exercise, or limited carbohydrate intake, the brain will use *ketone bodies* for fuel with a smaller need for glucose. The brain can also utilize *lactate* during exercise. The brain stores glucose in the form of *glycogen*, albeit in significantly smaller amounts than that found in the liver or skeletal muscles.

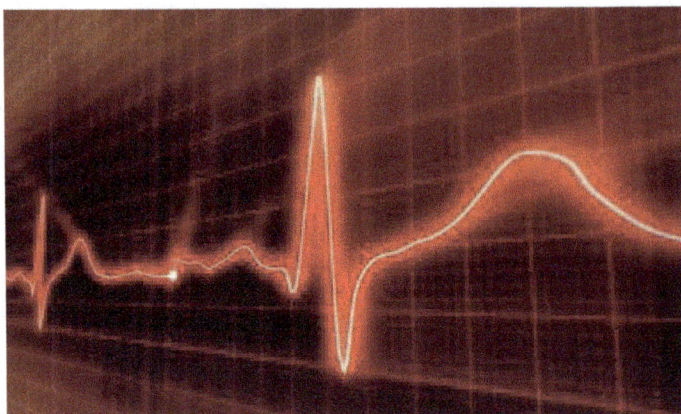

Although the human brain represents only 2% of our body weight, it receives 15% of the cardiac output, 20% of total body *oxygen* consumption, and 25% of total body glucose utilization. The brain primarily uses glucose for energy, and deprivation of glucose, as can happen in hypoglycemia, can result in loss of consciousness.

So why is the brain so important to our running? Before we go any further, let's take a look at some of the words we just encountered. All of the terms I am referring to, are as important for the brain as they are for muscles in your legs. These terms correlate directly to running efficiently and effectively. As you can see, the brain likes to hoard the bodily resources, such as blood supply and energy consumption. When you run, your brain can work with your body or can compete against it.

Your *metabolism* is the result of all the processes in your body working together to create the energy that keeps you going. Your metabolism is the rate at which your body's many processes function, and it can be low, high, or somewhere in the middle. When you're younger, your high metabolism makes it easy to lose weight, but as you get older, your metabolism slows down and you might put on a few pounds. Exercising speeds up your metabolism and can therefore result in faster and easier weight loss.

How Our Bodies Turn Food Into Energy

Just as a car needs fuels for its engine, our bodies need a carbohydrate fuel source to work efficiently. Our "car" is comprised of our muscles, brain and internal organs, and the fuel comes from the foods we consume. Food is converted to fuel by mixing it with the acids and enzymes in the stomach, which break down into a type of sugar called glucose.

Some will say that glucose is the same as *dextrose*. Chemically speaking, they are identical ($C_6H_{12}O_6$), but dextrose is actually a form of glucose and goes well beyond the scope of this book. In casual conversation, many of us use the words dextrose and glucose interchangeably. It doesn't matter what you call them, but it's important to note that both of the names are important to healthy running. In this conversation, we'll refer to both as glucose. This glucose is transported through the bloodstream to provide the much needed energy to our cells in the body and is sometimes referred to as a monosaccharide or "simple sugar."

Glucose is almost always your body's preferred energy source. It is easiest for your body to make glucose from carbohydrates like oatmeal, legumes, whole grains, nuts and yogurt, but if you provide your body with very few carbs, it will eventually be coerced to make glucose from the materials it does have available, such as protein or fat. (See **Chapter 10 – Nutrition** for information on "good" and "bad" carbs).

The stomach and small intestines absorb this glucose and subsequently release it into the bloodstream. Once it's introduced into the bloodstream, glucose can be immediately used for energy, or stored in our bodies as glycogen and used later. This is why it's so important to have a steady intake of glucose before, during and after physical activity.

To use or store the energy-laden glucose, our bodies require the use of ***insulin.*** Without insulin, the glucose can remain in the bloodstream, thus keeping blood sugar levels high. Insulin is a natural hormone made by beta cells in the pancreas. These special cells are normally used to monitor the glucose levels in the blood every few seconds, and are very sensitive to those levels.

The beta cells are designed to sense when they need to escalate or scale back the production of insulin in the bloodstream. When someone eats something high in carbohydrates, such as bread, rice, or pasta, the glucose level in the blood rises and forces the beta cells to trigger the pancreas to release more insulin into the bloodstream. All of these special functions keep the various hormones and chemicals balanced in our bodies. The ingestion of simple sugar gives us immediate energy once they're introduced and processed by the bloodstream.

As previously stated, glucose is the preferred source of fuel for our cells. And when the body doesn't need to use the glucose for energy, it's stored in the liver and muscles. This stored form of glucose is made up of numerous connected glucose molecules called **glycogen**. When the body needs a rapid burst of energy or even when the body isn't getting enough glucose from food, glycogen is broken down to release the required amount of glucose into the bloodstream to be used as fuel for the cells. We'll take a deep dive into glycogen in **Chapter 10 – Nutrition** and again in **Chapter 16 – Training Plans.**

Glycogen creation and storage is crucial for any type of racing because we have such a limited supply. While an experienced marathoner may be able to have enough natural glycogen stored up for an entire marathon, many sports physiologists suggest that a sprinter or short distance racer only has a 30 second supply if he or she runs at full speed.

The Importance of Carbohydrates

Carbohydrates often receive unjustified criticism, especially when it comes to weight gain, but it doesn't mean that all carbohydrates are bad. Because of their numerous health benefits, carbohydrates have a rightful place in your diet to allow the body to function well. That said, some carbohydrates are healthier for you than are others. In this section we'll try to understand more about carbohydrates and in **Chapter 10 – Nutrition**, we'll learn how to choose healthy carbohydrates.

> **Motivation**
>
> **"Your biggest opponent isn't the other guy. It's human nature."** — *Bobby Knight*

Carbohydrates are a type of nutrient found in most foods and beverages, and occur naturally in plant-based foods such as grains. Carbohydrates are also added by food manufacturers to processed foods in the form of added sugar or starch. Fruits and vegetables, milk, nuts, grains seeds, and legumes are all sources of naturally occurring carbohydrates.

There are three primary types of carbohydrates: *sugar, starch* and *fiber.*

The simplest forms of carbohydrates originate naturally in some foods including vegetables and nuts, milk and milk products. These naturally occurring sugars include fruit sugar (fructose), table sugar (sucrose) and milk sugar (lactose).

Starch is actually a complex carbohydrate comprised of many sugar units bound together and also occurs naturally in vegetables, grains, and cooked dry beans and peas.

Fiber can also be considered a complex carbohydrate and naturally occurs in fruits, vegetables, whole grains, peas and cooked dry beans.

Expressions such as "low carb" or "net carbs" sometimes appear on food product labels, but the FDA doesn't officially regulate these terms, so there's really no standard meaning. In most cases, "net carbs" indicates the amount of carbohydrates in a product, not including fiber and sugar alcohols. Another term you've most likely heard about is the *glycemic index.* The glycemic index classifies food with carbohydrates according to their potential to raise your blood sugar level.

If you use a weight-loss diet that is based on the glycemic index, it's usually recommended that you limit foods that are high on the glycemic scale. Starchy foods such as potatoes and corn, along with less healthy foods such as desserts and snacks are fairly high on the glycemic index rating. Most legumes, fruits, vegetables and low-fat dairy products are lower on the glycemic index.

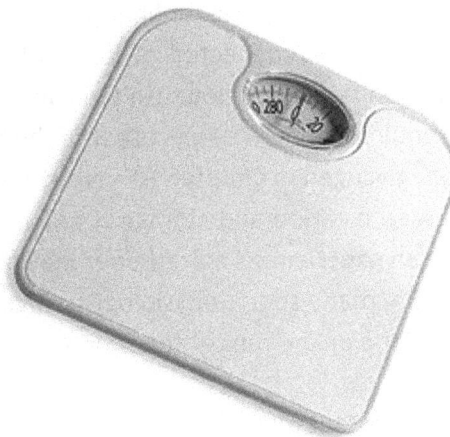

Carbohydrate Summary

Carbohydrates are especially important for runners because your body uses carbs as the primary fuel source. Sugars and starches are transformed down into simple sugars during the digestion process. Once absorbed into your bloodstream, they're known as blood sugar (glucose) and eventually, this glucose enters your body's cells, aided by insulin. Glucose is used for energy by your body, fueling all of your activities, whether it's going for a short jog or running a marathon. The spare glucose that isn't used immediately by your body is stored in your muscles, liver and other cells for later use, or is converted to fat.

The Importance of Oxygen

Oxygen is a colorless, odorless reactive gas, and the life-supporting element of the air we breathe. The earth's atmosphere is made up of about 20 percent oxygen, and is the most abundant element in the crust of our planet, mainly in the form of silicates, carbonates and oxides. All animal life needs oxygen to survive, but its importance is often disregarded when it comes to exercise capabilities and muscle performance.

Most biologists suggest that **Adenosine triphosphate (ATP)** is the most important component of energy production. ATP is a high-energy molecule that helps to store the energy we need to do just about everything we do.

Through a rather simple process known as **cellular respiration,** your muscles use oxygen to produce ATP energy. Typically, your body acquires oxygen from the air you breathe. As it enters your blood stream, it's then transported to your muscles, where some of it is available for immediate use, and the remainder is stored by a compound called myoglobin. Even when you're not exercising, the oxygen in your body is used to break down glucose and create ATP fuel for your muscles.

When you exercise, your muscles must work harder, which increases their demand for oxygen. This causes your breathing and heart rate to increase, and induces more oxygen into the bloodstream. As you continue to exercise, the oxygen that reaches your muscles never really leaves; instead, it works to immediately convert the available glucose into ATP.

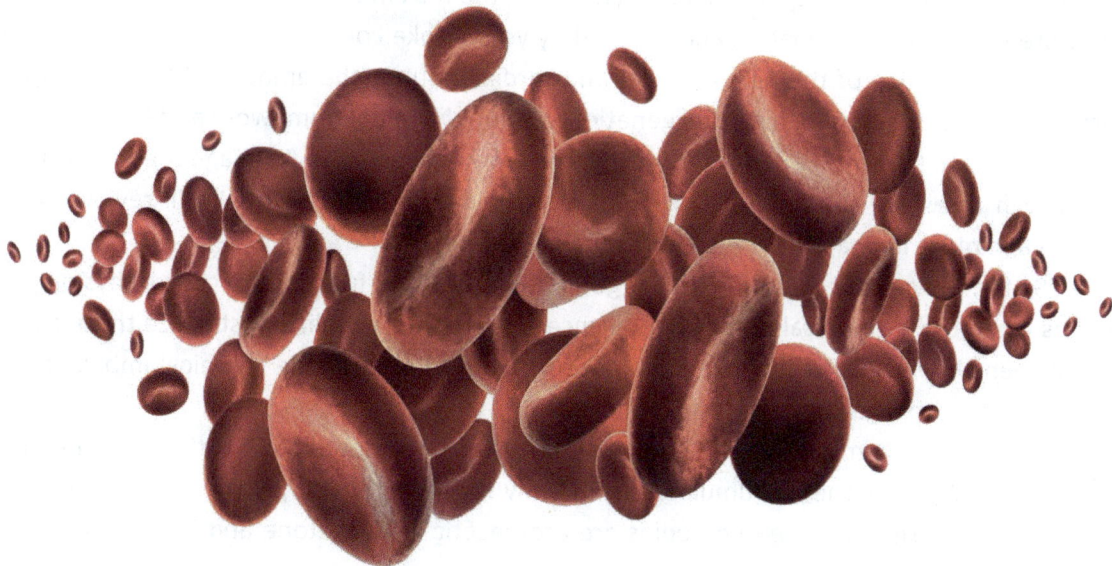

When your body runs out of oxygen, or your blood stream simply can't deliver enough oxygen to your muscles fast enough, your muscles begin converting glucose into lactate instead of energy. At this point, anaerobic exercise begins, your power output drops and fatigue sets in. Unfortunately, anaerobic exercise can only continue for a short period of time before your muscles run out of energy completely.

Motivation

"Nobody who ever gave his best regretted it." – *George Halas*

Oxygen also plays a role in the recovery of damaged or depleted muscles because it helps restore pre-exercise ATP levels and helps your liver break down lactate into simple carbohydrates. This emphasizes the importance of an effective "cool down" after a vigorous workout. A proper cool down helps to stabilize and return appropriate oxygen levels to your body. It doesn't matter how you view it, the more oxygen you have in your body while exercising, the better you'll perform and the faster you'll see a more complete recovery.

Since we're talking about oxygen, let's now discuss a new term: **VO2 max**. VO2 max is simply a measure of the maximum volume of oxygen an athlete can use. It is measured in milliliters per kilogram of body weight per minute (ml/kg/min). Okay, maybe it's not so simple. Let's take another shot without the math formula: As you increase your exercise effort, the consumption of oxygen used to produce energy also increases. However, there is a maximum level of oxygen consumption; basically a saturation point of the amount of oxygen your body can consume. This level of oxygen consumption is called the VO2 max or **maximum volume of oxygen**.

Some experts believe that VO2 max is the single most important physiological element of an athlete's performance, while other sports scientists maintain that the limits of an athlete's running performance are determined by many different factors, including adaptation and strength of muscles, **running efficiency**, **lactate threshold**, and your metabolism. They argue that VO2 max is just a measurement of oxygen that an athlete consumes at the maximum level of energy output. VO2 max is largely predetermined by genetics, and dictated by your stroke volume (the amount of blood your heart pumps per contraction of the left ventricle) and cardiac output (the amount of blood pumped by your heart per minute). Even though natural genetics give you the initial framework and baseline for your VO2 max, it is possible to increase your VO2 max in other ways, even as an "average Joe" runner. You can do this through **threshold training,** higher mileage and long interval training. We'll review these training methods and more in **Chapter 16 – Training Plans.**

So far, we've looked at some of the "good" chemicals and functions of sports physiology. But what happens when these chemicals are out of balance? How do we equalize or stabilize these chemicals and what happens if we can't? Let's take a look at some of the undesirable chemical imbalances and what effects they have in regards to healthy running.

Ketone is a chemical that the body manufactures when there are insufficient amounts of insulin in the blood. When ketones accumulate in the body for an extended period of time, serious illness or coma can result. (The three ketone bodies are acetoacetic acid, acetone and beta-hydroxybutyric acid, although the latter is technically a carboxylic acid.)

Lactate (when used as a noun), is a salt or ester of **lactic acid**. In the next few paragraphs, we'll take a detailed look at lactate, the effects of lactate, and how to increase your threshold for this very important component of running physiology.

Why do your muscles hurt after you run hard or far? There are theories and myths on this, some of which are accurate, and some of which are based on outdated and inaccurate findings. The first theory, which is accurate, is that you've torn muscle tissue during your activity. These tiny tears in the tissue are known as **micro-tears** or **micro-trauma**, which contribute to muscle soreness. The second theory is based on the buildup of **lactic acid** (lactate) in your bloodstream. Normally, micro-trauma will last much longer — hours, days or even weeks in some cases. However, the pain caused from lactate buildup is much shorter lived — anywhere from a few to 90 minutes after a race or difficult workout. While some of these theories are true, let's take a look at some myths and updated theories regarding lactate. For many runners, this section will be an eye-opener as it was for me when I was researching it.

MYTH: The body produces lactic acid during intense workouts.

MYTH-BUSTER: The body does *not* produce **lactic acid**, instead creates a very similar compound known as **lactate**. Lactic acid and lactate are sometimes used **interchangeably** even though they are technically different. Lactic acid is the joining of lactate with a hydrogen ion. It's the hydrogen ion in the lactic acid that contributes to the burning sensation in the muscles during exercise, not the lactate. For the rest of this discussion we will refer to lactic acid as lactate.

MYTH: When a runner burns too much oxygen, a waste product called lactate is produced. The acidic nature of lactate produces a long lasting burning sensation in the muscles.

MYTH-BUSTER: Lactate is not a caustic waste product at all. It is actually a fuel produced naturally and intentionally by your body's muscles. It is not produced from the absence of glucose, as originally thought, but is created by glucose itself and is used for fuel by the body.

MYTH: Lactate causes muscle fatigue.

MYTH-BUSTER: It is true that muscles become more acidic during intense or prolonged workouts, but this buildup of acid is not the cause for the fatigue. Lactate in the blood actually delays fatigue by mitigating a process called depolarization. The accumulation of lactate helps to counteract against depolarization.

MYTH: Lactate causes you to perform poorly.

MYTH-BUSTER: Without lactate, your fitness levels will not increase in response to training to the same degree you do with its presence. Lactate production during intense exercise stimulates a process called **mitochondrial biogenesis**. Mitochondria are known as the energy producers in our bodies where aerobic metabolism occurs. This process is used to break down the fats and glucose to produce energy in our bodies. When there is an increase in the concentration of mitochondria inside muscles, the body responds by improving the endurance performance. The presence of lactate is what makes the process possible. This is one of the reasons high-intensity interval training is such a potent performance booster.

MYTH: Lactate causes post-run soreness.

MYTH-BUSTER: The soreness you experience after a run is due to tearing (micro-trauma) of the muscles, inflammation and free radical damage, not from lactate.

Generally speaking, lactate build-up is completely normal and short-term in its effects, but can be reduced or eliminated by proper conditioning. This adaptation to lactate capacity is known as Lactate Threshold training.

Now that we've learned about metabolism, glucose, glycogen, oxygen, ketone bodies, VO2 max, lactate, and micro-trauma, we can finally see how each one influences the others, and how they all work together to help us become more fit by improving our lactate threshold. As we noted on the previous page, lactate is produced every time you use your muscles, and the lactate levels in your blood usually stay fairly level. During intense exercise, however, *lactate accumulates faster than it can be dissipated from your blood* — this is known as your **lactate threshold**. When you cross this threshold, you feel fatigued, and you might even feel a burning sensation in your muscles. Modern day sports physiologists now know that your lactate threshold can be increased with proper training methods. Athletes can train their bodies to use lactate more efficiently, so it takes longer to accumulate in the blood stream. Runners who are able to increase their lactate threshold can usually pick up their pace and get to the finish line faster.

Adapting to, and increasing your lactate threshold will increase your running success. As with any type of success, you must start with a plan — in this case, a lactate threshold training plan.

Tip

For most "average Joes," lactate threshold training is not required, but it's highly recommended, especially if you are seeking a personal record (PR), running distance races, competing to win a race or age group, or wishing to enhance your speed or endurance base.

Lactate threshold training could come in handy during the part of the race when you feel the need to compete, as in passing someone, or you need a sustained burst of speed to capture that PR! We'll take a more in-depth look into this area in **Chapter 16 – Training Plans.**

As mentioned in my "Tip" above, threshold training is not a requirement, and could actually lead to over-training, resulting in injury. Be mindful of this as you train, and listen to your body. I intentionally added this section in the book so you can be informed and make your own decisions regarding your training plans. If you decide to engage in lactate threshold training, here are some examples for 5k and 10k runners:

Generally speaking, lactate threshold pace is about 10 to 15 seconds per mile slower than your 5k race pace for slower runners. If using a heart rate monitor, *which I highly recommend*, the pace is about 75 to 80 percent of your maximum recommended heart rate. (See Zone Training on pages 198-203 for more information.) For highly trained and elite runners, lactate threshold pace is about 20 to 30 seconds per mile slower than 5k race pace, and corresponds to about 85 to 90 percent of the recommended maximum heart rate. The pace should feel "comfortably hard."

Motivation

"Some people say I have attitude – maybe I do...but I think you have to. You have to believe in yourself when no one else does – that makes you a winner right there. " — *Venus Williams*

Running Economy

Earlier in this chapter, we covered VO2 max and lactate threshold. Even though they don't apply to "average Joe" runners like us, as much as they do for elite athletes, we can still get some benefits from them. The third topic I'd like to touch on is *running economy*. Running economy (RE) is yet another component of overall *running performance*.

(VO2 max + RE) + lactate threshold = RUNNING PERFORMANCE

Conventional wisdom states that the runner with the highest aerobic capacity (VO2 max) will win the race. Sometimes, this is true, but in most cases it is not.

The runner utilizing the best *running economy* normally has the greatest chance to win the race. This runner will be able to use *less* oxygen and energy, just as a car uses *less* gasoline to improve its gas mileage.

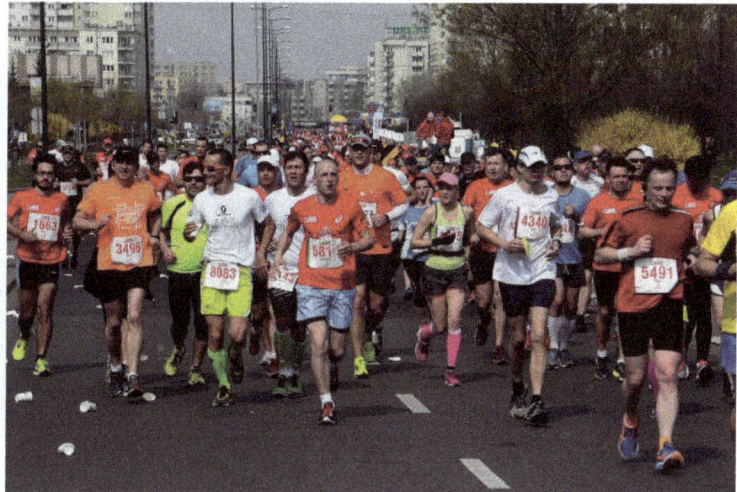

Some of the lesser informed "experts" say that running economy is directly related to *running form*, but in truth, it is more associated to those microscopic structures known as capillaries and mitochondria, which deliver oxygen to the blood. The densities of both improve with higher mileage. Higher mileage not only conditions the athlete for improved endurance, but also improves the running economy, biomechanics, and cardio fitness – all of which result in less oxygen consumption needed in a given time or distance run.

The most significant gains in running economy are realized with higher mileage, usually between 65 or 75 miles per week. Notably, this is about the same mileage where VO2 max seems to level off with only minimal advancements. Again, genetics most likely play a part in both VO2 max baselines and overall running economy. As noted earlier however, tempo runs, hill repeats and long intervals can all contribute to increased VO2 max and running economy.

Heavy lifting and plyometric exercises have also been known to increase muscle development and density, and can most certainly improve oxygen distribution in the body.

Motivation

"Winning has nothing to do with racing. Most days don't have races anyway. Winning is about struggle and effort and optimism, and never, ever, ever giving up." – *Amby Burfoot*

When Things Go Terribly Wrong

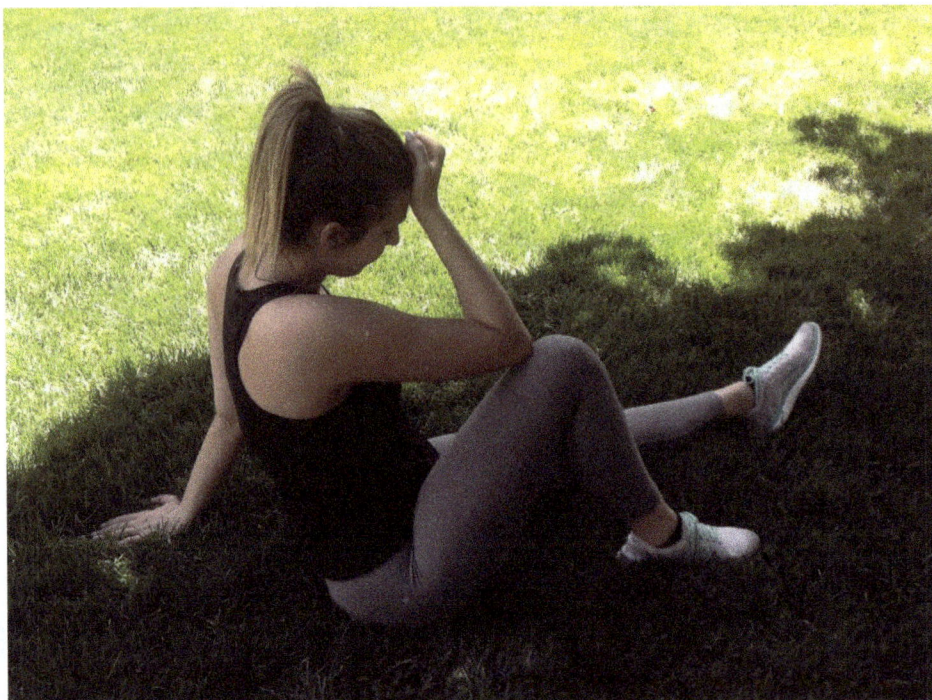

Prepare properly in your training sessions to avoid disasters

So far in this chapter, we've looked at theories, facts, numbers and definitions. But what happens when bad things happen to good people?

- What do we do when our bodies don't respond to our training?
- What happens when outside forces such as extreme weather conditions play into our training and competition?
- Why can a human run 26 miles and 345 yards, then completely fall apart within the last 30 or 40 yards?
- What happens when we get dehydrated or don't have enough nutrients?
- What happens when we have too much water?
- What if we think we're healthy enough to run, but find out we're really not?

We've all heard the question: Is running safe? And this question is truly justified, as we've seen runners go down, never to get up again. Normally, these stories draw a huge presence in the press, and rightfully so. Running *can* be dangerous, but *statistically* speaking, it is not. In almost all cases of runner deaths, there are underlying health reasons, or extreme weather conditions that can contribute to the death of a runner. This is a difficult topic to discuss, not only for the runners, but for the concerned friends and families of the runners, who might question our health (and sanity) in the first place.

Motivation

"It is not the size of the man, but the size of his heart that matters." — *Evander Holyfield*

Running a marathon is risky. So is walking across a street or shoveling snow. Life itself is full of risks, and we face them every day. For the several thousand people who die walking across the street or shoveling their snow each year, little is heard. But, if one person dies during a race, it quickly becomes front page, exclusive news. Runner deaths are both over-hyped and very infrequent, but they do occur. Statistically, runners are much healthier than non-runners, and potentially have fewer health risks.

In this section, we're going to look at the following topics and see if we can find ways to avoid or eliminate the most common risks of distance running.

Upcoming Topics

- Hydration
- Hyponatremia
- Postural Hypotension
- Heat Exhaustion
- Heat Stroke
- Cardiac Arrest

Hydration

For some reason, proper hydration is another topic that seems to be either ignored or underestimated by many runners. For any animal, hydration in the right amounts is paramount for the activity at hand, whether it's walking through a snow storm or running a marathon in Death Valley.

Many people overcomplicate this topic and try to turn it into rocket science, but when it comes right down to it, hydration is easy to understand: *When you run, you sweat. When you sweat a lot, your **blood volume** decreases, and the more your blood volume decreases, the harder your heart has to work.* While this may sound dangerous, it's really not, as long you monitor your situation. Very few athletes experience hydration conditions that cause serious health problems, but when they do occur, athletes may become temporarily weak, nauseous, or faint. The bigger and more common problem is that the athlete can forget her water bottle, or assume she doesn't need it because she's only doing a short run. Far too many people make false assumptions about proper hydration, whether it's over-hydration or under-hydration. Unfortunately, hydration-induced health problems arise when you're already under or over hydrated. Let's look at the differences.

> **Tip**
>
> There are many ways to carry your water. Choose a way that's convenient and one that meets your needs. Mix and match! If you have a fuel belt that has multiple bottles, fill a couple of them with plain water and use the other two for a sports drink. During hot weather, freeze your bottles overnight and they'll thaw while you're on your run the next day.

> **Motivation**
>
> **"Running should be a lifelong activity. Approach it patiently and intelligently, and it will reward you for a long, long time."** – *Michael Sargent*

Dehydration

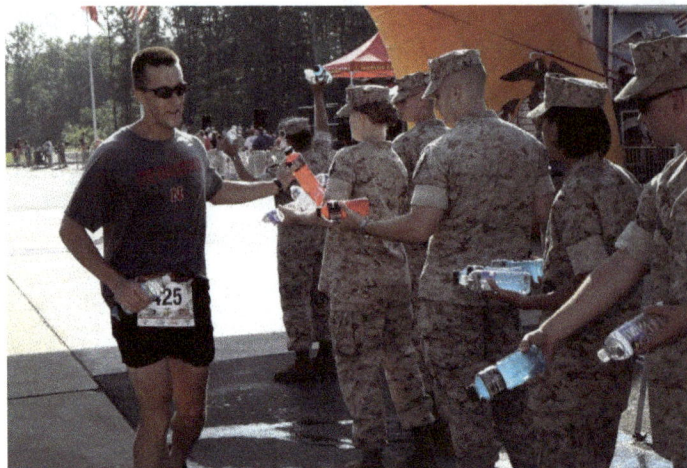

Simply put, dehydration occurs when you use or lose more fluid or salts than you take in, and your body doesn't have enough fluids to carry out its natural functions. Dehydration can worsen from fever or illness, a hot and dry climate, prolonged exposure to the sun or high temperatures. It can also occur by the overuse of diuretics or other medications that increase the normal output of urination. And of course, insufficient water intake can cause an imbalance in the delicate fluid and salt levels in our body. Water accounts for about 50% of a woman's body weight and about 60% of a man's weight.

Age and Dehydration

It's a known fact that many adults older than 60 years old don't get the hydration they need. And as some of the elderly persons move to warmer and dryer climates, the tendency for dehydration dramatically increases. All their lives, they only drank a certain amount of water, and now they're suddenly faced with dehydration problems. And of course, activities such as running and dancing only increase their difficulties.

Types of Dehydration

Mild dehydration is defined as the loss of no greater than 5% of the body's fluid. A loss of 5-10% is considered to be moderate dehydration and severe dehydration occurs with a loss of 10-15% of body fluids. Severe dehydration is a life-threatening condition that demands immediate medical attention.

Complications of Dehydration

If a person is severely depleted of fluids, **hypovolemic shock** can occur. Also known as **physical collapse**, it's usually recognized by pale, cool, clammy skin, shallow breathing and rapid heartbeat. If and when it does happen, blood pressure sometimes drops so low it can't even be measured, and skin at the knees and elbows may become blotchy.

Motivation

"I hated every minute of training, but I said, 'Don't quit… Suffer now and live the rest of your life as a champion." — *Muhammed Ali*

Causes and Symptoms

Strenuous activity, excessive sweating, overexposure to the sun and insufficient fluid intake all contribute to dehydration. Alcohol, caffeine, medications and diuretics that increase the output of fluid from the body can also impact dehydration levels.

Diagnosis

The patient's symptoms and medical history usually indicate dehydration. Physical examination may reveal rapid heart rate, shock, or low blood pressure. Blood tests can be used to check electrolyte levels and urine tests can be run to evaluate the severity of the issue. Other lab tests may be arranged to determine the underlying problem, such as diabetes or adrenal gland problems that may be the source of dehydration.

Treatment

For persons who are mildly dehydrated, drinking plain water may be all that's needed for treatment. An increase of fluid intake and replacement of lost electrolytes are usually all that's needed to sufficiently restore fluid balances in athletes who are moderately dehydrated. Adults who need to replace lost electrolytes can drink sports beverages and take in a little additional salt to help balance their body fluids. Commercial drinks such as Pedialyte can also help to alleviate the symptoms or conditions.

Medical Care

In cases of severe dehydration, intravenous fluids are almost always administered and the patient remains hospitalized until the condition improves. If an individual's blood pressure drops enough to cause the development of shock, medical treatment is usually required and intravenous fluids are administered to expedite normal hydration.

Tip

Never underestimate your training goals or overestimate your potential. Take your training seriously, and if you make a mistake, correct it before you try it again. Maintaining access to fluids during runs can be challenging. You can carry some fluid in a squeeze bottle stashed in a fluid belt worn around your waist, but you cannot always carry enough fluid in this manner to cover your longest runs. To ensure that you have enough fluid to cover these runs, either plan to return home midway through your run to refill your bottle or carry some money and refill your bottle at a convenience store. Wearing a fluid belt may slow you down a bit in your faster runs, so do these runs on a track or short circuit where you can stash a bottle at a convenient place and grab it for a quick drink as you pass by.

Motivation

"To give anything less than your best is to sacrifice the gift." – *Steve Prefontaine*

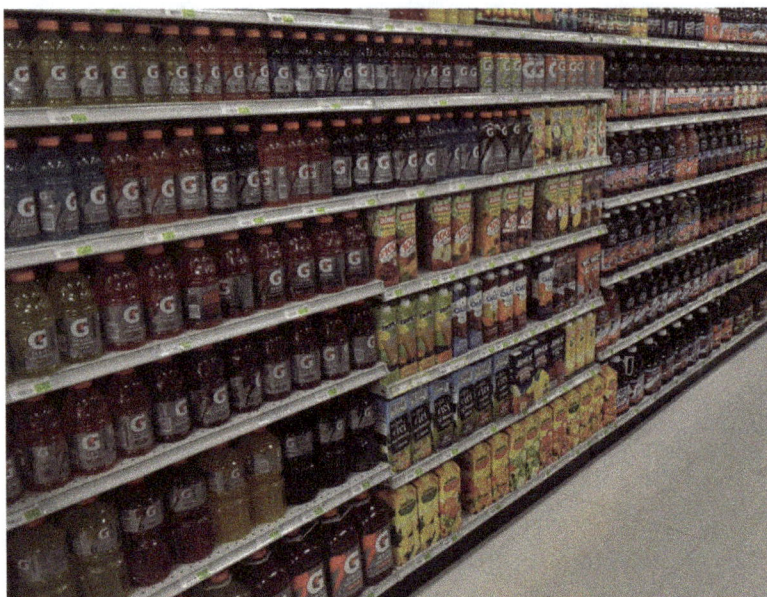

Hyponatremia

In the previous section, we looked at the causes and effects of dehydration, the danger signs, and ways to avoid it. Unfortunately, an opposing and potentially more dangerous problem lurks out there – that of *over hydration*, also known as **hyponatremia**, *hypotonic hydration or water intoxication.*

During a long-distance run, your body generates a significant amount of sweat, which may lead to dehydration. For many, there can be a temptation to drink large quantities of fluid before or during the run to prevent dehydration. While it can have the intended results, too much water can cause an imbalance characterized by low amounts of sodium in the blood. This condition is known as hyponatremia. Normally, the human body attempts to maintain a careful balance of sodium and fluid levels, but when you consume too much water, the sodium levels become diluted. These dangerous levels of sodium can lead to brain swelling and impaired hearing.

Description

Sodium is an atom or ion that carries a single positive charge and occurs as a salt in a crystalline solid. Sodium chloride, sodium phosphate, and sodium bicarbonate are commonly occurring salts. These types of salts can be dissolved in various fluids such as water or juices from foods. Dissolving these salts involves the complete separation of ions, such as sodium and chloride in common table salt.

About 40 percent of our sodium is contained in our bones and approximately 2 to 5 percent is contained within our organs and cells. The remaining 55 percent is in our blood plasma and other extracellular fluids. This specific distribution of sodium ions is essential for human life. Proper nerve conduction, blood pressure and the transit of nutrients into the body's cells are all dependent on the delicate balance of sodium in the system.

The body continually regulates its handling of sodium. The concentration of sodium in the blood plasma depends on two basic elements: the total amount of sodium, and the amount of water in the arteries, veins, and capillaries. The body uses separate methods to regulate sodium and water, but they work in unison to correct blood pressure when it's either too high or too low. An abnormally low concentration of sodium which, in effect, is the definition of hyponatremia, can be resolved either by increasing sodium or by decreasing the amount of water in the body.

Causes and Symptoms

Most cases of hyponatremia are caused by unusual consumption of fluids or abnormal amounts of sodium excreted by the body, either of which can render the body's ability to regulate properly.

Secondary causes are long-term low sodium diets, and, you guessed it, excessive sweating while on a long run. Long distance running, under certain conditions, can trigger hyponatremia, because the body can lose 2 to 2-1/2 gallons of water through sweating. This usually occurs in distances of marathon-length or greater, and normally in hot or humid weather conditions. Excessive consumption of beer, which is mainly water and naturally low in sodium, can also produce hyponatremia, especially when combined with a poor diet.

It should be noted that drinking pure water instead of a sports drink that contains sodium could exacerbate the symptoms of hyponatremia because it dilutes the sodium in the bloodstream. Severe hyponatremia can trigger neurological problems that require immediate emergency treatment.

Symptoms of moderate hyponatremia include fatigue, headaches, disorientation, nausea and muscle cramps. Severe cases of hyponatremia can lead to seizures, coma and death. These neurological symptoms are thought to result from the sudden increase of water into brain cells, causing them to swell and malfunction.

Diagnosis

Hyponatremia is diagnosed by running specific blood tests, preparing plasma, and using a sodium-sensitive electrode for measuring the concentration levels of sodium. Sometimes, additional tests must be run on the patient to determine if the sodium was lost through diarrhea, urination or vomiting.

Treatment

Severe hyponatremia is usually treated by infusing a solution of 5% sodium chloride in water into the bloodstream.

Tip

Don't be fooled! While hyponatremia occurs infrequently in runners, it is a very real and potentially life-threatening condition. It is more common due to health-related illnesses, but can still affect anyone that dilutes their sodium levels with too much water.

The same rule applies with dehydration. Drink when you're thirsty, but not in excess. If you drink so much fluid that you hear or feel it sloshing in your stomach, you've had enough. Whenever possible, drink electrolyte fluids such as Gatorade, instead of pure water, because it is more effective in keeping your sodium at the proper levels.

Motivation

"An ounce of prevention is worth a pound of cure." – *Benjamin Franklin*

Postural Hypotension

Earlier in this chapter, I asked the question: *Why can a human run 26 miles and 345 yards, then completely fall apart within the last 30 or 40 yards?"* I struggled with this question for quite a while until I experienced it myself. When the runner approaches the finish line, does the body produce a rush of "emotional" chemical releases that overwhelm the body? Are the legs acting as an auxiliary pump for the circulatory system, and when the legs stop, does the blood pressure drop? Are the natural body chemicals so depleted that it can no longer keep going? Why does this happen near the finish line?

Dehydration or improper nutrition prior to race day are sometimes caused by inexperience or over-confidence. But, some breakdowns aren't nearly as simple, and aren't just "mistakes." Some are very serious health issues and can be dangerous or even deadly. The final four topics in this chapter are ***postural hypotension, heat exhaustion, heat stroke*** and ***cardiac arrest.***

Have you ever stood or sat up suddenly and had a head rush or dizzy spell? This sudden change from a horizontal to vertical position can cause a rapid drop in blood pressure and can cause the dizziness. There are a number of issues or incidents that can complicate this condition, including dehydration, blood loss, heart disorders, diabetes and certain medications.

Unfortunately, this sudden loss of blood pressure can also occur in runners, particularly when a runner stops at an aid station or slows or stops at the end of the run. Physiologists originally thought this phenomenon was directly related to heat exhaustion, dehydration or worse yet, heat stroke. Confusion arose because postural hypotension is, in fact, more prevalent in hotter conditions.

In recent years, however, biologists and physicists have been able to determine that the legs are actually acting as an auxiliary pump and assisting the cardiovascular system with blood flow. As the leg muscles contract rhythmically, they force un-oxygenated blood out of the legs and back toward the heart and lungs. The elevated heart rate also contributes to increased blood circulation, allowing your heart to pump blood more quickly to the rest of the body. When the legs slow or stop, however, those two mechanisms cease to assist with the blood supply and the effect is immediate dizziness. Some experts believe that without the rapid heart rate and the contraction of the leg muscles, blood can get trapped in the legs – a condition typically referred to as blood pooling. This trapped blood is not capable of returning to the brain, heart and lungs in its current condition and this can cause a sudden collapse.

Treatment and Prevention

You can prevent the effects of this condition by walking for several minutes after finishing your race. If you don't feel good enough to walk, lie down and elevate your legs to foster blood return. This condition is rarely fatal, but it can certainly cause a patient to pass out or, at the very least, be very uncomfortable. Postural hypotension is not related to heat exhaustion or heat stroke, although elevated temperatures can certainly contribute to the frequency and severity of it. If you see a runner coming into the finish line strong, and they suddenly start to struggle or falter, chances are their "auxiliary" pump is slowing down and they are suffering from postural hypotension. Finish line race volunteers should watch for these victims and be prepared to help them either stay on their feet, or get them off their feet and elevate their legs as soon as possible.

Heat-related issues

There are actually five heat-related illnesses, but in the running context, we'll only talk extensively about **heat exhaustion** and **heat stroke**. The other three are **heat rash, heat cramps,** and **heat syncope.** *Heat rash* is defined as a skin irritation that usually occurs in hot, humid weather. It is caused by excessive sweating, and can lead to the blockage of sweat ducts. *Heat cramps* usually affect people who sweat profusely during strenuous activity, which depletes the body's fluids and salts. This low level of sodium in the muscles causes painful muscle cramps, usually following exercise. Heat cramps may also share symptoms similar to heat exhaustion. The third heat disorder is known as *heat syncope,* which is a fainting episode that occurs in the heat, either during prolonged standing or exercise, or when rapidly moving from a horizontal to vertical position. It typically occurs in individuals who are not accustomed to high temperatures and humidity. Dehydration can also contribute to this condition. Now, let's look at the two main heat-related illnesses with respect to running – heat exhaustion and heat stroke.

Heat Exhaustion

First of all, heat exhaustion and heat stroke are *not* the same things, although heat exhaustion can be a precursor to heat stroke. Both can be dangerous and uncomfortable, but heat exhaustion is usually temporary and rarely causes permanent damage or death.

Heat exhaustion is a condition with symptoms that may include a rapid pulse and heavy sweating (a result of your body beginning to overheat). The most typical causes of heat exhaustion are exposure to high temperatures, especially when combined with high humidity and vigorous physical activity. Without rapid treatment, heat exhaustion can initiate heat stroke, which is a life-threatening condition. In most cases, heat exhaustion is completely preventable.

In essence, heat exhaustion is the body's response to an excessive loss of fluid and salt contained in sweat due to strenuous physical activity, usually in a hot environment. The body temperature may be normal or mildly elevated, but not above 104° F degrees. It often occurs in individuals who are not acclimatized to running or exercising in the heat.

Most victims of heat exhaustion have minor complaints of headache or dizziness; however, they will not experience central nervous system problems as severe as those suffering from heat stroke. Most cases of heat exhaustion can be treated without hospitalization.

Warning signs of heat exhaustion include a normal or slightly elevated body temperature, heavy sweating, pallor, confusion, dizziness, fainting, fatigue, dark urine (also a sign of dehydration), nausea, vomiting, diarrhea and muscle or abdominal cramps. In some cases, if heat exhaustion is untreated and exposure to the heat continues, it may progress to heat stroke.

Treatment and immediate cooling measures that may be effective include the consumption of cool, non-alcoholic beverages, such as water and sports drinks, eating salty snacks, or rest in the shade or in a cooler environment. Taking a cool shower or bath, and loosening or removing restrictive clothing may help. Always seek medical attention immediately if conditions worsen or if there are underlying health conditions such as diabetes, heart diseases or other illnesses.

Motivation

"I never left the field saying I could have done more to get ready and that gives me peace of mind." *– Peyton Manning*

Heat Stroke

Heat stroke is a very dangerous and life-threatening condition if the body's temperature stays high for an extended period of time. Most experts agree that heat stroke will not occur until the patient's internal temperature reaches 104° F, or more.

Prior to the actual stroke, the patient will most likely suffer from nausea, lightheadedness, profuse sweating, and muscle cramps. If the patient experiences all of these symptoms and the temperature remains high, collapse is likely. Under the right conditions, heat stroke can happen at any time during the race. If you begin to feel any or all of the symptoms, you should stop immediately and seek medical assistance. While heat *exhaustion* can be just a minor inconvenience, heat *stroke* should ALWAYS be considered a medical emergency, requiring IMMEDIATE attention. Heat stroke is considered to be the most severe of the heat-related illnesses, and can lead to permanent disability or death.

Heat stroke takes place when the body's natural ability to regulate its internal temperature has faltered. In these conditions, the patient's internal temperature quickly rises above 104° F, leading to brain and internal organ damage. Normally, the extent of temporary or permanent injury depends on the duration of exposure and the peak temperature attained. Heat stroke is sometimes referred to as sun stroke.

While warning signs of heat stroke can vary from person to person, they almost always include an internal temperature of 104° F or greater. Symptoms include rapid heart rate, breathing difficulties, dizziness, headache, loss of balance and coordination, nausea, vomiting, restlessness, confusion, seizures, unconsciousness, coma or death. Even though sweating can occur, it should be noted that a patient doesn't always sweat because the sweat glands may have already malfunctioned. This means the patient has no functional cooling system and immediate aid is required.

If any or all of these conditions are present, it should be considered to be a life-threatening emergency. At this point, an emergency response is required – paramedics or medical experts must be called right away. Start by calling 911 and begin some type of cooling process, using whatever means you have available. If possible, immerse the patient in a tub or shower with cool water. Remove any restrictive clothing, spray them with a mist bottle and turn on a fan to cool their skin. Wet sheets in drier climates will also help with cooling the patient. Apply ice or cold packs if they are available. For best results, place the packs in the armpits, groin, and the head and neck areas. Constantly monitor the patient and remain vigilant with the cooling efforts, until the patient's temperature is 102° F or lower. Be aware that a patient in this condition can also be overcooled because some key internal functions have ceased to function. If the patient is conscious, give them cool liquids to drink.

Heat Stroke Avoidance and Prevention

To prevent heat stroke, wear sunscreen and sunglasses, stay hydrated, wear lightweight clothing that wicks sweat away from your body, and try to avoid running in oppressive heat.

> **Motivation**
>
> **"Don't let the past keep you, don't let the present stop you, and don't let the future scare you. Be bold."** – *Gordon "Fuzz" Watts*
>
> *Words from my father on my birthday, just three days before he passed away in 1984*

Cardiac Arrest

The final portion of this chapter deals with heart attacks during running or training events. While it is very rare that a person dies during a running event, it does occur. In 2012, the *New England Journal of Medicine* conducted a study related to "Cardiac Arrest During Long Distance Running Races." In 2010 alone, nearly two million runners ran marathons or half-marathons in the United States. The study was based on individuals who suffered cardiac arrest at the finish line, or within an hour of their finish.

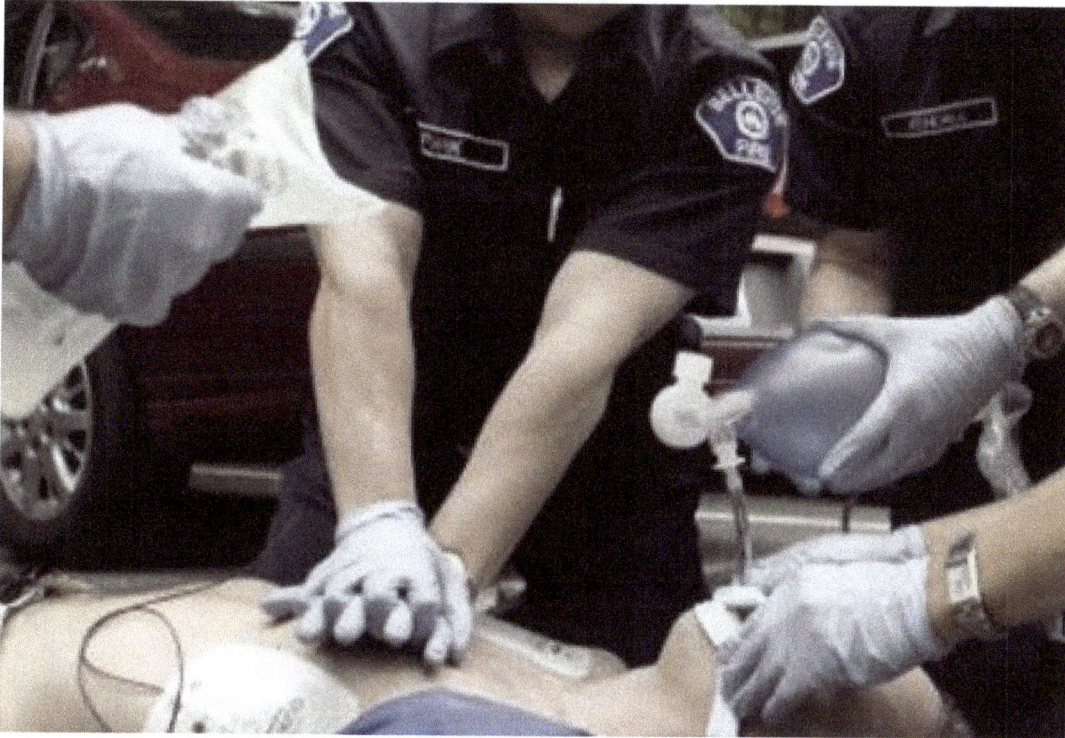

"Cases of cardiac arrest were defined by an unconscious state and an absence of spontaneous respirations and pulse, as documented by a medical professional. Non-survivors of cardiac arrest were defined as persons who were not successfully resuscitated in the field, or who died before hospital discharge. Survivors of cardiac arrest were defined as persons who were successfully resuscitated and subsequently discharged from the hospital." ** Source: New England Journal of Medicine*

The study included nearly 10.9 million marathon and half-marathon runners from various races around the country, and found that 59 people suffered cardiac arrest in the study period. Of those 59 people, 51 of them were men. This equates to an attack in one out of 184,000 runners, most of which occur during marathons (as opposed to half-marathons), and most of which are men as opposed to women.

Of the 59 people in the study, 41 were fatal, with 18 survivors. Medical history was available for 31 of the victims (survivors or non-survivors), and of the 31 runners for whom complete clinical data were obtained, 23 had died. Hypertrophic cardiomyopathy (in eight of 23) and possible hypertrophic cardiomyopathy (in seven of 23) were the most common causes of death. Notably, nine of the 15 non-survivors who had cardiac hypertrophy had an additional clinical factor or postmortem finding: obstructive coronary artery disease, myocarditis, aortic valve or coronary anomaly, or other serious cardiac defects.

The study found "that the incidence rates of cardiac arrest and sudden death during marathon and half-marathon long-distance running races were 1 per 184,000 and 1 per 259,000 participants, respectively." They estimated "that this translates into 0.2 cardiac arrests and 0.14 sudden deaths per 100,000 runner-hours at risk, using average running times of 4 and 2 hours for the marathon and half-marathon, respectively. Thus, event rates among marathon and half-marathon runners are relatively low, as compared with other athletic populations, including collegiate athletes (1 death per 43,770 participants per year), 23 triathlon participants (1 death per 52,630 participants), 24 and previously healthy middle-aged joggers (1 death per 7,620 participants.)"

Source: New England Journal of Medicine

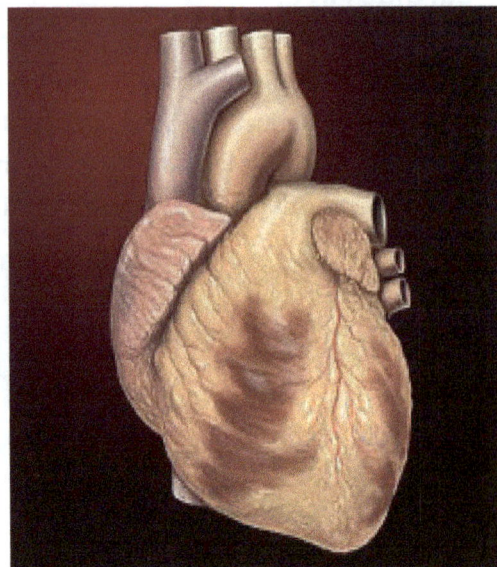

FINAL CONCLUSION: These data suggest that the risk associated with long-distance running events is *equivalent to* or *lower* than the risk associated with other vigorous physical activity.

Challenge!

The importance of a physical evaluation

Before embarking on a new physical activity such as running, you should always seek a medical professional to assess your health. In the past, most medical groups encouraged an annual health exam. More recently, however, the American Medical Association and other similar groups have migrated away from the annual exam. They now suggest that medical checkups or "Periodic Health Assessments" should be executed every five years for adults between the ages of 18 and 40, and every one to three years thereafter. The frequency for these health checks increases for those taking prescription medications.

Most men and women younger than 40 years of age are typically free from serious illness or disease that could be diagnosed by a physical examination alone. In this age group, major health problems usually display specific signs or symptoms that might prompt you to seek your doctor's advice. Additionally, much of the testing that was done routinely in the past is not cost effective and, in some cases, causes pointless and unnecessary additional testing and anxiety. Your challenge: *See your health professional before you start your training program!*

Chapter 7 – Dealing with Injuries

My Story

As I mentioned in Chapter Three, your **foot strike type** can be the cause of injuries, particularly if you're a heel striker like I was. Likewise, an injury can force you to modify your foot strike. From 2005 to 2008, I ran no fewer than 50 races, 30 of which were the full marathons. I was convinced that I could run one marathon, plus another 275 training miles each month. I pushed myself to the limit, loaded up with unnecessary miles, and put in training sessions that contained no plan or methodology. I became the king of "junk miles" – running too many miles with no purpose. I thought if I ran more, I'd get stronger but soon found out that it was quite the opposite. At some stage, I hit the point of diminishing returns. I fatigued my body to the point that I was now much weaker, and my times were slowing down dramatically. I went from my "average Joe" marathon time of 4 hour marathons to 4:15's, 4:30's and 4:45's… then it happened.

A small pain emerged in my left foot. Thinking I could "run through the pain," I continued my gluttony for self-punishment. Sharper, more direct pain ensued – and I still refused to listen to my body. I ran the Colorado Marathon in Fort Collins and it took well over five hours. In May of 2007, I ran the Colorado Colfax Marathon, and it took over SIX hours to complete. Finally, I acknowledged the fact that I was injured and needed to drastically cut back the miles, or stop completely. I reduced the mileage down to about 10 miles per week, barely enough to sustain even a moderate level of fitness. Eventually, I started to feel better, *gradually* increased my mileage, and managed to run a Boston qualifying time of 3 hours and 30 minutes at the Denver Marathon in October of that year. During the winter of 2007-2008, I averaged only about 20 miles per week, but was still able to land a couple fast times in shorter distance races of the five and ten-mile variety.

On April 5th, 2008, while at the Eisenhower Marathon in Abilene, Kansas, I was about 20 miles into the run, enduring the usual pain I had been accustomed to. Loaded up with Ibuprofen, I was clicking off eight minute miles, with a predicted finish time of 3:30, a time that would have again qualified me for Boston. The Eisenhower Marathon was supposed to be my warmup for the Boston Marathon, which was only 16 days away. Rounding a corner at mile 20, a surge of pain shot up from my foot and brought me to a complete stop on the course. I hobbled through the next 6 miles at an 11:30 minute per mile pace.

…continued

Motivation

"A champion is someone who gets up when he can't." – *Jack Dempsey*

My Story... continued

In tears because of the pain, I finished with a 4 hour and 21-minute time. It was a setback for me, but my stubbornness prevailed and two weeks later, I ran the Boston Marathon. Of course, Boston was a disaster for me – I hadn't listened to my body and my pride led me into something I shouldn't have done.

When I returned to Colorado, X-rays showed that I had three stress fractures in the fourth and fifth metatarsal bones of my left foot. At this point, I was fitted with a soft cast and quit running altogether.

Just eight weeks later, I began to run again, but because of fear of reinjuring myself, and a bit of lingering pain, I started running on the soft trails in the foothills west of Denver. I immediately noticed that I spent a lot more time running on my toes and balls of my feet. And if you really think about it, it's nearly impossible to run flat-footed, either up or downhill. When running uphill, you can't be a heel striker – it just doesn't work. It's like going up the stairs on your heels instead of your toes.

Eventually, I started mixing in runs on the hard concrete and asphalt streets of Denver. Again, I noticed a change in my *biomechanics*. No longer was I a heel striker, but had unknowingly converted to a mid-foot striker. My foot strike type had magically changed in six short months, partially due to my injury and partially because of my hill running. On October 19th of 2008, I ran the Denver Marathon in 3 hours 14 minutes, my fastest marathon yet.

Feeling like I was "back," I attacked the Colorado Trail, with mountain running on soft, single track trails, reaping the benefits of altitude training, along with hill climbing. The Colorado Trail is a 480+ mile trail that stretches from Denver to Durango, Colorado. Running many of the lengthy segments on this very steep terrain, I increased my fitness well beyond what I could ever imagine, all the while becoming much stronger and faster.

In 2009, after finally listening to my body, my efforts paid off, and I ran my four fastest marathons, with times of 3:00.09, 3:11.00, 2:59.01 and 2:59:17.

So what are the lessons here?

- Listen to your body! You cannot "run through" an injury. Take the necessary time to heal when you do have an injury.
- Strengthen with hill work and various forms of cross-training.
- Don't be afraid to change your running style if your normal biomechanics will allow it. It may take time, but it can be done.

Motivation

"The will to win means nothing, if you haven't the will to prepare." – *Juma Ikangaa*

Common Injuries

At some point during your training or racing, you will most likely have some sort of injury. This could be a nagging pain that might be a mere annoyance, or it could sideline you for months. Most of your running injuries occur when you push yourself too hard. Your biomechanics and physical stature may also play a role in why and how often you become injured.

There are a number of ways that a runner can become injured, but to avoid re-writing entire medical journals, we'll focus on the most common ones. We'll start with "shin splints," the most common injury for new runners just beginning a training program. This is most likely the injury that causes people to quit running shortly after they begin.

Shin Splints

Tibial stress syndromes, frequently known as shin splints, often occur in runners who have recently increased or changed their training routines. Shin splints are caused when the connective tissue (muscles and tendons) to the bone become agitated, stressed or mildly torn by the increased activity. You'll know when you have shin splints if you have tenderness, soreness or pain, along the bones of your lower leg. You may also experience minor swelling from the damaged tissue.

By the very nature of their activities, runners are most at risk of shin splints, especially new runners. Other characteristics that may cause or worsen shin splints are running on hard surfaces, especially with sudden starts and stops; running on uneven surfaces such as hills; or if you have flat feet or very high arches.

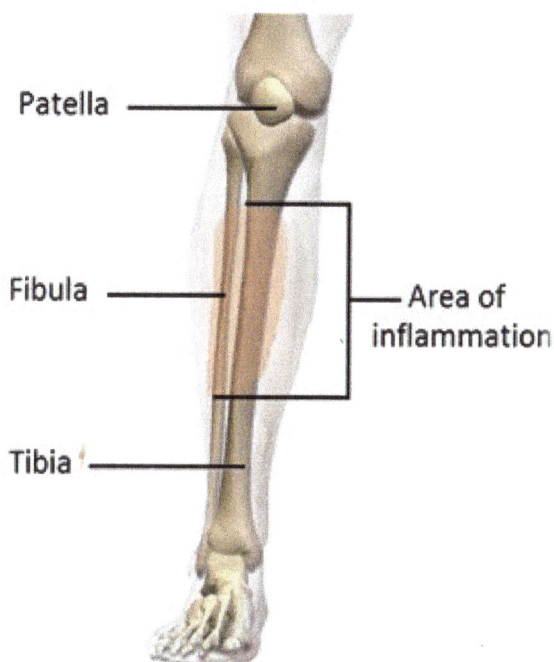

If you don't heal in a reasonable timeframe, you should see your doctor because you may actually have stress fractures, which are sometimes mistaken for shin splints. You should also modify your routine so you don't reinjure yourself.

Motivation

"Courage doesn't always roar, sometimes it's the quiet voice at the end of the day whispering 'I will try again tomorrow.'" — *Mary Anne Radmacher*

If you are new to the running sport, please make the following considerations before you begin your training. Go to a running store and get fitted for the correct shoes. Replace them every 400 to 500 miles or sooner if you see unusual wear. If you know that you have arch problems, either too high or too low, make sure that you have the correct fitting shoes with optional arch supports. Start your training with a conservative plan. Practice the walk/run technique (use the Galloway method described earlier in this book) and limit yourself to short runs. Utilize cross-training activities that place less impact on your body, such as swimming, walking or biking. Finally, add strength training to your routine. Implement toe raises, calf stretches and leg presses. Do not progress to heavier weights until your current regimen feels easy.

Knee Injuries

"Runner's knee" is probably the second most common complaint among runners, especially for runners who are new to the sport. As the name suggests, runner's knee is usually described as an aching pain around the kneecap. Runner's knee isn't really a condition itself, but a collection of symptoms specific to other disorders with various causes. Runner's knee is also called patellofemoral pain syndrome.

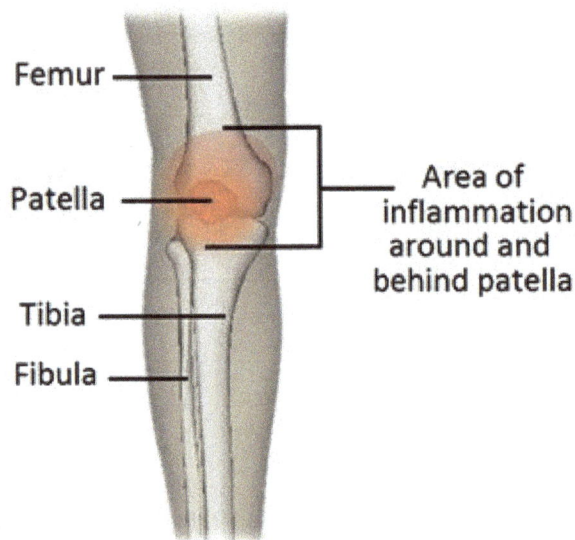

Femur — Patella — Tibia — Fibula —
Area of inflammation around and behind patella

Patellofemoral Pain Syndrome or Runner's knee results primarily from *overuse*. Repeated knee flexion can irritate the nerves of the kneecap, along with overstretched connective tissue (tendons and cartilage) of the knee. *Direct trauma* such as a fall or blow to the knee can also cause pain. Physical problems such as *bone misalignment, problems with the feet,* or *weak leg muscles*, particularly in the thighs, can contribute to runner's knee. Symptoms of runner's knee are pain when flexing the knee, when walking, kneeling, running or even sitting for long periods of time.

The pain could worsen when you go up or down stairs or hills. Pain around the kneecap becomes prevalent, especially where the kneecap and thigh bone meet. Other symptoms include a popping or grinding sensation or swelling of the knee.

Accurate diagnosis of runner's knee may include a trip to the doctor for a physical examination, X-ray, MRI, or CT scan. Runner's knee is always a good candidate for the **RICE** therapy treatment – *(Rest, Ice, Compression* and *Elevation).*

Motivation

"Only he who can see the invisible can do the impossible." – *Frank L. Gaines*

If you are diagnosed with runner's knee, or you suspect that you have it, rest your knee as much as possible. Most runner's knee injuries will heal on their own with the proper amount of rest. Ice your knee to reduce inflammation 3 to 4 times per day, for 2 to 3 days in succession, or until the pain is alleviated. For extra support, use an elastic bandage or soft knee brace and elevate your leg on a pillow when you're sitting or lying down. If you have a known alignment or low arch problem in your feet, make sure you get the proper supports for your shoes. From an over-the-counter medicine perspective, taking Non-steroidal anti-inflammatory drugs (NSAIDs), like Advil, Aleve, or Motrin, will help with pain and swelling.

Severe cases of runner's knee may need surgery. A surgeon could remove damaged cartilage or rectify the position of the kneecap so that stress will be distributed evenly and recovery time depends on each particular case. While you recover, try out a new activity that won't aggravate your runner's knee. For instance, if you're a jogger, do laps in the pool instead. Don't return to your old level of physical activity until your pain has subsided, and your knee feels as strong as your uninjured knee.

Prevention of runner's knee includes correction of your arch or alignment issues, strengthening your thigh muscles, and avoiding runs on hard surfaces such as concrete. For obvious health reasons, stay in shape and stay at a healthy weight. Avoid intense workouts as much as possible and make progressive changes in your workout routine. Know when to discard old shoes!

Runner's knee is the most common knee injury, but certainly isn't the only knee injury. I won't go into great detail of the more serious knee injuries, but I will list them here with a very brief description, for informational purposes.

ACL Injury – An anterior cruciate ligament, or ACL injury is the tearing of one of four ligaments that connect your femur (thighbone) to your tibia (shinbone). ACL injuries are especially common in people who play basketball, football, soccer or other sports that involve sudden changes of direction.

Torn Meniscus – The meniscus is a durable, rubbery cartilage that acts as a cushioning shock absorber between your femur and tibia. It can be torn by sudden twisting or flexing of the knee while bearing weight on it. *(See more about a torn meniscus on page 76 in the upcoming section.)*

Knee Bursitis – Some knee injuries cause inflammation in the bursae, the small sacs of fluid that cushion the outside of your knee joint so that tendons and ligaments glide smoothly over the joint.

Patellar Tendinitis – Tendinitis is best described as irritation and inflammation of one or more tendons. Tendons are the fibrous, thick tissues that attach muscles to bones. Skiers, runners, cyclists and those involved in jumping sports and activities are more prone to develop inflammation in the patellar tendon, which connects one of the quadriceps muscles on the front of the femur to the tibia.

Foreign Object or Loose Body – Injury or degeneration of bones or cartilage can often cause a piece of bone or cartilage to break and float in the space between the bones. Sometimes this creates problems when the loose body or object interferes with knee movement.

Motivation

"Adversity causes some men to break, others to break records." — *William A. Ward*

Dislocated Kneecap – Dislocation of the kneecap occurs when the patella that covers the front of your knee becomes dislodged, usually to the outside of your knee. In some cases, the kneecap may stay dislodged and you'll be able to see the dislocation.

Hip, Leg or Foot Pain – If you're having problems with your feet, legs or hips, it's possible that you may change the way you walk to alleviate the pain, but this altered gait can place even more stress on your joints. Be aware of your injuries and treat them accordingly. Don't try to "run through" your pain.

Iliotibial Band Syndrome

Iliotibial band syndrome (IT band syndrome) is usually caused from overuse of the tissues located on the outer part of the thigh and knee. This can be very tender and painful in those areas, especially just above the joint of the knee. Iliotibial band syndrome is very prevalent in runners and bicyclists, especially early in the training cycle. Heel strikers are more likely to have IT band syndrome than mid- or fore-front runners.

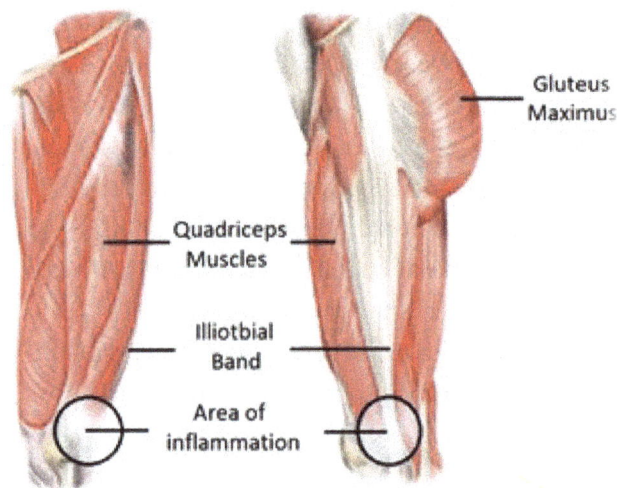

Anatomically speaking, the iliotibial band runs along the lateral or outside portion of the thigh and is an important feature that stabilizes the outside of the knee as it extends and flexes. The iliotibial band is a thick, fibrous band of tissue that begins at the iliac crest in the pelvis and traverses the outer part of the thigh, eventually crossing the knee to attach into the top part of the tibia.

Functionally, the IT band helps to stabilize the outside part of the knee throughout its range of motion. IT band pain occurs when the ligaments which extend from the outside of the tibia to the outside of the pelvic bone become so tight that they rub against the outer portion of the femur. Long distance runners and trail runners are especially susceptible to iliotibial band syndrome when long periods of stabilization are required.

When the knee is flexed, the IT band should be located behind a small, bony outcropping of the femur at the knee. When the knee is extended, the IT band moves forward across this bony structure. In a healthy knee there is a sac (bursa) that allows the ligament to gently glide across this outcropping, but if the area becomes irritated or inflamed, the increased friction from repetitive rubbing of the iliotibial band across the bone can cause pain, especially along the outer area of the knee joint. Ignoring the symptoms can lead to further inflammation and scarring can occur in the bursa, decreasing the range of motion in the knee. Most IT band injuries can be prevented by maintaining leg and core strength and flexibility.

As with most soft tissue injuries, *RICE* therapy treatment (see previous section) and anti-inflammatory medications are first-line treatments. Physical therapy may also be helpful but for some rare cases, surgery may be required if therapy fails.

Achilles Tendinitis

Achilles tendinitis is a very painful inflammation of the Achilles tendon, and is similar to other soft tissue injuries that are normally caused from sudden overuse.

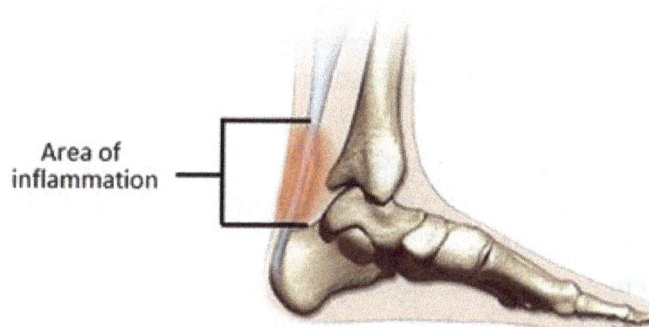

Area of inflammation

The Achilles tendon is a strong, fibrous band of tissue that connects the muscles of the lower leg (calf) to the bone of your heel. Achilles tendinitis is most common in runners who have abruptly increased the duration or intensity of their workouts. In most cases, this tendinitis is usually treated with fairly simple, home care that your doctor can prescribe. Decreased duration or intensity usually expedites the healing process and prevents recurring episodes. Serious instances of Achilles tendinitis can lead to tendon tears (ruptures), and painful bone spurs that require surgery.

Achilles tendinitis can cause pain and stiffness in the area of the tendon, as shown in the diagram above. It is moderately painful in the morning but can hurt worse with increased activity. As with most tendon issues, repetitive stress and overuse is the primary reason for the tendinitis. Adding too much distance to your running routine can cause tendinitis, along with tight calf muscles. The symptoms commonly associated with Achilles tendinitis usually begin with mild aches in the back of the leg or just above the heel. Pain is most noticeable immediately following a run or intense workout. Stairclimbing and hill running can exacerbate the pain.

Middle-aged men, overweight people of either gender or those with tight calf muscles or flat feet are more prone to this injury. Other high risk factors include those who have diabetes or high blood pressure.

Activities that can contribute are increased intensity in your workout, running more in colder weather and hilly terrain, and running in shoes that have expired. Finally, certain types of antibiotics, called fluoroquinolones, have been associated with higher rates of Achilles tendinitis.

Diagnosis is fairly simple with an MRI, X-Ray or ultrasound procedure. Home treatments are usually very successful with **RICE** (Rest, Ice, Compression and Elevation) therapy. Effective over-the-counter medications such as ibuprofen (Advil, Motrin) or naproxen (Aleve) usually work well for these injuries.

Prevention usually includes daily stretching exercises, strengthening of the calf muscles, cross-training to work other muscle groups, increasing your training regimen gradually and choosing your shoes carefully.

> ### Motivation
>
> **"You're never a loser until you quit trying."** – *Mike Ditka*

Muscle Pulls

A muscle pull is defined as a small tear in your muscle, also called a muscle strain. It's often caused by overextending a muscle or overuse of a muscle in conjunction with heavy lifting or pulling, or rapid movement of a muscle or ligament.

When you pull a muscle, you may experience a popping sensation when the muscle tears. The tearing of the muscle can also damage small blood vessels and capillaries, causing local bleeding and bruising, and pain caused by irritation of the nerve endings in the area.

Common muscle pulls are normally short-lived in nature if you implement immediate simple *RICE* therapy treatment. More serious muscle tears can take weeks or months to heal, and may require surgery, although these are fairly rare for runners.

The most common muscle pulls are the Hamstrings, quadriceps, calf and groin areas. Normally, the larger the muscle affected, the longer it takes to heal. Once again, as with other soft tissue injuries, effective over–the-counter medications such as ibuprofen (Advil, Motrin) or naproxen (Aleve) are recommended.

Upper Leg Muscle Pulls

The "Quadriceps" muscle is actually made up of four different muscles: the *vastus medialis, vastus intermedius, vastis lateralis and rectus femoris*, thus the "quad" moniker. Therefore it is a "muscle group," rather than one large muscle. Usually, when a runner complains of quadriceps pain, it's usually a strain to the Rectus femoris, the largest of the four muscles. Because it is connected to both the hip and the knee, it is very prone to injury. Strains are also common in the *gluteus maximus*, the largest and strongest muscle in the human body. It's the main connecting point to the torso and legs and is prone to pain from too much activity and overuse. Finally, the hamstring is also a group of muscles and tendons and easily injured from overuse. It's comprised of the *Semitendinosus, Biceps femoris short head, Biceps femoris long head, Seminmembranosus*. Portions of the *Adductor magnus* are considered to be part of the "hamstring."

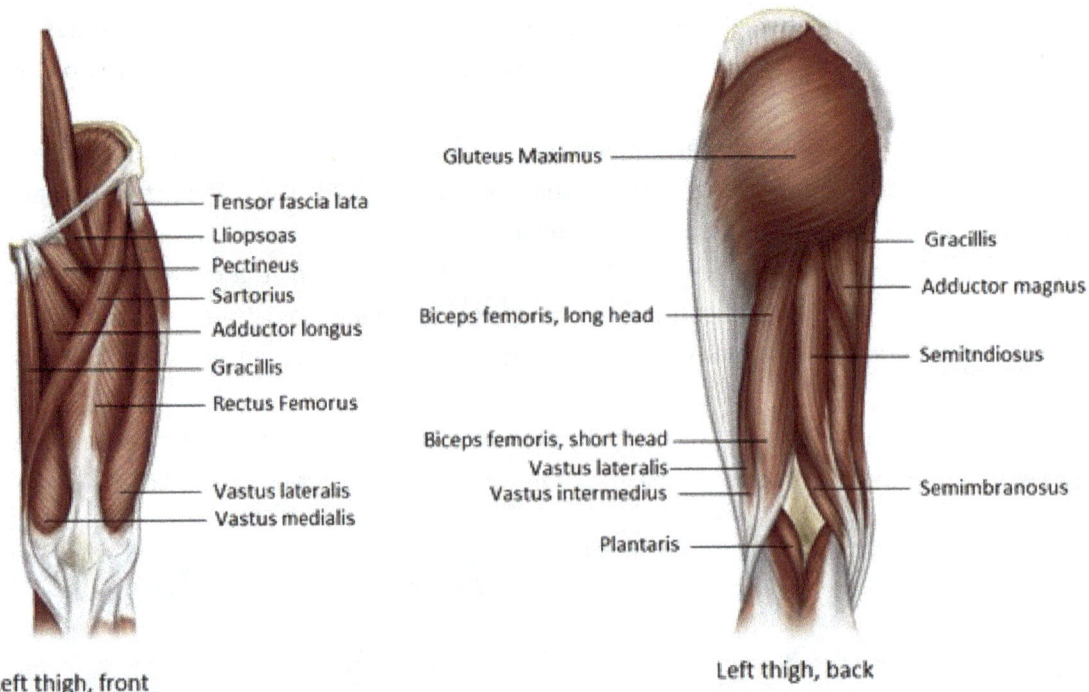

Left thigh, front

Left thigh, back

Lower Leg Muscle Pulls

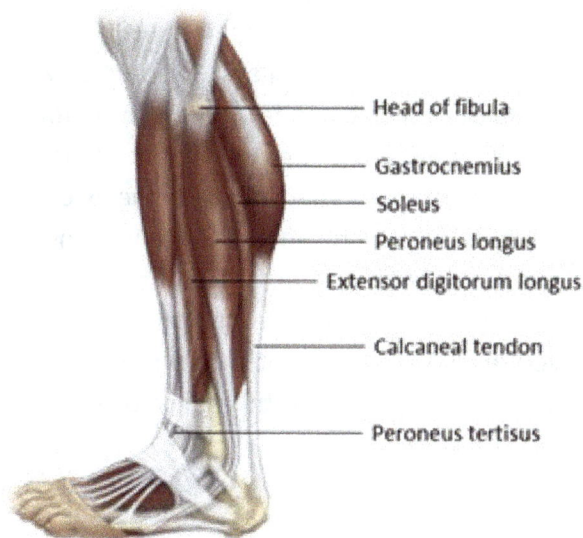

Head of fibula
Gastrocnemius
Soleus
Peroneus longus
Extensor digitorum longus
Calcaneal tendon
Peroneus tertisus

Once again, the calf muscle is another muscle group made up of the *gastrocnemius*, and *soleus.* These two muscles provide power and balance for the lower leg. They're connected to the *Achilles tendon*, the area most common for muscle tears. Another source for pain, and far less severe as a tear, is a muscle cramp. A cramp is a spasm in the leg that is usually short-lived, but can be very painful. Some spasms can be severe enough to cause bruising within the muscles. Runners sometimes experience these at night while in bed, and the pain can be excruciating even though it only lasts a few seconds.

Plantar Fasciitis

Plantar fasciitis is one of the most common causes of heel and arch pain. It involves inflammation and pain of a fibrous band of tissue known as the plantar fascia. This band of tissue runs nearly the length of the bottom of your foot and connects your toes to your heel bones. Plantar fasciitis generally causes very sharp pain that usually occurs with your very first steps in the morning. Once the foot limbers up a bit, the pain usually decreases, but there may be a reoccurrence of pain after long periods of sitting or standing. Plantar fasciitis is very common in the running community.

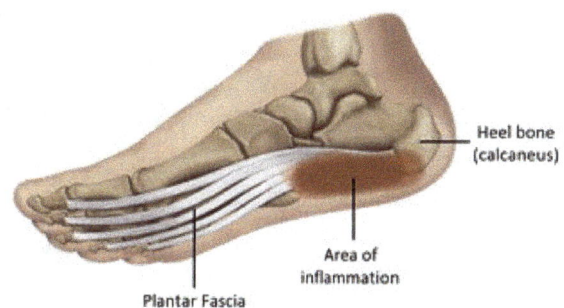

Heel bone (calcaneus)
Area of inflammation
Plantar Fascia

Normally, your plantar fascia acts as a shock-absorbing bowstring that supports the arch in your foot. If tension on that fascia becomes too great, small tears develop. Repetitive tearing and stretching causes the fascia to become inflamed or irritated. Plantar fasciitis is most common in persons between the ages of 40 and 60 and is not gender specific. The most common contributors are a sudden increase in activities that place abnormal stress on your heel and attached tissue such as long-distance running and hill running. Other contributors such as faulty foot structure or mechanics, like flat feet, or excessive limping, can cause plantar fasciitis.

Other causes may be related to uneven weight distribution, such as bearing weight on one foot more than the other one. Finally, obesity or a sudden onset of weight gain can cause tearing or inflammation of the plantar fascia.

Complications of plantar fasciitis can occur if you ignore the pain and symptoms. This may result in chronic heel pain that hampers your normal activities. Changing the way you walk to minimize the pain of plantar fasciitis can also cause the development of foot, knee, hip or back problems.

The diagnosis of plantar fasciitis is fairly straightforward. Normally, X-Rays, CT scans or MRIs are only ordered to find out if there are other problems besides the plantar fasciitis, such as torn heel ligaments or bone spurs. Most people who suffer from plantar fasciitis recover with a conservative treatment plan in just a few months, although some cases may take years depending on the extent of the damage and condition of the patient. Pain relievers such as ibuprofen (Advil, Motrin IB, others) and naproxen (Aleve) may ease the pain and inflammation associated with plantar fasciitis.

Strengthening and stretching exercises, combined with the use of simple, yet specialized devices may provide symptom relief. A physical therapist can show you special exercises that stretch the plantar fascia and Achilles tendon, along with strengthening your lower leg muscles. All of this helps to stabilize your ankle and heel.

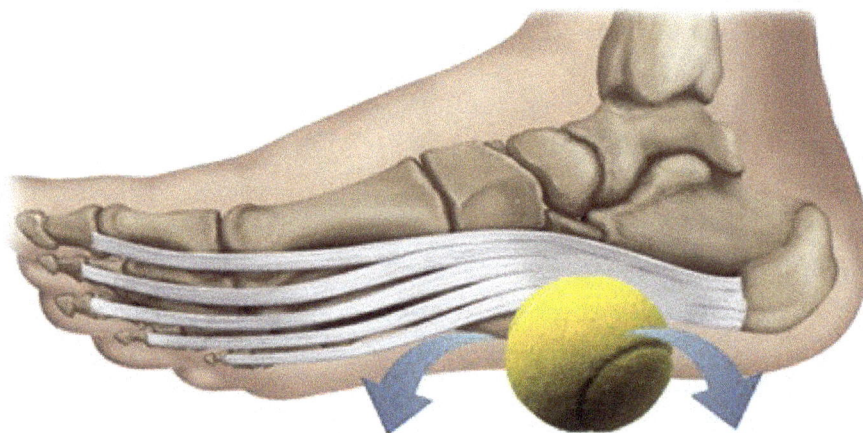

Home remedies may include rolling a tennis ball, baseball, or frozen water bottle on the bottom of your feet, several times per day for about 10 minutes each time. Ice can help alleviate the pain and rolling a bottle or ball can help stimulate the fascia and return much needed blood supply to the injured area, critical for the healing process. Your physical therapist or doctor may recommend wearing a "Strasburg sock" or splint that stretches your calf muscles and the arch of your foot while you sleep. This helps to hold the plantar fascia tendon and Achilles tendon in a lengthened position overnight and facilitates proper stretching of the fascia.

Custom-fit arch supports (Orthotics) may also be prescribed to help distribute the pressure more evenly. These are usually prescribed for those with weak or flat arches.

Motivation

"You miss 100 percent of the shots you don't take." – Wayne Gretzky

---

When conventional treatment doesn't work, your doctor might recommend **extracorporeal shock wave therapy.** Extracorporeal shock wave therapy consists of sound waves being directed at the area of heel pain to help stimulate healing. This special therapy is usually reserved for those with chronic plantar fasciitis in which more conservative treatments have failed. This procedure may cause swelling and bruising, along with pain, numbness or tingling—and it's not always an effective treatment plan. **Steroid shots** can provide temporary pain relief, but use caution. Repetitive or multiple injections in a six-month period are not recommended because they can weaken your plantar fascia and possibly cause it to rupture or damage the fat pad covering your heel bone.

Runners beware: Do not run for at least 10 days after steroid injections or you may risk rupturing the fascia! In extreme cases, some people require surgery to detach the plantar fascia from the heel bone. This should be considered as a final option only when the pain is severe and all other treatments have failed. Side effects include a weakening of the arch in your foot and it could end your running career.

Stress Fracture – A stress fracture is a minute crack in a bone that causes pain and discomfort. For runners, it's most prevalent in the shins and metatarsal bones of the feet. Linked to overuse or from a sudden change in activity, the pain usually gets worse with an increase of activity and improves with rest. Rest is important, because continued stress on the bone can lead to a complete fracture of the bone.

Sprain or Strain?

What's the difference between a sprain and a strain?

A ***strain*** is the tearing or injury of the ***muscle*** and/or ***tendon***. The tendon is the fibrous band of connective tissue that connects muscle to bone. This is the same as a muscle "pull" described in the previous pages. Typical symptoms include pain, muscle weakness, muscle spasms, inflammation, and cramping. In severe strains, the muscles or tendons are partially or completely ruptured, often debilitating the individual. With a mild strain, the muscles or tendons are stretched or pulled, but only slightly. Some muscle function is lost with a moderate strain, where the muscles or tendons are overextended and slightly torn.

A ***sprain*** is the tearing or injury to the ***ligaments,*** the fibrous bands of tissue that connect the end of one bone to another.

The most common sprains include the knee, ankle and foot, and the intensity can vary from case to case. Bruising, pain, and inflammation are common in all three categories of sprains: mild, moderate, and severe. The runner will usually sense a pop or tear in the joint. A severe sprain can produce excruciating pain at the moment of injury, as ligaments tear or separate from the bone. This damage makes the joint nonfunctional. A moderate sprain consists of a partial tear of the ligament, producing swelling and instability of the joint. A ligament is stretched in a mild sprain, but there is no joint loosening.

Ankle Sprain – An ankle sprain is best defined as the stretching or tearing of ligaments surrounding the ankle. This injury can occur when the foot rolls or twists inward and is common for trail runners.

> ### Motivation
>
> **"Go fast enough to get there, but slow enough to see."** *– Jimmy Buffet*

Knee Sprains of the external (medial and lateral collateral) or internal (anterior and posterior cruciate) ligaments or injuries of the meniscus may result from knee trauma. Symptoms include pain, instability with severe sprains, joint effusion, and locking of the joint with some meniscal injuries. Use the **RICE** therapy or sprains and strains.

Torn Meniscus

A tear of the meniscus is also one of the more common knee injuries. Activities that cause you to abruptly rotate or twist your knee, especially with pressure of your entire body weight, can lead to a torn meniscus. Each knee has two menisci, C-shaped sections of cartilage that act as a shock-absorbing cushion between your tibia and femur. A tear of the meniscus causes pain, swelling and stiffness and full extension of the knee is difficult. Conservative treatment includes RICE for minor tears, as they can heal on their own; however, in more serious cases, surgery is the only option.

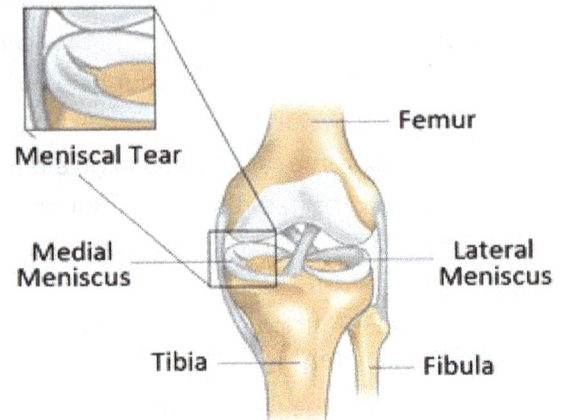

Meniscal Tear
Femur
Medial Meniscus
Lateral Meniscus
Tibia
Fibula

Foot Care – Blisters

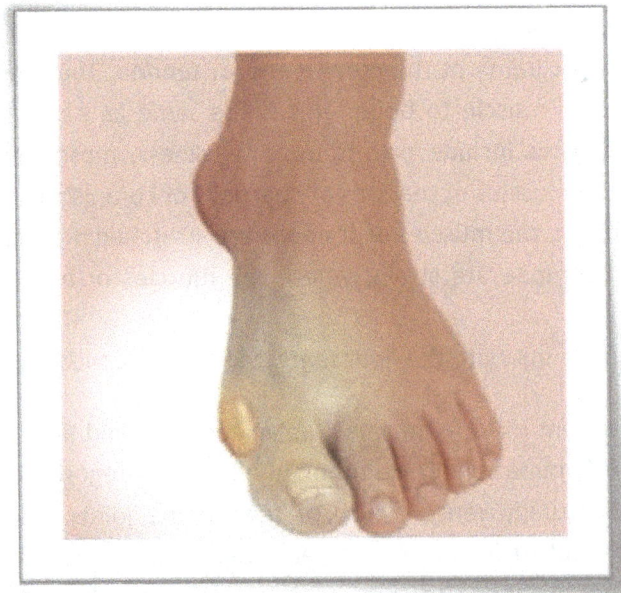

What is a Blister?

A blister is best defined as a small bubble on the skin caused by heat or friction and filled with serum. This damage causes the outer layers of the skin to rub together, separate, and fill with fluid. For the ordinary person, the formation of a blister isn't much of a deal. Non-runners can deal with them immediately by changing the footwear they have on, or changing the socks they wear. Unfortunately for runners, we don't always have that option available, especially on a long run, where a blister can seem to appear at will and grow exponentially. The source of the blister can be anything from new shoes or poorly fitting shoes, wet feet, or something as small as a pebble. Heat can also be a big contributor to the formation of blisters. At some point, a blister is likely to form and it may cause quite a bit of pain. In this section, we'll learn how to deal with blisters and how to avoid them altogether.

Ignoring a blister can cause unnecessary pain and the potential for a nasty infection. Without the proper treatment, you can acquire a life-threatening infection called sepsis. Sepsis has the ability to leave the localization of the wound and infiltrate the bloodstream and body tissue around the blister.

Diabetics can be more susceptible to blisters as a result of diabetic neuropathy, and should be very careful to prevent infection. Yes, a simple blister can kill you if untreated.

How to Deal with Blisters

When dealing with blisters, always keep the blister and the area around the blister clean. If the blister is small and isn't too painful, it's always best to leave it intact to prevent the risk of infection. Minor blisters will usually heal quickly on their own without intervention.

You may relieve the pressure of larger blisters by popping them with a sterile needle. Long distance runners, such as marathoners and ultramarathon runners may have to keep medical supplies with their running gear and deal with them on their run. If you need to pop a blister, always look for pre-existing signs of infection. Blisters can develop quickly and can get infected almost as fast. If you notice yellow or green pus, a sure sign of infection, treat it immediately or see your doctor or trainer.

If popping the blister is the only choice, make sure you follow these steps:
- Keep the blister and the area around it clean.
- Make sure your hands are clean – use antibacterial soap, iodine, alcohol and plenty of clean water.
- Use a small needle to poke a hole in the edge of the blister from the side. Do not poke the top of the blister! It will heal more quickly if the drain hole is on the edge of the blister. Press lightly on the blister to drain as much of the fluid as possible, and apply an antibiotic ointment.
- Cover it immediately with a bandage or gauze pad.

How to Avoid Blisters in the First Place

Healthy, moist feet are happy feet. Let your feet dry out, or get them too wet, and you will be prone to blisters. Sweaty skin with abrasive salt is also a key contributor to friction which can cause blisters. On a daily basis, apply skin creams and lotions to keep your feet healthy and moist.

Runners should never wear cotton socks for extended periods of time. Cotton may work fine for short races or cooler climates, but a good synthetic sock will work much better.

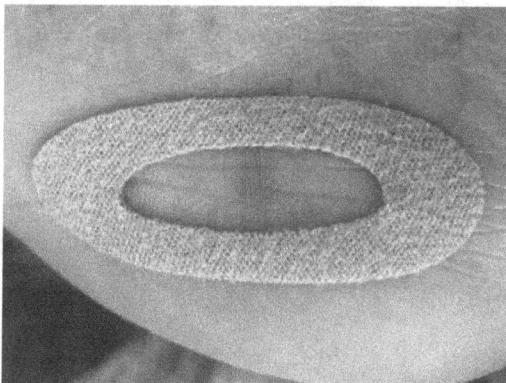

Moleskin works as a great protective barrier for treatment of burgeoning blisters. If possible, try to catch the sore while it's still a red "hotspot" and before it fills with fluid.

When dressing a blister, make sure the bandage or moleskin protects the injury by placing it around the blister and not on top of the blister. Pressure, heat and moisture will make a blister worsen.

Synthetic socks wick moisture away from your skin, keeping your feet free of too much moisture. I've never tried it, but some runners actually coat their feet, especially between the toes, with a lubricant such as Vaseline.

Proper fitting shoes and socks are the most important element to prevent blistering. Shoes that are too big will allow your socks to bunch up in your shoe, causing friction that can cause blisters. Shoes that are too tight can cause blisters around the toes and heel areas.

Professionals are available to help fit your shoes properly at most running stores. They can recommend shoes that will help with blister prevention if you're prone to getting blisters. Don't wear untested shoes on race day! I like to get at least 20 miles on a new pair of shoes before I run any sort of distance in them. When buying socks, make sure you buy synthetic socks that allow wicking and breathability for the foot and toes. Some socks have extra cushion in the heal area and fore-front portion of the sock.

There are also a number of commercially sold foot products, in the form of creams, powders, tapes and bandages that can help reduce the formation of blisters. See your doctor, pharmacist or running store professional for advice.

Toenail Loss

It's very common for runners to develop black or bruised toenails. The loss of toenails can be a non-event or they can be very painful, depending on how you got them in the first place and how you treat them.

The two most common causes for toenail loss are **downhill** running and **long distance** running. Combine the two, and you have a very good recipe for toenail loss, or bruising of the toenails and cuticles. In most cases, the friction in the toe box of the shoe presses on a toenail that is either too long or rubs constantly within the shoe.

Warm weather can also cause the tissue to soften and your feet to swell, adding to the likelihood of a black toenail.

If you damage your toenail, try to leave it alone. Usually, a new toenail will start to grow underneath the damaged one within a week or two and force the other one to fall off within four to six weeks. Avoid taking the toenail off unless it's infected. You may need a doctor's help if it does get infected.

Prevent black toenails by wearing properly fitting shoes. For some long distance and ultramarathon runners, this may include getting a pair of shoes that are slightly larger, as the feet may swell, causing more friction within the shoe.

Make sure your toenails are trimmed. Your toenails should never stick out longer than the toe. Keep them short! Also, keep your shoestrings tight, particularly for downhill running. This will keep your feet from excessive movement in the shoe.

Motivation

"The principle is competing against yourself. It's about self-improvement, about being better than you were the day before." — *Steve Young*

Morton's Neuroma

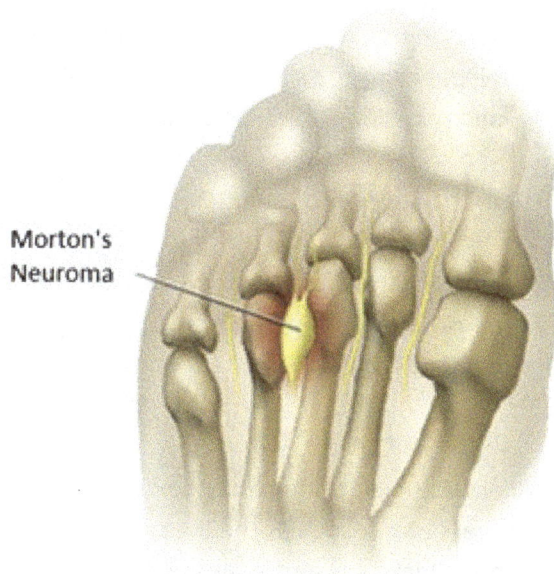

Morton's neuroma is swelling of the tissue surrounding the nerves that lead to the toes. This is a painful condition that can affect the ball of your foot. Another symptom is the sensation that you have a small rock in your shoe or bunching of the sock. Severe cases feel like a sharp, burning sensation in the ball of your foot. Additional symptoms may include toes that sting, burn or feel numb. Women who wear high heeled shoes are more prone to this condition. Some relief can be realized by wearing shoes with lower heels and wider toe boxes. In some cases, corticosteroid injections or surgery may be needed to reduce the swelling.

In most cases, there are no visible signs such as redness or swelling on the outside of the foot. If you have pain for more than a few days, you should see your doctor. This is especially true if you've already changed your shoe type or decreased your physical activities.

The prescribed treatment will depend on the severity of your symptoms. Your health professional will most likely recommend a very conservative approach at first. He may suggest arch supports or foot pads that fit inside your shoe and help to reduce pressure on the nerve. These can be purchased over the counter or your doctor may prescribe customized inserts designed specifically for your feet. If there is no positive resolution with conservative treatment, your doctor might suggest:

- **Injections** – Steroid injections may be recommended to help reduce the inflammation around the nerve.
- **Decompression Surgery** – In some instances, surgery may relieve the pressure on the nerve by cutting nearby structures, such as the ligament that holds the bones together at the front of the foot.
- **Removal of the Nerve** – Surgery to remove the growth may be needed if conservative treatments fail to provide relief. Although surgery is normally successful, the procedure can result in permanent numbness of the affected toes.

Motivation

"You can motivate by fear, and you can motivate by reward, but both of those methods are only temporary. The only lasting thing is self-motivation." — *Homer Rice*

Other Pains and Ailments

Side Stitches

Side stitches (side cramps) are a very common problem among runners, particularly for new runners. Even though they're really not considered to be a sports injury, they can certainly affect the most serious of runners. A side stitch usually manifests as a stabbing, aching, or sharp pain in your abdomen, just below your ribs. It's usually prevalent on just one side, and occasionally will be accompanied by pain at the tip of your shoulder on the same side.

While it's not known exactly what causes side stitches, there are a number of theories, any of which are possible based on survey and science.

One survey infers that eating a large meal or drinking concentrated, sugary fluids like fruit juice or sports drinks just before the run begins will increase your risk of developing a stitch. Science however, contradicts this by stating that proper nutrition and hydration have a defensive effect from side stitches.

Irritation on the Ligaments and Abdominal Pain

From one biological viewpoint, some theorists believe that a side stitch may be due to pulling on the ligaments or membranes that support and connect internal organs, such as the liver. This theory may hold true for athletes that perform in a vertical position, but swimmers and equestrian riders are also known to develop side stitches while performing. Based on these findings, it's hard to assign hard facts to this theory.

Diaphragmatic Ischemia

Another long-standing theory for the development of side stiches is a decrease in blood flow to the diaphragm, the muscle which expands and contracts your lungs. This decrease in blood flow is known as *ischemia*.

This theory also supports the opinion that certain foods or fluids seem more prone to causing side stitches. The theory suggests that more blood is required by the stomach for digesting certain foods and liquids, and may potentially pull more blood away from the diaphragm. Several opposing, but inconclusive studies have provided evidence against the theory of "diaphragmatic ischemia."

Irritation of the Spinal Column

Finally, a fourth line of reasoning connects side stitches with irritation of the spinal column. Studies have found that kyphosis, (also known as round-back), a condition in which the upper spine is more sharply curved than normal, is related to an increased risk of experiencing side stitches. This theory is further supported by some patients who experience pain at the tip of the shoulder. Both of the nerves – the nerve that runs to the diaphragm and the one that runs to the tip of the shoulder, commence from the same vertebra level.

> ### Motivation
>
> **"All progress takes place outside the comfort zone."** *– Michael John Bobak*

Furthermore, it can *also* explain why runners, horse riders, and swimmers experience higher rates of side stitches, but cyclists do not. Horseback riding and running involve a vertical jolt of the spine, while swimmers use a rotational twisting motion, all of which place additional stress on the upper spine. Comparatively, cycling involves little vertical spinal stress.

Suggested Preventive and Treatments

The true origin of side stitches remains a mystery, but they do indeed exist and can impact a runner's performance, although usually only for a brief time. If you are prone to side stitches, there are a few things you can do to mitigate the impact.

- Studies suggest that stretching the stomach, deep breathing, and contracting your abdominal muscles can all help alleviate a side stitch. Do these before you begin your run.
- For long-term prevention, make sure your core – your hip flexors, back and abdomen — are strengthened with proper exercise and conditioning.
- Take note of the food and drink you consume on days when you develop side stitches, and see if you notice a pattern or particular food that correlates with your side stitches. Avoid the foods or drinks that might contribute to your side stitches.
- If you have chronic side stitches, it may be worth having a physical therapist or chiropractor examine your spine to see if there is truly a dysfunction or alignment problems that could be irritating or worsening your side stitches.

Things That Happen That No One Wants to Talk About
Chafing in Sensitive Areas

Chafing of the skin is very common for runners, especially for long distance runners. It's normally caused from skin rubbing on loose clothing or other skin. Unfortunately, chafing can occur in the most sensitive areas such as the groin area of both men and women, along the bra line for women and under the arms of either gender.

Braces, elastic bandages, fuel belts, hydration bladders with shoulder straps – all are potential contributors to chafing. As we've seen throughout this book, improper hydration can also accelerate chafing. Body salt and drier skin can contribute heavily to this condition. Some runners, usually men, get chafed or bleeding nipples, which can be extremely painful. When men run, their nipples rub constantly against their clothing. Over the course of a long run, the nipples can be irritated to the point of bleeding. Because women usually wear tight-fitting sports bras, this usually isn't an issue for them.

Motivation

"We run, not because we think it is doing us good, but because we enjoy it and cannot help ourselves... The more restricted our society and work become, the more necessary it will be to find some outlet for this craving for freedom. No one can say, 'You must not run faster than this, or jump higher than that.' The human spirit is indomitable."
— *Sir Roger Bannister*

To help avoid chafing, do the following:

- Stay hydrated
- Wear tight fitting clothing – loose clothing will rub more frequently
- Wear wicking material, like Coolmax, Dri-Fit or other synthetic fabric. Cotton will cause more friction, especially if it gets wet from rain or sweat. Once cotton gets wet, it stays wet much longer than synthetic fabric.
- Apply a skin lubricant like Vaseline or Body Glide to sensitive or chafe-prone areas.
- Make sure your gear is fitted properly – fuel belts, braces, etc.
- Men – wear bandages like Nip Guards or Band-Aids to protect the nipples.

Leaky Bladder

Female runners can sometimes have issues with urinary incontinence, especially if they've previously given birth. Of course men can leak urine too, but the problem is much more common in women. There seems to be many causes for incontinence, but the most common is loss of strength of the pelvic and sphincter muscles. Pregnancy and childbirth can worsen this condition. Extra internal pressure that builds suddenly can also be cause for leakage, such as sneezing, coughing, laughing, or making abrupt moves.

For females with incontinence problems, Kegel exercises can help to strengthen the pelvic floor muscles and it doesn't require any equipment. To exercise the correct muscles, attempt to stop the flow of urine without using your stomach, butt or leg muscles. Contract these muscles for 10 seconds, rest for about 10 seconds, and repeat this process 10 times. For best results, do this three to four times per day. After several weeks, your incontinence issues should improve and you'll experience better bladder control. Obesity problems can also put additional pressure on your bladder. By losing weight, you may be able to alleviate some of the pressure and regain complete control of your bladder. See your doctor if you continue to have bladder problems, as surgery may be required in severe cases.

Acne and Skin Problems

Acne problems are common for runners, especially on the back, chest, and upper arms. Women seem to be more affected by acne than men when it comes to running. This could be the result of covering the skin with tighter fitting clothes such as sports bras. The combination of friction from clothing, along with sweat, which irritates the skin, increases the likelihood for acne. Furthermore, sunscreen and makeup seem to clog the pores even more, but that can be remedied by proper cleansing of the skin after a run. To prevent exercise-induced acne, you should shower as soon as possible after your exercise activities. Make sure you clean areas susceptible to acne thoroughly, with a soap that's specifically designed for acne. Try to avoid wearing make-up when you run and select an oil-free sunscreen. If you can, use a sunscreen gel in lieu of a cream-based lotion for the rest of your body.

Motivation

"The master has failed more times than the beginner has even tried." – *Stephen McCranie*

Hemorrhoids

Hemorrhoids, which are an enlargement of the anal vein, are somewhat common to runners, especially those who are in their pregnancy, have recently given birth, or have had digestive issues. The symptoms of hemorrhoids can range from mildly irritating to bleeding. Any physical activity, especially running or biking, can be painful and may actually worsen your condition.

If you're dealing with hemorrhoids, your best bet is to check in with your health care professional before you continue to run. Your doctor or nurse will most likely recommend an over-the-counter topical cream or ointment to give you some relief. Stage 3 and stage 4 hemorrhoids almost always require surgery because they are external to the body and cannot be pushed back in.

Gastrointestinal Issues

If you're prone to intestinal problems, make sure that your training includes proper diet and planning before you run. During your training, keep track of your meals in your runner's log, and record which foods cause problems for you. Always make sure that your bathroom needs are met before you go out on a long run. Get to know your body and the way it processes food. For instance, a marathoner should know how many hours it will take for the pasta to process before tomorrow's marathon. If your food usually takes 12 hours and the race begins at 6:00 a.m., you should eat before 6:00 p.m. the night before. Your nutritional needs and bodily functions should be tracked and practiced before race day. Make this part of your training!

There are a couple of other things you can do to avoid intestinal issues:
- Cut back on foods that cause excessive gas, especially two to three hours before your run. The list includes sugar-rich and high-fiber foods such as fruits, vegetables, bran, and beans.
- Chew your food well and don't rush through your meals. Proper digestion is important to the next day's success.
- Don't overeat.
- Drink plenty of water and make sure you're staying well-hydrated, since water is an essential part of the digestion process.

If intestinal issues continue, consult your health care professional to determine whether there is a medical reason for it. See **Chapter 10 – Nutrition** for more information.

Women's Issues

Read **Chapter 9 – Women's Running** for more information on specific issues that women deal with, such as pregnancy, special dietary needs, menstruation, and more.

Challenge!

When it comes to any sport, pain and injury are inevitable, but if you deal with them properly, you can minimize the downtime. Your challenge: *ALWAYS listen to your body, and do not try to run "through" an injury. Utilize the treatment that your doctor prescribes to you, and take the necessary time to heal.*

Chapter 8 – Benefits of Running

My Story

When I first began to run, I was looking for a quick fix for my failing health. I was living in the present, and had absolutely no long-term goals. I felt lousy and wanted to feel better – right now! I soon realized that the *shorter* path to better health and fitness was not the *better* path. My immune system quickly broke down, and I began to feel sick from such a sudden drop in weight. About three months into my weight loss program, I realized that the magic was not going to happen overnight, and I would see no benefits at all if I stayed on the current path. At that point, I made a conscious decision to back off on the weight loss and slow my running down a bit. It wasn't until then, that I finally started to experience the benefits of running, which included weight loss at a *healthy* rate, better quality of sleep, and normal vital statistics. This chapter touches on the various benefits of running from physical and emotional benefits to social networking with your friends. As you go through this chapter, make notes of the benefits that you notice as you progress through your training.

Why do we run? What are the benefits of running? In this chapter, we'll take a look at four different types of benefits that running can offer us.

- Health and physical benefits
- Mental and emotional benefits
- Social benefits
- Availability and convenience

Health and Physical Benefits

Can exercise be considered a *medicine?* By most accounts, exercise is a form of medicine, with running arguably being the most effective when it comes to good health. Studies show that running can help prevent heart disease, high blood pressure, stroke, Type 2 Diabetes, and obesity.

Obesity Prevention – As I mentioned in the prologue of this book, there are many reasons why people choose to run, but the most common reasons are to attain a certain level of fitness and reach an ideal body weight. This can be achieved through a good diet plan and regular exercise – for about 30 minutes per workout, 5 days per week, or 150 minutes.

Running is a great way to burn calories. The average human burns around 100 to 110 calories per mile when jogging or running. Remarkably, the speed at which a person runs has little effect on how many calories they will burn. As you progress in your training, the composition of your body will change and you'll begin to see "a whole new you." Coupled with proper nutrition, exercise will trigger the loss of body fat and a proportional increase of lean muscle tissue. We'll discuss this in great detail in **Chapter 10 – Nutrition.**

The human body burns 2,000 to 2,500 calories per day, even *without* exercise. If you add a five mile run to your activities, you can burn an extra 500 calories. Furthermore, if your caloric intake meets the FDA's minimum of 2,000 calories per day, you've achieved a net loss of 1,000 calories or more!

The Magic Number is 3500

By the numbers, the human body requires an excess of 3500 calories in order to gain a single pound of fat. Likewise, we must have a deficit of 3500 calories to lose a single pound. That said, a 180-pound person who runs five miles each day will lose about five pounds per month. As the person continues his weight loss, he becomes lighter and will burn fewer calories per mile. Eventually, a runner's weight will stabilize or *plateau*. This can change, of course, if the runner intensifies his training or consumes fewer calories. As a runner, you should always set a reasonable, attainable goal for your weight loss program. Once you get to your ideal or goal weight, a consistent running schedule will help keep you at your desired weight.

We all know that exercise burns calories, but did you know that calories continue to burn *after* your workout? This process is known as *Excess Post Oxygen Consumption* (EPOC) and your workout does not have to be an intense one to reap the benefits of EPOC.

Heart and Lung Health – Another common reason for running is increased health and decreased risk of impact on the cardiovascular system – our heart, arteries and veins. Nearly all studies suggest that running for just an hour per week can reduce the risk of heart disease by approximately half compared to non-runners. Running is a natural way to regulate healthy blood pressure, and the results can happen in just a few shorts weeks. Running helps to lower blood pressure by maintaining the elasticity of our veins and arteries and strengthens our heart muscle. As a person runs, his arteries expand and contract more often, creating more elasticity in the veins and arteries. This elasticity allows the arteries to relax more between each heartbeat, thus keeping his blood pressure low. Finally, the inactive person's heart beats *36,000 more times per day* than that of a runner!

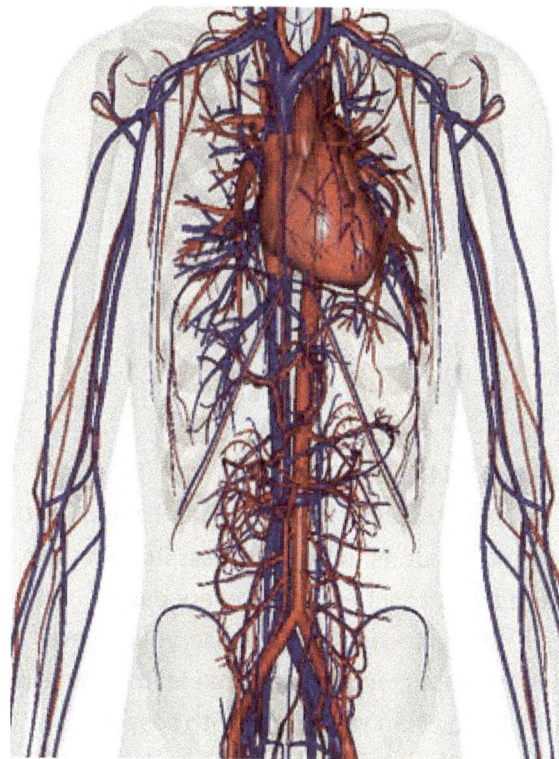

Running also maximizes the lungs' effectiveness, increasing our lung capacity and efficiency by keeping them strong and powerful. Running regularly will improve stamina, making workouts more productive and enjoyable.

Bone and Joint Health

How many times have you heard that running is bad for your knees? If you're like me, you've heard it over and over – and it usually comes from non-runners! Unless you have a predisposed condition such as poor leg and knee alignment, running and other weight-bearing exercise helps to build strength in your bones by increasing the bone density. This is especially beneficial for young adults, whose bones are still developing. In adults, it may help to slow down the natural loss of bone density that occurs with the natural aging process. Studies show that running does not contribute to osteoarthritis either.

Reduction of Risk for Cancer

Of course, running cannot cure cancer, but studies show that exercise is associated with a lower risk of certain types of cancer. Furthermore, if you already have cancer, running can help to improve your quality of life while you're undergoing chemotherapy or other treatments.

Give Yourself More Time

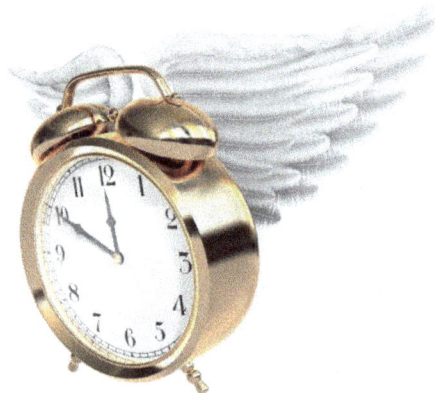

It's a proven fact that runners have fewer doctor visits, fewer disabilities and remain active much longer than their sedentary counterparts. Furthermore, running may add years to your life by improving your quality of life, physically, emotionally and mentally. Studies also show that both genders of active people are less likely to develop colon cancer. Women who regularly engage in intense workouts like aerobics and running reduce their risk of breast cancer by up to 30 percent.

Other Health Benefits

Older runners maintain their balance better than their non-running peers, protecting their bones, joints and tendons in the process. Running can improve core muscles, providing better coordination, posture and strength to make every day activities easier and more pleasant.

Running can also increase your overall skin health, by flushing sweat through your pores and cleansing those clogged pores that lead to acne breakouts. Running can boost your natural oils, so it's also important to clean your pores with soap and water *after* your workout to keep them clean.

Finally, runners tend to sleep better by keeping routine and consistent schedules. This can help them maintain a higher performance level.

Motivation

"Somebody may beat me, but they are going to have to bleed to do it." — *Steve Prefontaine*

Mental and Emotional Benefits

Runner's High

Most of us have heard about it – the "runner's high" that some athletes experience during or after a good workout. It's been noted that it really doesn't matter what our previous mood was like – whether we were in a good mood or a foul one, the **Endocannabinoids** – hormones that give us the "runner's high" – are released in the body during our workouts. These powerful hormones can elevate our moods and feelings almost instantly and they usually last for the entire day. Research shows that these hormones can even kick in after a very short workout of 30 minutes or less.

Various studies have also shown that running causes the same kind of neurochemical adaptations in the brain that are shared by some addictive drugs. It's also been noted that exercise helps diminish anxiety and stress, and can help people cope with everyday life.

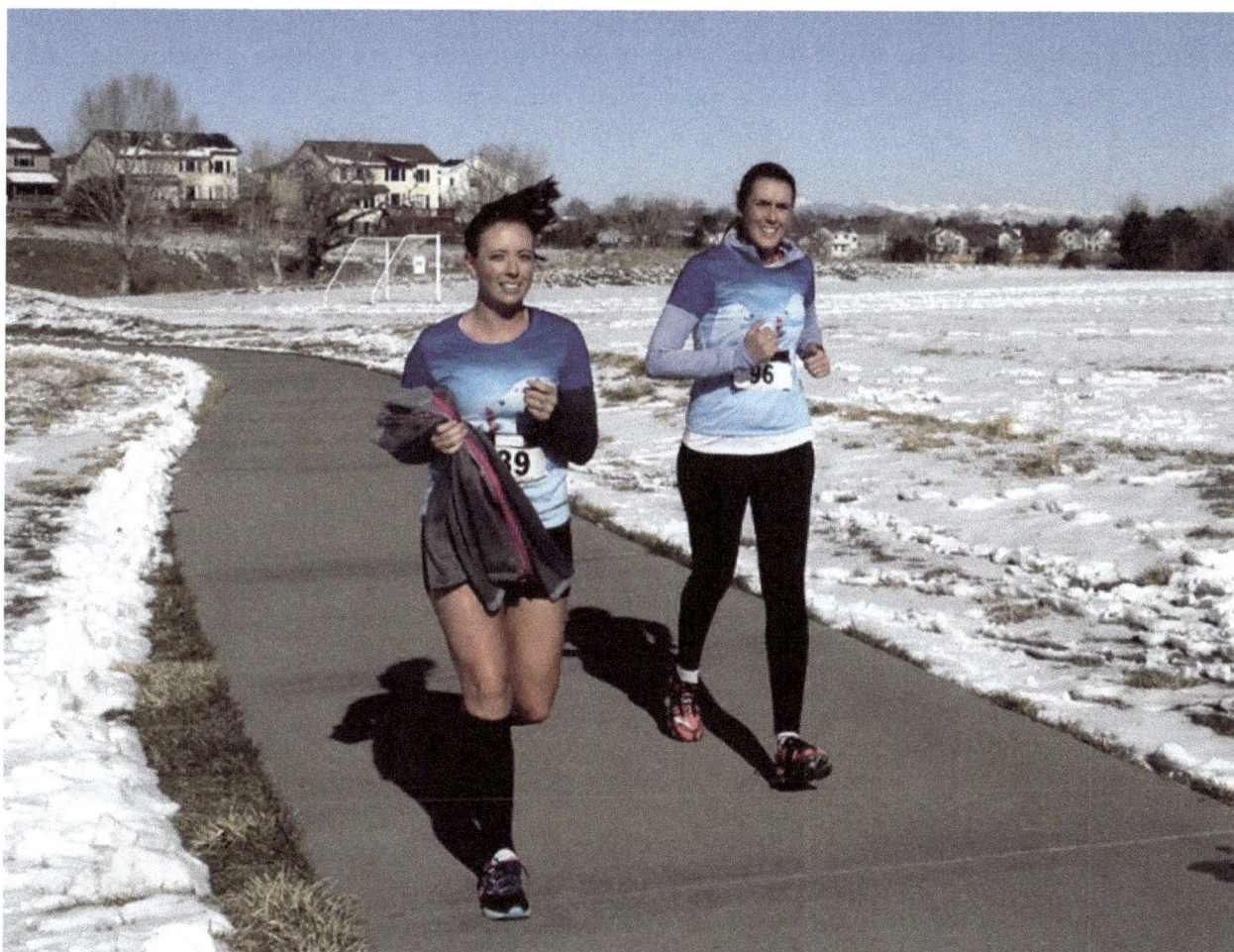

For an emotional lift, run with friends

Motivation

"Never let your head hang down. Never give up and sit down and grieve. Find another way." – *Satchel Paige*

Running is Good for Your Mind

Running can benefit some people more for its psychological values than its physical values. Running can be used to benefit others through charity, or it can help your own mental and emotional state. For years, psychologists and other medical professionals have claimed that physical activities can help lift your spirits and even ward off bouts of clinical depression and other disorders.

Many runners participate to help with their psychological issues and alleviate the stressors in their lives, but running can also aid in the mental anguish related to addictions, such as alcohol or drug abuse. Some runners have been able to overcome addiction issues with physical activity, replacing the urge for a drink or a high, with an urge for a run.

Finally, even if you don't have psychological issues or addiction problems, running can simply allow you to get out and clear your head!

According to some studies, aerobic exercises such as cycling and running can elevate the Serotonin levels in your brain. Serotonin is a chemical that helps move instructions through the nervous system and aids in many functions, including regulating moods, appetite and sleep cycles. Increased Serotonin levels help you deal with stress more effectively. Running outside has also been shown to increase self-esteem, give you peace of mind and create a more optimistic outlook for the things that you do.

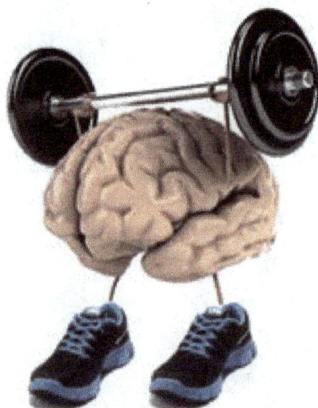

Several studies concluded with overwhelming evidence that routine exercise can help slow or overcome age-related mental decline, particularly functions like attention disorders, multi-tasking and memory retention. Physical activities have been shown to help keep the mind focused and could even decrease symptoms of some mental illnesses.

Recent studies also found that older adults with better fitness levels achieved higher scores regarding cognitive function than their less fit counterparts.

Studies suggest that people who set and meet long-term fitness goals are more committed and satisfied with their exercise routines than those who don't commit to goal setting.

Motivation

"Inspire and motivate yourself – winners are made when you're by yourself and no one is watching." – *Bill Watts*

Social Benefits

Friends for Life

If you're just getting into running, you may lack motivation, and joining a running club may help you attain and sustain your motivation. Friendly competition with other runners of similar skills can help you train harder and achieve your goals much faster than training alone. Group members can also benefit from group rates when entering relay races or benefit races. Running with others can create a sense of belonging, and helps to keep each other motivated and accountable when training. Running clubs are also great for team building at your place of employment. Some runners choose to participate in fun runs, mud runs, trail runs or marathons. If you are interested in competing with other runners, contact your local running club.

Family Ties

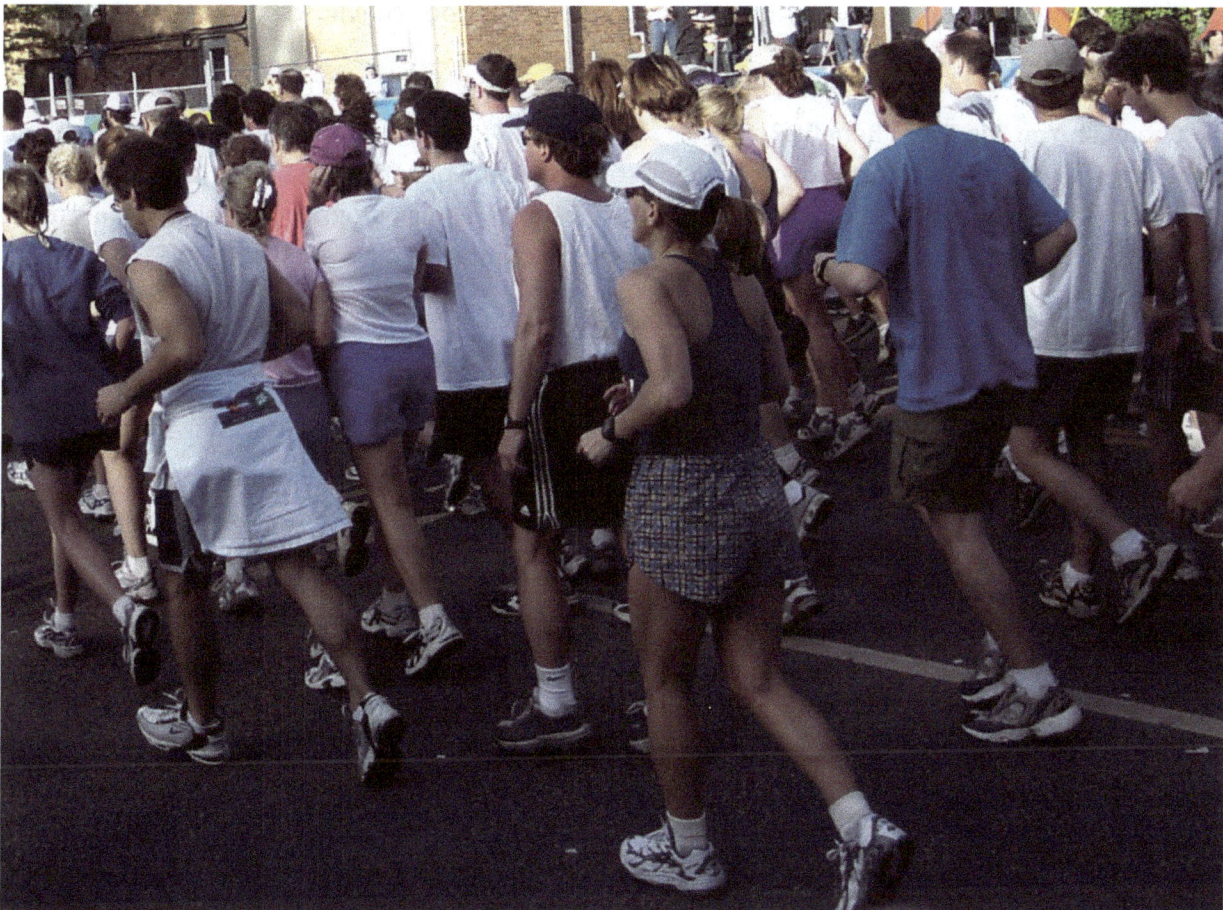

Stay connected by running with family members

Motivation

"Set your goals high, and don't stop until you get there." – *Bo Jackson*

Running can be a great bonding experience for families as well as friends. I know of a number of couples, fathers or mothers with kids, and entire running families. They train together, compete together, they laugh and they cry together. Running can bridge generational gaps and allow families to communicate in ways that they normally might not achieve in this fast-paced world.

Availability and Convenience

Running has many advantages compared to other sports or hobbies. You can run just about anywhere, whether you're at the beach or on a mountain trail. You can run indoors or outdoors, on your lunch hour, or while you're on vacation – and you can do it all year around if you have the right equipment. Outdoor running allows you to interact with nature, even when it's raining or snowing. (Be smart about severe weather!) Running has been described as the world's most accessible sport.

You don't need a club membership to benefit from running – you simply lace up your shoes and put one foot in front of the other. If you have a dog, you can also include your pet in your running route. This is another great way to stay motivated and it's good for your canine friend as well! Running is accessible, practical and inexpensive.

How Soon Can You See These Benefits?

It's very difficult to predict how soon you'll start to see the benefits of running. As always, you get out of it what you put into it. Generally speaking, if you begin a running program, you should start to see results in 10 to 20 days. These results can be measured in a number of different ways:

- You start to lose weight
- Your routine starts to become easier
- You're able to increase your pace or distance
- You have less pain than you did when you first started

Of course, the more expectations you have, the more effort you'll need to put into your workouts. For instance, if you plan on running a marathon in October, and it's already August, you should probably consider moving your marathon to a springtime race, and work on 5k or 10k distances for your autumn race. You simply won't be able to run a marathon *effectively*, after only a month or two of training. Refer to **Chapter 16 – Training Plans** on how to set your goals and plan your races around those goals.

The realization of your training benefits may seem inconsistent at times. The ebb and flow of your fitness level will vary, especially when it comes down to how your body responds to the type and duration of your workout, the intensity level, your recovery schedule and your body's rate of adaptation. Age, weight and basic health will most certainly factor into how quickly you see the benefits and start achieving your expected fitness level. **Chapter 15 – Setting Goals** will help you with these expectations.

> **Motivation**
>
> **"It's not whether you get knocked down, it's whether you get up."** – *Vince Lombardi*

Tip
The Point of Diminishing Returns

We all know that running or any other physical activity can be good for the body, mind and soul, but when is it too much? At what point do we start to see a regression in benefits, and when does the physical activity start to work against us?

It's long been recognized that running can quickly become an obsession, or even an addiction. When this happens, it can be dangerous for the athlete, because you don't want to give up what you think is making you feel good. Many "average Joes" have been through this phase, including myself. You tend to ignore your minor aches and pains, only to get a more serious injury. Or you tend to come back too fast after an illness or injury, because you don't want to lose your fitness level. It's at this point where you need to have patience and logic, neither of which are easy to come by when you're obsessed or addicted to the activity. We tend to try to "run through the pain," and trust me, it rarely works. If it's a minor injury or illness, you normally won't reduce your fitness level by missing 15 to 20 days of running. I've had several illnesses or injuries that lasted a week or two, and it was actually fairly easy to get back to the original level of fitness. A number of times, the lengthy rest actually put me back on track faster, because my body was fresh once again. This doesn't work in all cases, however. If the illness or injury is severe enough, you may need to take additional time, sometimes for several months. To avoid starting all over, engage in cross-training such as non-impact activities like running in a pool, walking or cycling. During this recovery period, work on your free weights and upper body workouts, combined with full-body stretching.

Finally, don't become obsessed with mileage only, as this will most certainly result in an overuse injury. Mix up your running with fartleks, strides, intervals, hill running, long runs, and make each type of run, in each workout, a definitive and achievable plan. Junk miles are easily accumulated, but rarely meaningful. See **Chapter 13 – Training Basics** for more information.

To reap the benefits for your mind and body, keep your running in perspective and enjoy it as part of a full, active lifestyle.

Challenge!

At the beginning of this chapter, I suggested that you take note of the benefits that you experience in your running program. Is your health improving? Are your personal relationships better? How are your stress levels and your self-esteem?

Challenge: *When we get into "logging" your runs later in this book, write down your feelings from physical and emotional viewpoints. Make adjustments accordingly so you can reap the full benefits of healthy living.*

Chapter 9 – Women's Running

Jane's Story

Throughout this book, the general theme has been "Running for the Average Joe." But, what if you happen to be a woman – an "average Jane"? If so, CELEBRATE - REJOICE! Embrace the fact that you're a woman – and know that you don't have to choose between being a runner and simply being a woman. You can be both!

Jane was a young woman in her late twenties and was married to Todd, an athletic young man whom she met in college. Both had "career" jobs, but had recently begun talking about raising a family. Todd and Jane ran together regularly, but she feared that if she became pregnant, she would have to stop running, and possibly break one of the strong bonds that she had with Todd. She desperately wanted to have children, but didn't want to choose between running and being a woman.

This chapter will disclose some of the differences between men and women runners, but it will also reveal the similarities between them. Aside from some physiological disparities, women should be considered athletes, just as much as men. And as we'll see, women may be better suited for some aspects of running, especially when it comes to endurance!

Earlier in this book we noted that there were no women entered in the first modern Olympic Games in 1896. It wasn't until the 1900 Games in Paris that 22 women competed in tennis, golf, sailing croquet, and equestrianism. In 1967, race official Jack Semple tried to rip off Katherine Switzer's bib during the "men only" Boston Marathon. Of course, his attempt to remove her from the race encouraged more women to run and forced the rules to be changed to allow women to participate.

For years, women were unjustifiably excluded from sporting events, treated as though they were not athletes at all. In recent years, however, we've found this to be quite the opposite; women are quite capable of any sporting event, including sports as punishing as boxing. Physiologically speaking, women may even be better suited than men for endurance sports such as ultramarathons.

By the numbers, women are approximately ten percent slower than men at all distances, but that may be due to several biological and physiological differences from their male counterparts. Men tend to have stronger muscles and denser bones, which may be related to the effects of testosterone. Wider hips in women may account for less leverage when it comes to running. Finally, women generally have less cardiac output and less hemoglobin per blood volume, in addition to less overall blood volume than men of comparable size.

While it may be possible that women could overtake men in overall speed, it's not likely to happen for some time because of these factors. Does this mean that women are less competitive than men? Not at all! As a matter of fact, Paula Radcliffe, the world record holder in the women's marathon, is faster than 99.9% of the men on the planet. While they might not be as fast as men, women actually have some advantages when it comes to running, particularly in long distance races. For one thing, women burn calories at a slower rate than men and aren't as prone to "hitting the wall" in long races.

Furthermore, women sweat less so they don't lose as many bodily fluids during a race and research also shows that they dissipate heat more efficiently. Because of these factors, women are more likely to hold their pace for the duration of a long run.

What it comes down to is this: Men and women are equally worthy of being categorized as athletes, but their biological differences separate them in many ways. We can generalize many topics when it comes to running, but we also have to mention the specific differences between the genders. And that brings us to this chapter – a portion of the book dedicated to women.

Aside from the obvious physical differences, women have other aspects to consider in regards to **health, nutrition, equipment** and **safety.** We'll take a look at each of these general categories as we go through this chapter.

As I mentioned several times already, runners should always undergo a physical examination before beginning a running regimen and women are no exception to this rule. Before you begin, always consult your physician. Many women decide to start running because of obesity concerns, and these should always be monitored. Obesity contributes to heart disease, which kills 10 times more women than breast cancer does each year. Proper exercise can lower your blood pressure, decrease your resting heart rate, elevate your good cholesterol levels and help you maintain a healthy weight.

For years, estrogen, a natural hormone in the woman's body has been thought to cause cancer when found in unhealthy quantities. Women who begin menstruating early or start menopause late in life produce more estrogen in their lifetime and therefore a have a higher propensity for developing breast and uterine cancer. Research has also shown that women who run produce a less potent form of estrogen and cut their cancer risks nearly in half by staying healthy and active. Additionally, diabetes risk is cut by nearly 66% in women who exercise frequently, as compared to their sedentary peers. Other benefits of running include healthier skin, better circulation and a healthier outlook on everyday life.

Pregnancy and Running

In the past, most doctors urged their pregnant patients to cut back or give up their running and exercise regimen entirely, fearing that it may have a negative impact on both the mother and child. Today, however, we know that this is not the case according to most medical professionals. In fact, most state that physical exercise has many benefits associated with pregnancy. For instance, a physically fit mom usually has a shorter labor period, and an easier time in labor when the moment does arrive.

As we did in other sections of this book, we analyzed yesterday's myths with today's truths. As we did in those chapters we'll confront the issues head-on.

MYTH: If you were running before you became pregnant, you must stop running during your pregnancy.

MYTH-BUSTER: The truth is, in most cases, you can safely continue your running program but ONLY if your pregnancy is in good health – that is, both you and your unborn child are safe and healthy. In fact, if all is well, you should be able to run all the way up until you are full-term. If your doctor says it's okay to run, it doesn't mean you should be doing *competitive* running – it means that you may jog in a healthy manner, without overdoing it. You shouldn't even consider any personal records at this time. And of course, always listen to your body – if you sense there is something wrong with you or your child, stop immediately and consult with your doctor!

MYTH: If you exercise too much, you'll take too many nutrients away from your unborn child.

MYTH-BUSTER: By nature, the baby will get its nutrients before you do. If anything, you'll be cheating yourself out of your nutrients, vitamins and minerals. What's more, your baby will most likely be healthier at birth, by being leaner and stronger.

MYTH: It's not safe to do core workouts when pregnant.

MYTH-BUSTER: Not only is it safe but it's probably one of the best things you can do for your overall health, as it will be very beneficial at delivery time. Recovery will be quicker and it will mitigate potential posture problems during and after your pregnancy. However, most doctors will suggest that you avoid exercises that you do on your back, after the first trimester.

MYTH: Pregnancy can leave you predisposed to some specific fitness injuries.

MYTH-BUSTER: While intense workouts can cause injury, it's best to stick to simple warm-ups and stretches, and avoid exercises that involve deep muscle or joint movements. Stay away from exercises that push the limits of the hips, such as squats, lunches and deadlifts.

MYTH: You can do the same exercises throughout your pregnancy.

MYTH-BUSTER: This isn't always correct. All of your past and current exercises should be evaluated to assure you that you have the proper strength and balance in all three trimesters. Any exercise that causes a jolt or sudden movement should be avoided. Modify your regimen accordingly.

MYTH: If you didn't run or exercise before your pregnancy, it's okay to start now.

MYTH-BUSTER: Wrong again – maybe. Even though you weren't a fitness fanatic before your pregnancy, it doesn't mean that you should start now. But, it also doesn't mean you should be a couch potato. Like everything else in this world, moderation is the key. You don't have to start jogging at the park or track, but a good, robust walk a couple of times per day can have huge benefits. Be smart about what you do and how you do it, and ALWAYS consult your physician if you're thinking about starting an exercise program.

Motivation

"I think sports gave me the first place where this awkward girl could feel comfortable in my own skin. I think that's true for a lot of women—sports gives you a part of your life where you can work at something and you look in the mirror and you like that person."
– *Teri McKeever*

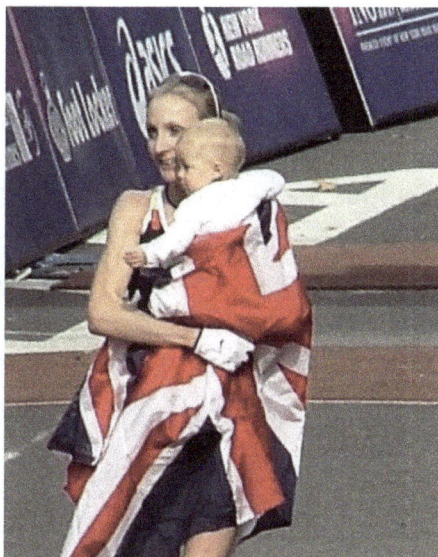

Paula Radcliffe and her daughter after winning the women's division in the 2007 NYC Marathon

Only nine months after giving birth to her daughter, Great Britain's **Paula Radcliffe** won the women's division of the 2007 New York City Marathon. At that time, some experts thought it was ludicrous for her to even try to run the marathon, let alone the training she did during her pregnancy. Radcliffe included two-a-day workouts with laborious hill workouts, strenuous long runs, all while being criticized and scrutinized by her peers and the so-called-experts.

In 2014, 31 of the elite women in the New York City marathon had already given birth. University of Colorado alumni and professional marathoner, **Kara Goucher**, thought she would have to make a tough choice when it came to motherhood, but after seeing Radcliffe's success, she quickly changed her mind: "I watched Paula win New York, basically leading from the starting gun to the finish tape, and afterward she picked up her baby." Goucher, one of the top American runners, then added, "I realized I can do both, and I want to do both."

For these elite runners, timing and scheduling is everything to them when planning their next big race. This includes pregnancy, especially when an Olympic title or corporate sponsorship is on the line. Between the World Championships and the Olympics, most elite women have a very small window of opportunity – usually less than 18 months. As professional athletes on corporate contracts, this could mean living without pay while they are away from competition. Most are bound to contracts that require them to run competitively every six to twelve months. Furthermore, as "contractors," they don't always enjoy the same benefits as blue collar workers, such as enhanced insurance and leave of absence programs. Federal laws do protect them with FMLA programs, but their contracts may not honor their payroll based on some stipulations. For example, a contract may explicitly state that if the woman becomes pregnant, they may terminate the contract. Professional runners must be very careful when signing long term commitments with corporate sponsors.

Motivation

"Without self-discipline, success is impossible – period." – *Lou Holtz*

Women's Physiological Differences

Men tend to have a fairly stable hormonal structure and environment, and aren't as sensitive to frequent changes as women are. Because of the physiological differences, women's hormones fluctuate greatly in regards to the amounts of **estrogen** and **progesterone** during intense exercise. The greatest fluctuations are usually a direct result from a menstrual cycle. A lot of women become concerned with the thought of running and dealing with the monthly cycle. The good news is that other than the discomfort and inconvenience that goes along with this, their running should not be impacted whatsoever. Women shouldn't be afraid to run during this time, and may actually find that running helps to improve their moods. Some women have set personal records or even world records during various parts of their menstrual cycle.

Bone Health

Of course, with good news comes some bad news. A woman's bone density relies heavily on the presence of estrogen in the body. Many women athletes develop menstrual irregularities, especially if they are in an intense training program, have very low body fat, and are not taking in the proper nutrients. These irregularities can reduce the amount of estrogen, which negatively affects bone density. This can help explain why athletic women are more prone to osteoporosis and stress fractures. Worse yet, because of their intense activities, they may end up missing their cycles completely, a condition known as **amenorrhea**. If you are an at-risk athlete for amenorrhea, you need to make sure you keep your bones healthy in other ways, including adequate doses of calcium and vitamin D, strength training, and optionally, oral contraceptives which contain estrogen. You should always consult your health care professional and monitor your estrogen levels, as amenorrhea can lead to other issues like stress fractures and even infertility.

Endurance Performance Effects

In most cases, females can expect to perform better in the menstrual cycle when estrogen is the prevailing hormone and perform the worst when progesterone is at its peak. For comfort and confidence, it's usually best to avoid intense workouts during your period. It might also be a good idea to plan your training run during your period to help alleviate your fear and nervousness in case your race does fall during your cycle. Be sure to keep your feminine products in your running kit or fuel belt.

Your Body's Internal Thermostat

A woman's body temperature changes rhythmically throughout the menstrual cycle, peaking in response to the surge in progesterone. Because of this phenomenon, your body's "set-point" increases and changes the threshold for dissipation of heat. This makes it more difficult for the body to cool, a very undesirable problem on a hot, humid day. Conversely, estrogen has the opposite effect, decreasing body temperature, which explains why body temperature is lower during the estrogen-dominant follicular phase.

> **Motivation**
>
> **"Progress is rarely a straight line. There are always bumps in the road, but you can make the choice to keep looking ahead."** – *Kara Goucher*

Metabolism and Muscle Glycogen

With the increased amounts of estrogen, women rely more on fat than men when running at the same pace, which in some cases can give women an advantage during long endurance events, such as ultramarathons.

Breathing

Lung function can be affected during the menstrual cycle, too. Perceived effort is greater when progesterone is the dominant hormone. Because of this, a female runner may tire sooner or feel more winded when progesterone levels are highest. This can also lead asthmatic runners to increased asthma attacks, which can negatively affect her performance during training or in a race.

Thirty-three to fifty-two percent of asthmatic women report a premenstrual worsening of asthma symptoms, and an additional twenty-two percent report that their asthma is worse during their periods.

Special Nutrition and Vitamin Supplements

For running, you need the same types of daily vitamins as your non-running friends; however, you have a greater need for nutrients that move oxygen through your system and focus on bone strength. I've listed the over-the-counter products here, but we'll look at them from a food-source perspective in the next chapter.

Vitamin E

Every day, your body naturally produces a compound known as ***reactive oxygen species***, or ***ROS***. These important compounds are a byproduct of the normal metabolism of oxygen within our bodies, and aid in homeostasis and cell signaling. ROS levels are elevated significantly during times of stress, however, which can result in substantial damage to structures of the cells. This process is known in the medical field as oxidative stress. During vigorous or extensive exercise, your body consumes up to 200 times more oxygen than when the body is at a rest. Studies suggest that a considerable amount of cumulative ROS can increase the risk of chronic diseases and vitamin E has been shown to fend off ROS, diminishing their harmful effects. To meet the recommended daily requirements, you should take 22.5 international units (IU) of vitamin E every day.

Vitamin C

Similar to vitamin E, vitamin C helps to protect your cells from damaging compounds that circulate through your body. Vitamin C helps to improve *nonheme iron absorption*, but its absorption effects are much greater when combined with vitamin E.

Nonheme iron is a category of iron that originates from plant foods and is the main component found in hemoglobin. The presence of nonheme iron drastically improves the absorption rate that is so important for athletes. It distributes life-nurturing oxygen from your lungs to the tissues of your muscles. Women should take about 75 milligrams of vitamin C on a daily basis.

Iron

Iron is also very important to any runner, but especially for women during their menstrual cycle. Women should take 18 milligrams each day.

Vitamin D

Running puts a tremendous amount of stress on your skeletal system and increases the risk of stress fractures. To optimize your bone density, focus on vitamin D supplements. Vitamin D helps your bones absorb calcium which will increase your bone strength. Look for supplements that contain D-3 instead of D-2, as D-3 is better for stress fracture prevention. Take 600 international units (IU) per day.

Vitamins B-6 and B-12

The B vitamins 6 and 12 are critical for oxygen functions. These vitamins help synthesize hemoglobin, which further improves oxygen delivery to cells as you run, and aid in metabolizing proteins into smaller, more manageable molecules called amino acids. Nearly every cell in your body use these highly specialized amino acids to help convert proteins into energy when your glycogen stores are depleted. The suggested amount of B-6 is 1.7 milligrams for men and 1.5 milligrams for women. Both genders should take 2.4 micrograms of B-12 on a daily basis.

Injuries and Cross-Training

Men and women are just as likely to suffer from injuries but the types of injuries vary from one gender to the other. Women are more likely to suffer from stress fractures and minor sprains while their male counterparts are more likely to injure large muscle group connective tissue problems such plantar fasciitis and Achilles and knee tendinitis.

Safety Concerns

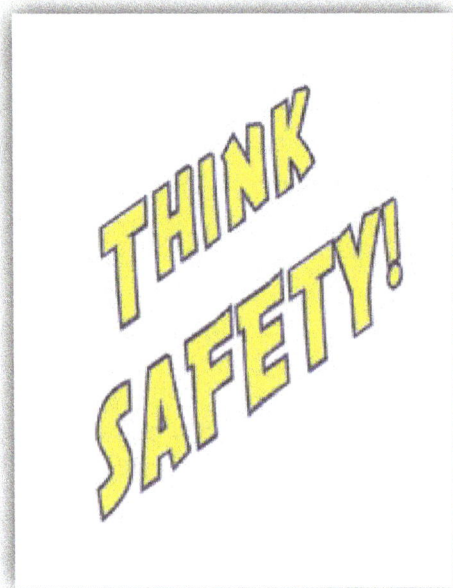

For women, safety can be among the toughest, if not THE toughest issues a woman can confront. Because of this fear, many women stay completely away from exercise and fitness programs. In this day and age, a woman should be able to move about freely with little or no concern for her safety. Unfortunately, that's not always a "real world" possibility. Every alley, every forested area, and every early morning run can expose a woman to a possible attack. In this section we'll take a look at the risks and ways to eliminate potential encounters with trouble. As a woman, what can you do to protect yourself from becoming another statistic?

> ### Motivation
>
> **"I am building a fire, and every day I train, I add more fuel. At just the right moment, I light the match."** – *Mia Hamm*

Keeping You Safe

Face it, staying safe in today's world is tough enough for either gender. But a lone woman in the early dawn hours, wearing minimal clothing in a high-risk neighborhood, increases the risk for a woman runner.

The numbers are frightening. As a woman, however, there are many ways to protect yourself from harms' way, and most of them are easy and logical. Let's take a look at some of the ways you can avoid getting into a scary situation.

Safety in Numbers

Most of us like to run alone because we don't have to worry about other people's schedules and we can run (or walk) at our own pace. Running with one or more people is much safer than running alone. If you can get your husband, boyfriend or one of your girlfriends to run with you, by all means, do it. Statistically, your chances of being attacked are reduced tremendously.

Safety Belt

Just like a carpenter has a tool belt stuffed with the tools of his trade, you, as a woman, should also be prepared with your collection of tools and necessities. I highly recommend one of the popular "fuel belts" with an accessory pouch, not just for toting your water and gels, but also to carry your defense systems too.

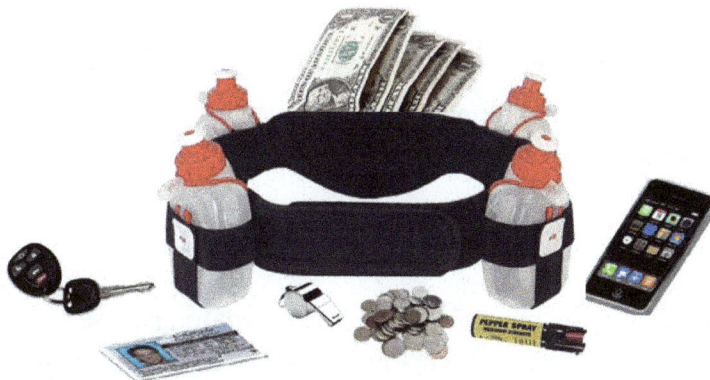

Besides carrying your water bottles, you should have:

- Cell Phone
- A can of Mace or pepper spray
- A whistle
- A spare car key
- Driver's License or ID

- SMALL amounts of cash
- Feminine products
- Chap-stick, sunscreen
- Band-Aids

> **Motivation**
>
> **"Look in the mirror – that's your competition."** – *Unknown*

Flight or Fight?

Even if an attack is unlikely, you should always be aware of your surroundings. Know where you are, where you've been and where you're going at all times. Before you start your run, make sure that SOMEONE knows your route, how long you expect to be out running and what you are wearing. This may seem a bit paranoid, but in this case, it really is better to be safe than sorry.

Don't engage in casual conversation with a stranger and don't run the same route at the same time every morning. You have a number of options if you feel someone is stalking you. One of the best ways is to pretend like you're talking on your cell phone and make eye contact with the person that is approaching you. Let him know that you see him. Take note of what he's wearing and what physical attributes he has because there is no "certain look" an attacker has. They can be in blue jeans or a three-piece suit. There really isn't a way to "profile" them. The best thing you can do is keep moving.

Theories suggest that women have an enhanced ability to read facial expressions and emotions. As a woman, you're much more likely to pick up on subtle emotional messages and read things like body language and tone of voice much better than men. As they say, a women's intuition is one of the strongest forces. Trust what you hear or see, and never, EVER ignore your instincts!

Unplug and Listen to Nature

If you're like me, listening to music can be very motivational and allows you to get into, and stay in your "zone." But it can also allow a predator to surveille you and make moves on you, if you can't hear him coming. If you must listen to music, use just one earbud and leave the other available for hearing the sounds of the great outdoors – as well as anything or anyone else.

Social Benefits

There are a number of benefits when running with others. Most importantly is the fact that you're much safer than when running alone. A running club can help you plan your runs with friends and allow you to make new friends, as well. This will give you a chance to bond with other club members in a group setting.

Run With Your Pet

One of the most discouraging things for a would-be predator, is to see a woman running with her canine friend, and the bigger the dog is, the more disinclined that predator would be to attack you. If a suspicious guy stops you and asks you if he can pet your dog, always warn him that "this dog might bite – he's not a friendly dog." That statement by itself could be enough to ward off a would-be attacker. Your dog can keep you safe. That said, you need to make sure that your best friend is kept safe by keeping him cool and hydrated. He can't tell you if or when he overheats, so you need to ease him into his training program like you did with yours, and make sure that you work as a team!

> ### Motivation
>
> *"For an athlete, the biggest pressure comes from within. You know what you want to do and what you're capable of."* – Paula Radcliffe

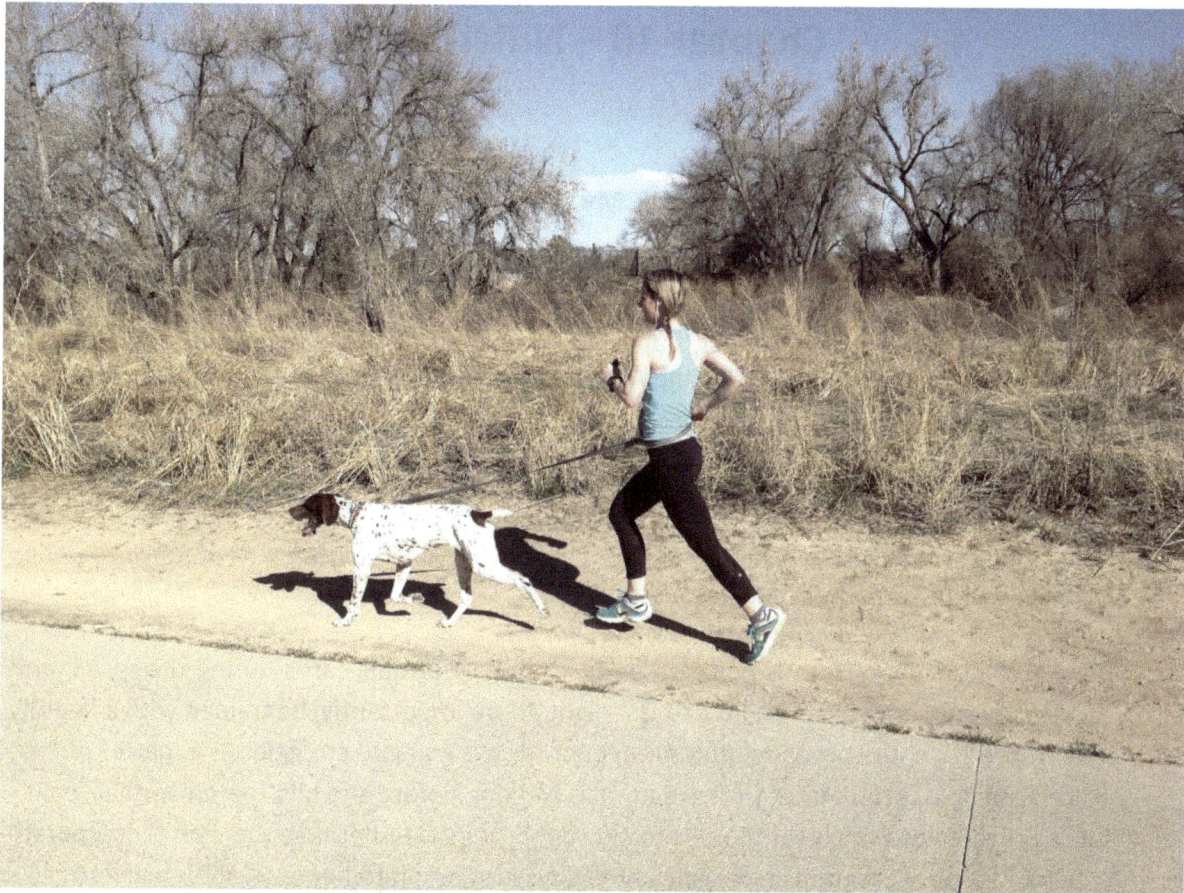

Running with your canine companion can literally save your life

Challenge!

As a woman, know that you're just as much of an athlete as a man. Just because he may be stronger, you still have the edge when it comes to consistency late in a race, especially a long distance endurance race.

Your challenge: *Be aware of your body and know how it adapts under varying circumstances during your training. Learn how to fuel your body with the proper vitamins and supplements. Finally, don't be forced to make a choice between being a runner and a woman. You CAN BE BOTH – and you can do it with great success! Run BECAUSE you are a woman!*

Motivation

"Never set limits, go after your dreams; don't be afraid to push the boundaries. And laugh a lot - it's good for you!" – *Paula Radcliffe*

Chapter 10 – Nutrition

My Story

Instead of telling my story, let's listen to Tom and Alice's story…

It seems like a no-brainer to most, but you'd be surprised at how many times I've heard a conversation like this before. Tom and Alice are at the start line of their marathon, and they trained together for months.

Tom: *"Alice, are you ready for the race?"*

Alice: *"I was so worked up for the past few days, I really didn't eat much. I get so nervous before each race; I just can't eat."*

Guess what? Tom is going to be just fine. He ate his carbs during the week, and loaded up with extra pasta and bread last night. More importantly, he trained with a healthy diet during his entire program. But, Alice, poor Alice is going to struggle. As a matter of fact, Alice is going to drop out of the race at mile 14, long before she hits the proverbial "wall." Alice prepared physically for months to get to this point, but because she didn't incorporate a healthy dietary program, especially in the days leading up to her race, she's going to have a rough time. Next time she'll incorporate a *nutritional* plan along with her *training* plan. Alice will learn a tough lesson, but she'll plan accordingly for her next race.

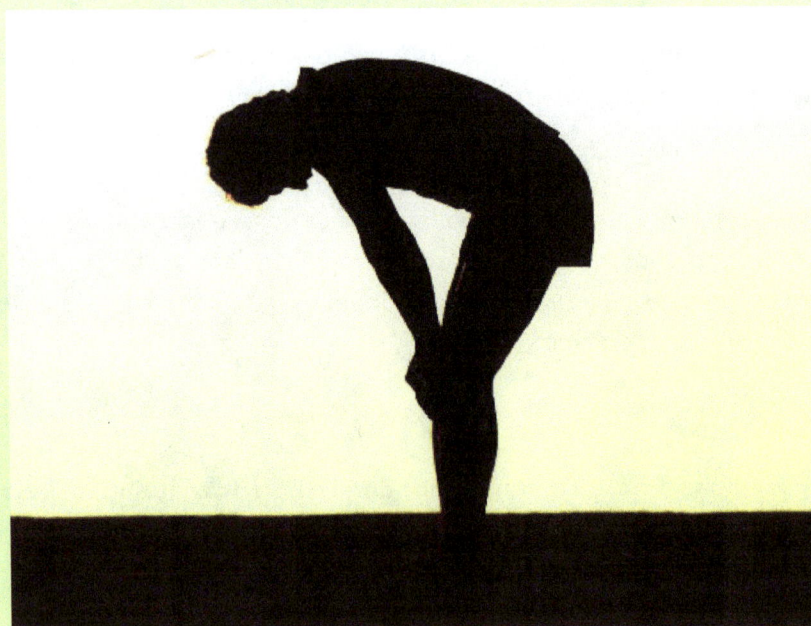

This story can be told over and over again - different people, same results. For some strange reason, many runners ignore one of the most important parts of running – one of the most important parts of life: proper nutrition. In the prologue of this book, I told my story of unruly weight gain, unhealthy diets, and overall disregard for my health. As Alice did in her story, I also learned valuable lessons around diet and nutrition. Many people overlook proper diet and nutrition in regards to running. They put a majority of their efforts into the physical aspects of their training and not enough into their nutritional program. And then they wonder why they struggle when it comes time to race.

As a runner, you cannot underestimate the importance of proper nutrition, whether you're a "comfort food" person, a vegetarian, or even a vegan. And depending on the type of nutritional lifestyle you commit to, it's important to know where your healthy energy sources lie. I'm not here to criticize or scrutinize any of the choices you make, meat-eater or not; I'm here to preach the importance of stocking up your energy sources without polluting your body. I've tried vegan and vegetarian lifestyles, I've tried high and low carbohydrate diets, high and low protein diets; I've tried breadless sandwiches, and yes, even wrap-less wraps.

I can honestly say that when done properly, any of these lifestyle choices or diets can work if you find the correct food sources or supplements to get all of the proper nutrients. It requires research and commitment, and sometimes, it can be expensive. But the important part is that you know where to find these nutrients and that you keep them balanced. If your food sources don't have the proper vitamins and minerals, you may have to rely on supplemental natural and synthetic sources.

Proper Nutrition

In this chapter, we'll take a brief look at the building blocks for proper nutrition relevant to running. As you'll see, these formulas depend on *nutritional needs, energy sources, nutritional lifestyles,* and popular *diet plans*. I'm emphasizing these four categories because they'll each have important sub-categories that are linked to them. As an example, your nutritional lifestyle may be far different than your *social, economic, religious, political, health* or *cultural* lifestyles. Conversely, it may also be possible that one of these lifestyles has a direct impact on the choice you make for your nutritional lifestyle. For instance, you may have a specific conviction towards animal rights and choose a *vegetarian* or *vegan* diet. Or, you may have celiac disease that requires the need for a *gluten free* diet.

Likewise, your *nutritional preferences* may vary greatly from your running friends, thus your *energy sources* will likely be different too.

The purpose of this chapter is not to persuade you into one type of diet and I'm certainly not going to try to influence you with my personal preferences. My goal is to briefly break down each of the five major nutritional lifestyles to find out how to optimize or enhance your intake of vitamins, minerals, and food energy sources made up of carbohydrates, proteins and fats. As with any new diet or lifestyle change, you should always consult your health care professional.

As we go through this chapter, I'll describe each category and the subcategories within. In the final section of this chapter, I'll give some examples of each type of nutritional lifestyle and make comparisons between them. We'll look at the five most popular nutritional lifestyles: *Vegan, Vegetarian, Paleo, Gluten-free, and Omnivore.*

Running and Diet

For the most part, runners monitor their food and nutrition more than non-runners and try to maintain a diet that's low on fats. Most athletes understand the importance of a balanced diet fueled primarily by carbohydrates. As we noted in chapter six, carbohydrates are especially important for runners because muscles need the glycogen that comes from them in order to produce energy for your body. Most health professionals agree that carbohydrates should supply about 55% of nutritional intake among runners. In order to enhance their energy stores, most distance runners practice ***carbo-loading*** before their races. It's common practice to eat a carb enriched diet during training, but most runners elect to increase a diet high in complex carbohydrates, such as pastas, breads and potatoes, just before a race or long run.

To some folks, carbo-loading might seem to be the most effective way to enhance performance, but it's really only a small part of your overall training. Carbo-loading does, however, allow you to store more fuel just before your race or long run. It should also be noted that running does not increase appetite. In fact, exercise tends to diminish it, acting as a suppressant. Many runners, like me, have to force down food the morning of a marathon. Even though I don't feel hungry on race day, I know the importance of the fuels that are available from the food. For many years, clinical dieticians have known that a fatty diet doesn't allow muscles to work well and intake of fat should not exceed 30% of your diet plan. Aside from carbohydrates, proteins can also supply energy and should make up about 15% of the calories in a runner's diet. Most importantly, fluids are necessary to allow blood to transfer glucose to the muscles and aid in flushing out metabolic waste. Moreover, insufficient fluids hinder your ability to sweat, an important function of our bodies during intense activities.

Sports Drinks

While the most effective and crucial fluid is water, I also recommend sports drinks like Gatorade ®, POWERADE ® and a plethora of other electrolyte filled beverages. Some people have a preference for energy drinks with caffeine, but I prefer the ones containing additional electrolytes. Electrolytes are minerals - sodium, calcium, phosphorous, chloride, potassium and magnesium, all of which you naturally lose when you sweat.

Electrolytes ensure proper muscle function during times of excessive sweating and need to be replaced as fluids are lost through our sweat glands. Electrolytes are also lost during moderate levels of exercise that last for more than an hour. One of the fastest ways to restore electrolyte levels is to consume sports drinks rich in potassium and sodium.

Some people like to consume sports drinks even when they're not working out intensely, but there's really no benefit since their loss of electrolytes is so low. Finally, most sports drinks provide a solid source for carbohydrates in the form of simple sugars. For athletes exercising longer than 60 minutes, these carbohydrates absorb quickly and convert readily into fuel.

Most sports drinks are considered "isotonic," meaning they're composed of a six to eight percent carbohydrate solution. This specific percentage of carbs takes advantage of fluid absorption and energy conversion because the concentration of salt and sugar is similar to that found in the human body. Studies suggest that isotonic drinks help to improve the body's ability to oxidize carbohydrates during exercise, and may enhance athletic performance. Sports drinks with one to three percent carbohydrates provide less energy, but do help with fluid absorption. Drinks that contain more than ten percent carbohydrates, including soda and some energy drinks, may cause digestive distress and slow your rate of rehydration.

Of course, many will subscribe to sweetened drinks with caffeine added, such as highly sugared teas before a marathon or long run. These can help boost energy and stamina during an intense or lengthy run.

And then there's beer. Beer does indeed contain water and carbohydrates, but unfortunately, most of the calories are from alcohol and alcohol cannot be converted into glycogen. Because of this, beer can actually dehydrate a runner, so I recommend saving the beer for the post-race celebration. Beer is still one of the favorite finish line consumables and many runners say that it helps to reduce the lactate buildup, but there is absolutely no science to this as we saw in chapter six. I do agree, however, that a beer or two can elevate your mood and dull your senses a bit.

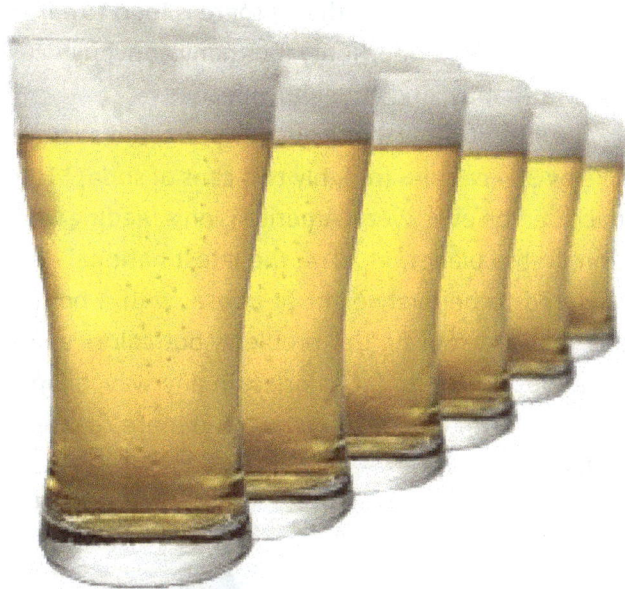

Long distance runners realize that it's important for them to maintain an abnormally low body weight in order to run their fastest and minimize the strain on their muscles, joints and cartilage. Some runners attempt to stay 10 to 20 pounds under their normal body weight. Some of the elite male marathon runners for instance, with an average height of 5'8," can weigh little more than 120 pounds.

It's not surprising that many runners have eating disorders, especially among women. The desire to stay thin often prevents the intake of the calories they desperately need. This can be a vicious cycle for many runners, and intervention is sometimes required.

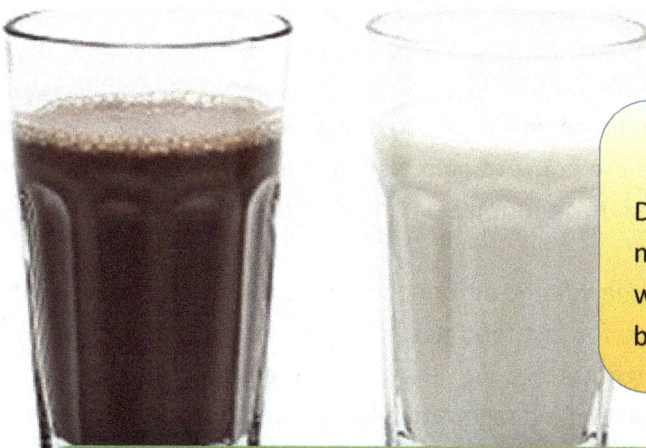

Tip

Did you know that chocolate and white milk are some of the best foods for post-workout recovery? They provide a good balance of protein and carbohydrates.

Motivation

"Keeping busy and making optimism a way of life can restore your faith in yourself."
– Lucille Ball

Nutritional Needs

In order to survive, all animals need water and food, along with shelter, habitable living space and air (oxygen, hydrogen, nitrogen, etc.) Most people in Western civilization are primarily concerned with *which* foods to eat, rather than *if* there is food to eat. Too much of the wrong food, too many calories, too much fat, too big of portions, too many conveniences! Too much of everything provides a grossly over-caloric, fat-happy, and unhealthy lifestyle.

Did you know that in just 25 years, the average American has increased their average daily calorie intake by 304 calories (roughly two cans of soda)? Theoretically, that's enough to add an extra 31 pounds to each person every year. America is on a feeding frenzy, literally, and has quickly become the most obese nation on the planet. In 2014, the latest national health surveys show that 68 percent of Americans are considered to be overweight or obese, with a body mass index greater than 25. And it's not just fatty foods that are causing the problem, but calories in general. Those two cans of soda I just mentioned contain absolutely no fat calories, in any way, shape or form, but they can certainly *change* your way, shape and form! *Calories, calories,* and more *calories.* Runners, it's time to take control – control of your health and your life.

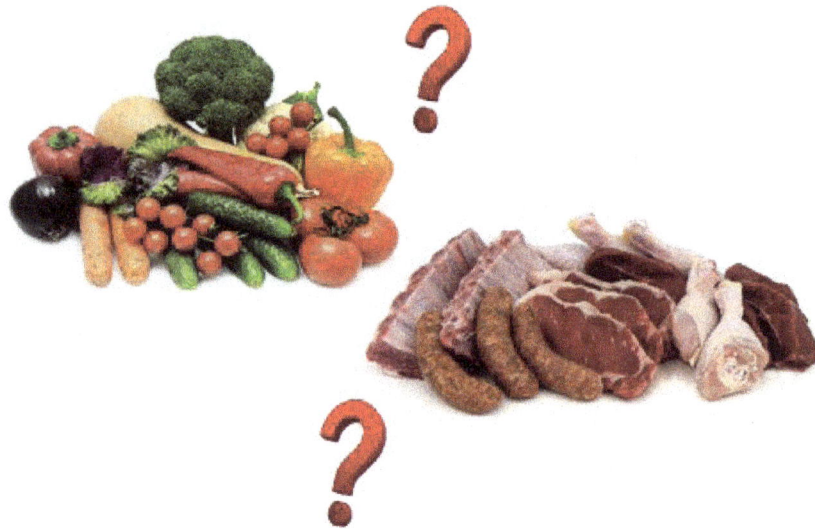

We consume either too many calorie-dense foods, or simply too much food. Early dieticians knew that if we take in more calories than we burn, we are going to gain weight. Guess what? None of the science, facts or modern technologies have changed those formulas. Decades later, it still holds true, just as two plus two still equals four.

Not only are we pouring on the calories or the volume of food, but we're also taking in unhealthy amounts of the wrong kinds of food. America's love for fast food has increased our rate of obesity, and sometimes with deadly consequences. The FDA suggests that we should eat at least two to five cups of fruits and vegetables per day, yet statistics say that the average American eats only three servings per day, and a whopping 42 percent eat fewer than two servings per day. Worse yet, frequent consumers of fast food, and financially challenged people, tend to eat less than one serving of fruit and vegetables every few days.

There are several good ways to see if you're overweight or even obese. The Body Mass Index (BMI) calculators found on internet are a great way to quickly find out if you're pushing your height/weight ratios.

The Convenient Truth

The root of our demise is both individual and cultural. The fast food market has made convenience their top priority. Faced with heavy workloads and a shortage of time, we've bought right into their marketing schemes and accept their unhealthy ways, along with their abhorrent prices. Much of this really comes down to how addicted to convenience we've become as a nation.

Convenience also comes with a hefty cost. As an example, let's pick on coffee. What should a cup of coffee really cost? If you go to your local gas station, it might cost you 69 cents. If you go to the convenience store up the street, you might have to pay 99 cents. Go to your local fast food restaurant, and the price doubles up to about $2.00. Now go see your favorite barista at the high-end coffee establishment and pay between $5.00 and $7.00 (without the espresso). You are now paying 10 times the amount of money for that same cup of coffee. Multiply your $5.00 cup of coffee over a 30-day period, and you've just spent $150.00 per month, or more, simply because you favor convenience over brewing it yourself. Folks, I'm no mathematician, but my calculator tells me that it adds up to $1,800.00 per year. Ah, the price of convenience. Oh, I forgot to mention that you don't even need to get out of your car to get that high dollar beverage. That's right, just sit there in your idling car, burn even fewer calories, and maybe add a little whipped cream and a few chocolate sprinkles. Yum.

So, how about this? Why not invest in a good quality home coffee brewing system, sleep a little later and avoid the wait at the coffee shop? I can almost guarantee that you'll save both money and time and wonder how in the world you survived without it.

One more example before I continue: Let's take a healthy peanut butter and jelly sandwich on whole wheat bread, a banana and a couple handfuls of fresh trail mix. This combination makes a very healthy lunch, and prep time is just a few minutes. Overall cost is probably less than $2.00 per meal. Compare that with a trip over to the fast food hamburger joint where you'll spend more time in your car and pay $7.00 to $10.00 on average. And don't forget to add in the price of gas for this little "convenient" trip. Make an attempt to start thinking about how much food you really eat, and how much of it may be unhealthy. Then find alternative ways to save money and decrease your junk food intake.

Portion Distortion

Large portions equal large amounts of calories. Our Western diet and culture has taught us to eat larger quantities on larger plates. Do we really need these larger portions? Of course we don't! In this world of "super-sizing," we've become advocates of "more is better" and in fact, it couldn't be further from the truth. Larger portion sizes are NOT better for your health or your budget.

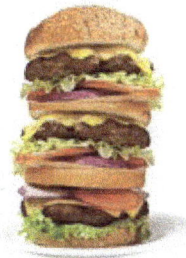

> **Motivation**
>
> **"See other competitors as your friends. Your only real competitor is yourself. The idea is to beat the distance, not the person next to you. So hang in there, stay positive, and take positive energy from everyone around you."** – *Kara Goucher*

Minimum Requirements

The history of **the Food and Drug Administration (FDA)** can be traced back to 1813 when the short-lived **Vaccine Act of 1813** was implemented to regulate the contents and sale of domestically produced foods and pharmaceuticals. In 1906, President Theodore Roosevelt signed into law the Food and Drug Act to prohibit the interstate transport of food that had been modified from its "standard of strength, quality or purity." Several more variations occurred in the 20th century, including the name change to **The Food, Drug and Insecticide Organization**, and ultimately the current Food and Drug Administration in 1930. This branch of the government regulates drugs, cosmetics, food safety, tobacco products, dietary supplements, vaccines, blood transfusions, electromagnetic radiation, medical devices, animal foods, veterinary products, and of course, our food labeling system. And that's the empahsis of the next portion of this book. While it may seem unrelated or even a bit technical, I'm trying to help you understand how to read food labels so you know exactly what's going into your body.

1. Portion Information

2. Calories listed here

3. Limit these

4. Meet these requirements

5. Footnotes

6. % of Daily Values

These are the recommended daily values for each nutrient.

5% or less is LOW

20% or more is HIGH

Nutrition Facts
Serving Size 1 cup (228g)
Servings Per Container 2

Amount Per Serving

Calories 250   Calories from Fat 110

% Daily Value*

Total Fat 12g — 18%
Saturated Fat 3g — 15%
Trans Fat 3g
Cholesterol 30mg — 10%
Sodium 470mg — 20%
Total Carbohydrate 31g — 10%
Dietary Fiber 0g — 0%
Sugars 5g
Protein 5g

Vitamin A — 4%
Vitamin C — 2%
Calcium — 20%
Iron — 4%

* Percent Daily Values are based on a 2,000 calorie diet. Your Daily Values may be higher or lower depending on your calorie needs.

	Calories:	2,000	2,500
Total Fat	Less than	65g	80g
Sat Fat	Less than	20g	25g
Cholesterol	Less than	300mg	300mg
Sodium	Less than	2,400mg	2,400mg
Total Carbohydrate		300g	375g
Dietary Fiber		25g	30g

Stay in charge of your health and learn how to read a food label

Motivation

"A goal without a plan is just a wish." *– Herm Edwards*

In the most condensed version I can come up with, I've provided a list of the FDA's advertised **Daily Nutritional Requirements**. These are based on the FDA's recommended intake of 2,000 calories per day.

Nutrition Values (These are listed on the **top half** of the **Nutrition Facts** label)

- You should get **no more** than:
- 65 grams (g) of total fat
- 20 g of saturated fat
- 300 milligrams (mg) of cholesterol
- 2,400 mg of sodium

- You should get **no less** than:
- 50 g of protein
- 300 g of carbohydrates
- 25 g of dietary fiber

Vitamins (These are optionally listed on the **bottom half** of the **Nutrition Facts** label)

Your diet needs to provide you with a certain amount of vitamins every day. Food labels must list the percentage of the daily value of each vitamin, based on the FDA's minimum values. The FDA lists the minimum daily values, meaning the **least amount** you should have in your diet.

- 5,000 International Units (IU) of vitamin A
- 60 mg of vitamin C
- 400 IU of vitamin D
- 30 IU of vitamin E
- 80 microgram (mcg) of vitamin K
- 1.5 mg thiamine
- 1.7 mg riboflavin

- 20 mg niacin
- 2 mg vitamin B6
- 400 mcg folate
- 6 mcg vitamin B12
- 300 mcg biotin
- 10 mg pantothenic acid

Minerals (These are optionally listed on the **bottom half** of the **Nutrition Facts** label)

Your diet also should provide you with necessary minerals. The FDA recommends you get **at least**:

- 1,000 mg of calcium
- 3,000 mg of potassium
- 3,400 mg of chloride
- 18 mg of iron
- 400 mg of magnesium
- 1,000 mg of phosphorus
- 150 mg of iodine

- 70 mcg of selenium
- 15 mg of zinc
- 120 mg of chromium
- 75 mcg of molybdenum
- 2 mg of manganese
- 2 mg of copper

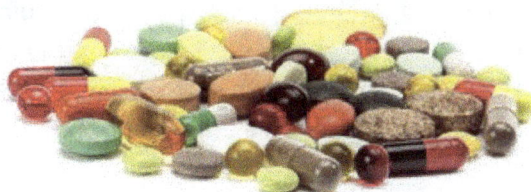

Nutrient Sources

Now that we've reviewed how to read an FDA food label, and what we need to maintain a healthy diet, let's examine the various ways to get all of those nutrients, vitamins and minerals.

The table below displays *animal-based* and *plant-based* availability sources for the nutrients you need. As an example, someone on a vegan or vegetarian diet will not be able to get adequate amounts of cholesterol or vitamin B12 from fruits or vegetables. These two diets will require vitamin B12 supplements. Likewise, if you live primarily on animal-based nutrients, you should supplement your dietary fiber, folate, chloride, chromium and manganese with natural vegetables.

Nutrient	Animal-based	Best sources	Plant-based	Best sources
Protein	Yes	Lean meats, fish, poultry, turkey, Greek yogurt, cottage cheese, milk, eggs.	Yes	Soy milk, navy beans, dried lentils, peanut butter, mixed nuts, tofu, edamame, green peas, wheat germ, and quinoa.
Carbohydrates	Yes	Yogurt, milk, ice cream, fat-free cheese.	Yes	Bananas, blueberries, strawberries, brown rice, oatmeal, whole grain bread, whole wheat pasta, potatoes, yams.
Fat	Yes	Fish, butter, margarine, mayonnaise, sour cream, salad dressing, cream.	Yes	Seeds, nuts, avocado, coconut, peanut oil, olive oil, safflower oil, soybean oil, grain-based desserts.
Cholesterol	Yes	Eggs, liver.	No	None
Dietary Fiber	No	None	Yes	Whole or cut grapefruit, oranges, most brans, beans, most berries, most whole grains, peas, greens, most nuts and seeds, kale, cabbage, broccoli, potatoes.
Vitamin A	Yes	Beef liver, tuna, sturgeon, mackerel, oysters.	Yes	Sweet potatoes, carrots, dark leafy greens, squash, romaine lettuce, dried apricots, cantaloupe, sweet red pepper, mango.
Vitamin C	Yes	Beef liver, oysters, cod, pork liver, goat milk, cow milk.	Yes	Kakadu plum, rose hip, black currant, red pepper, guava, kiwi, broccoli, papaya, strawberries, oranges, cantaloupe, grapefruit, mango, dark berries.
Vitamin D	Yes	Salmon, tuna, mackerel, beef liver, cheese, egg yolks.	Yes	Orange juice (fortified).
Vitamin E	Yes	Shrimp, sardines, salmon, cod.	Yes	Sunflower seeds, almonds, spinach, avocado, peanuts, turnip greens, asparagus, beet greens, mustard greens

Nutrient	Animal-based	Best sources	Plant-based	Best sources
Vitamin K	Yes	Pasture-raised chicken and eggs, grass-fed beef and lamb, shrimp, sardines, tuna and salmon.	Yes	Kiwi, blueberries, prunes, grapes, kale, spinach, mustard greens, collard greens, beet greens, basil, cilantro, sage, oregano, black pepper.
Thiamine (B1)	Yes	Trout, salmon, tuna, shad, mackerel, pork.	Yes	Macadamia nuts, sunflower seeds, wheat bread, green peas, squash, asparagus, soy beans, navy beans.
Riboflavin (B2)	Yes	Goat cheese, feta, Roquefort, brie, grated parmesan, lean beef and lamb, mackerel, eggs, pork, squid.	Yes	Almonds, raw brown Italian mushrooms, portabella, dried shiitake, sesame seeds, sunflower seeds, chia seeds, spinach, beet greens, asparagus.
Niacin (B3)	Yes	Tuna, chicken, turkey, salmon, lamb, beef, sardines, shrimp.	Yes	Peanuts, root vegetables and leafy greens, brown rice, cantaloupe, barley, sunflower seeds.
Vitamin B6	Yes	Tuna, turkey, beef, chicken, salmon.	Yes	Sweet potatoes, potatoes, spinach, sunflower seeds, bananas.
Folate	Trace	Very few folates can be found in poultry, eggs, seafood and some dairy products.	Yes	Lentils, pinto beans, garbanzo beans, asparagus, spinach navy beans, black beans, kidney beans, turnip greens, broccoli.
Vitamin B12	Yes	Sardines, salmon, tuna, cod, lamb, scallops, shrimp, beef, yogurt, milk.	No	None
Biotin	Yes	Salmon, eggs, milk, some meats.	Yes	Peanuts, almonds, sweet potatoes, onions, oats, tomatoes, carrots, walnuts.
Sodium	Yes	Cured meat, fish and bacon, fish sauce, cheese.	Yes	Salad dressings, soy sauce, steak sauce, BBQ sauce, relish, pickles.
Pantothenic Acid	Yes	Chicken, turkey, yogurt, eggs, dairy products.	Yes	Mushrooms, shiitake, avocado, sweet potatoes, lentils dried peas, broccoli.
Calcium	Yes	Sardines, yogurt, cheese, cow's milk.	Yes	Tofu, sesame seeds, collard greens, spinach, turnip greens, mustard greens, beet greens.
Potassium	Yes	Tuna, salmon, cod.	Yes	Lima beans, sweet potatoes, potatoes, soybeans, spinach, avocados, pinto beans, lentils, bananas.
Chloride	No	None	Yes	Seaweed, rye, tomatoes, lettuce, celery, olives.

Nutrient	Animal-based	Best sources	Plant-based	Best sources
Iron	Yes	Liver, kidneys, red meat, poultry, oysters, clams, eggs.	Yes	Soybeans, lentils, spinach, sesame seeds, garbanzo beans, olives, lima beans, navy beans, kidney beans.
Magnesium	Yes	Beef, cheddar cheese, caviar, cod, herring, perch, pollock, salmon, sardines, and tuna.	Yes	Pumpkin seeds, spinach, soybeans, sesame seeds, quinoa, cashews, black beans, sunflower seeds, navy beans.
Phosphorus	Yes	Scallops, sardines, cod, tuna, salmon, shrimp.	Yes	Soybeans, pumpkin seeds, lentils, Tofu, oats, green peas, broccoli.
Iodine	Yes	Scallops, cod, shrimp, sardines, salmon, cow's milk, eggs, tuna.	Yes	Sea vegetables, strawberries.
Selenium	Yes	Tuna, shrimp, sardines, salmon, turkey, cod, lamb, chicken, scallops, beef, eggs, milk.	Yes	Shiitake, asparagus, mustard seeds, Tofu, brown rice, sunflower seeds, sesame seeds, flaxseeds, cabbage, spinach, garlic.
Zinc	Yes	Beef, lamb, turkey, shrimp.	Yes	Sesame seeds, pumpkin seeds, lentils, garbanzo beans, cashews, quinoa.
Chromium	Trace	Very little found in eggs, cow's milk and some meats.	Yes	Broccoli, barley, oats, green beans, tomatoes, romaine lettuce, black pepper.
Molybdenum	Yes	Eggs, yogurt.	Yes	Lentils, dried peas, lima beans, kidney beans, soybeans, black beans, pinto beans, garbanzo beans, oats, barley.
Manganese	Trace	Very little found in some muscle meat.	Yes	Cloves, oats, brown rice, garbanzo beans, spinach, pineapple, pumpkin seed, rye, soybeans.
Copper	Yes	Shrimp, sardines.	Yes	Sesame seeds, cashews, soybeans, shiitake, sunflower seeds, lentils, garbanzo beans, walnuts, lima beans.

Tip

Top Five Nutritional Tips for the Modern Athlete

Number Five: Replace lost electrolytes

Number Four: Drink fluids early and often

Number Three: Go easy on the fat intake

Number Two: Get enough protein, but don't overdo it….

… and **Number One**: Load up on carbohydrates

Nutrients from Synthetic Sources

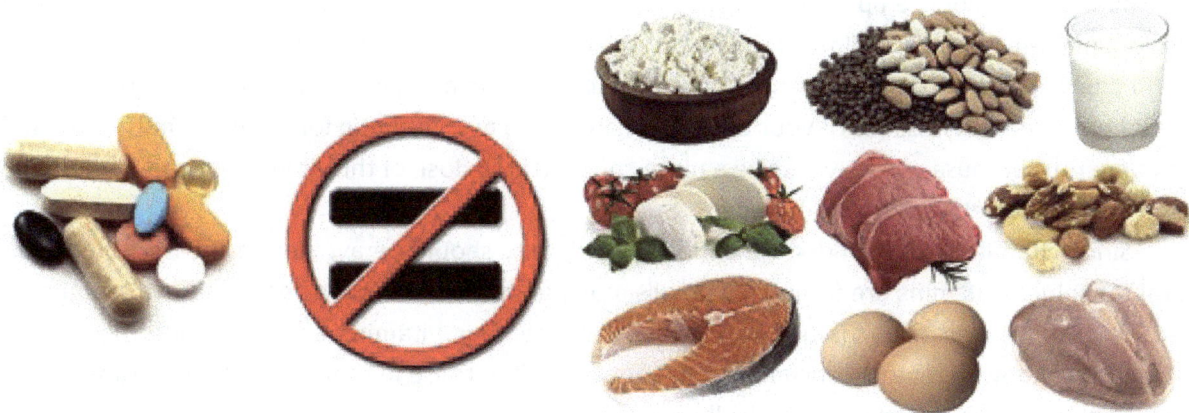

Differences Between Natural and Synthetic Vitamins

We just took a long look at natural vitamins and minerals from plants and animals. We can also get vitamins from our sun. No matter what the source is, vitamins and minerals are crucial to our health and the functions of our bodies. Without vitamins, we may suffer from confusion, depression, organ malfunction and weight problems from anorexia to obesity. What about synthetic supplements? Are they effective? Are they safe?

Synthetic Vitamins

From a dietary perspective, we should be able to get enough nutrients from our normal food sources. As humans, we choose what to eat, thereby limiting the vitamins and minerals our bodies can absorb. Because we don't all share the same diet or lifestyle, some of us miss out on many of the important nutrients we need. Supplements can help bridge the gap when we don't eat what we should.

Good News, Bad News

The benefits of good quality supplements are numerous and can help us with some of the deficiencies that we confront. The problem with these synthesized nutrients is that many of them lack the quality we need because they don't come straight from their natural sources. They're manufactured with the intent to impersonate the way that natural vitamins perform in our bodies. Unfortunately, a number of them lack the transporters and helper molecules associated with naturally-occurring vitamins because they have been "isolated." Most experts emphasize that isolated vitamins cannot be used or even recognized by the body in the same way as the natural form of the nutrient.

Many of the lower quality synthetic vitamins are also lacking the essential nutrients to be absorbed by the body and are simply excreted. Unfortunately, more than 95 percent of the vitamin supplements on today's market are categorized as synthetic. What's worse is that current regulation allows the manufacturer to state that it's a "natural" vitamin even if only 10 percent of the nutrient is actually derived from a biological material. This means that up to 90 percent of your "natural" vitamin may be synthetic.

Are Synthetic Vitamins Healthy?

There has been a great debate for years whether or not synthetic vitamins are healthy. Many of them, including the "D" form of vitamins have true, natural food sources, but the ones that are labeled as the "l" moniker may not live up to their reputation and may in fact be toxic to our systems. To add to the confusion, manufacturers are allowed to use "dl" which might suggest that it's still natural, however this just isn't true. Finally, fat soluble vitamins in their synthetic form are particularly dangerous because they can build up in the fatty tissues of your body and cause toxicity. Synthetic forms of the nutrients can be more dangerous because you may receive a more concentrated dose of the vitamin instead of the normal amount that you'd get from a food-based form.

Since vitamins A, D, E and K are all fat soluble, they should be avoided in their synthetic form. Natural fat soluble vitamins are found in fish, oils, nuts, leafy greens and butter, and extra amounts are stored in the liver and fatty tissues of the body. These four vitamins are hot sellers because the manufacturers know that most consumers don't get enough of these in their natural form. Most of the B Vitamins and Vitamin C are also synthetically manufactured.

Tip

Common Synthetic Vitamins to Avoid:
Look for these clues on your vitamin's label that display the origin of the vitamin:

- Biotin: d-Biotin
- Vitamin A: Acetate and Palmitate
- Vitamin B1 or Thiamine: Thiamine Mononitrate, Thiamine Hydrochloride
- Vitamin B2 or Riboflavin: Riboflavin
- Vitamin B6 or Pyridoxine: Pyridoxine Hydrochloride
- Vitamin B12: Cobalamin
- Folic Acid: Pteroylglutamic Acid
- Choline: Choline Chloride, Choline Bitartrate
- Vitamin C or Ascorbic Acid: Ascorbic Acid
- Vitamin D: Irradiated Ergosteral, Calciferol
- Vitamin E: dl-alpha tocopherol, dl-alpha tocopherol acetate or succinate
- Pantothenic Acid: Calcium D-Pantothenate
- PABA or Para-aminobenzoic Acid: Aminobenzoic Acid

It should be noted once again that any "dl" form of any vitamin is synthetic.

Other Toxic Ingredients to Avoid In Supplements

- Carnauba wax (used in car wax and shoe polish)
- Magnesium stearate (or stearic acid)
- Monosodium Glutamate (MSG) and can be disguised as "natural flavors"
- Titanium dioxide is a known carcinogen

Energy Sources: Protein, Carbohydrates & Fats

In **Chapter 6 – Running Physiology**, we touched briefly on the fuel sources we need for our bodies, not only for everyday activity, but for intense workouts, speed and endurance, too. Let's take a deeper glance at the fuels our bodies need – *proteins, carbohydrates and fats*.

Energy Source Percentages

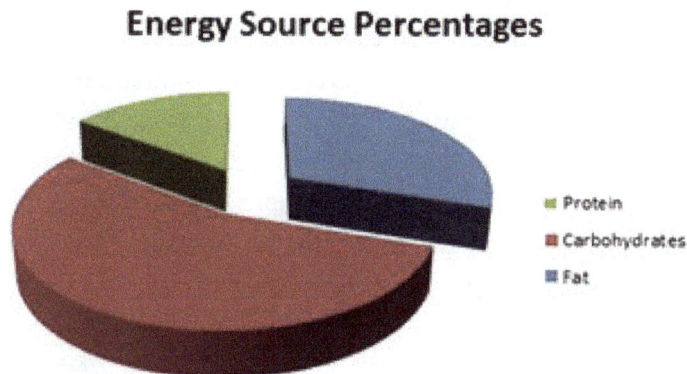

Most health experts recommend a caloric intake of 55% carbs, 30% fats, and 15% proteins

Carbohydrates

Carbohydrates are the body's principal source of energy. There are three types of carbohydrates: simple, complex starchy and complex fibrous carbs.

- **Simple carbohydrates** are found in vegetables, fruits, milk products, honey, fruit juice, candy, syrup, soft drinks and other foods with high sugar contents. Simple carbohydrates have a 'simple' molecular structure and are made up of just 1 or 2 sugar molecules. The simplest form of carbohydrate is glucose. Simple carbs that are found in common foods include sucrose (table sugar), fructose (fruit-based), and lactose (dairy-based). Many of these carbs serve a dual role when it comes to healthy foods. Foods such as milk, cottage cheese and other non-fat dairy products are powerful sources of calcium. Fruits and vegetables are excellent food sources for weight loss.
- Within the simple carbohydrates, there are several sugar types known as **"kCaloric Sweeteners"** and are comprised of the following:
  - **Glucose** is the primary type of simple sugar and is the vital source of energy for all living things. Glucose supplies the body with immediate energy. It occurs naturally in many vegetables and fruits and is also produced in the body by breaking down other foods into glucose. Glucose is sometimes known as blood sugar, sometimes as grape sugar. Almost all plant foods contain glucose.
  - **Sucrose:** commonly known as table sugar, beet sugar, or cane sugar. Sucrose occurs naturally in many fruits and some vegetables.
  - **Fructose:** known as fruit sugar. Most plants contain fructose, especially fruits and saps.
  - **Maltose:** known as malt sugar and is found in grains.
  - **Lactose:** commonly known as milk sugar. It is the principal carbohydrate found in milk.

- **Complex starchy carbohydrates** are found in breads, cereals, pasta, rice, beans and peas and starchy vegetables such as potatoes, green peas and corn. Similar to simple carbohydrates, complex carbohydrates are also made up of sugars, but the sugar molecules are laced together to form longer molecule chains. This type of carbohydrate includes peas, beans and whole grains, which are all rich in fiber, minerals and vitamins. Unfortunately, complex starchy carbohydrates are often refined by machinery that's used to remove the high fiber part – the germ and bran, from the grain. When this happens, all the properties that make it "healthy" are lost in this process. This basically changes its properties to that of a simple carbohydrate and the body uses it in that way. White flour and breads, white rice, pasta, sugary cereals and all other foods that are made from white flour all take on these characteristics. Try to avoid these highly refined carbohydrates. Instead, stay with unrefined complex carbohydrates because they still contain the complete grain, including the germ and bran. Because these foods are high in fiber, they can aid in the digestive process and help you to lose weight.

- **Complex fibrous carbohydrates** are most commonly found in green, leafy vegetables like kale, lettuce, cabbage, artichoke, broccoli, nuts and nut butters, eggplant, whole grains and raspberries. Eating food with high fiber content can help prevent stomach or intestinal issues such as constipation. Studies suggest that these foods may also help lower blood pressure, cholesterol and blood sugar. Most dieticians agree that your carbohydrate intake should be between 45 and 65 percent per day, with an average of 55 percent. Fibrous carbohydrates are plentiful sources of phytochemicals, minerals, vitamins, and other nutrients. Green vegetables make up a large percentage of these foods and they're loaded with fiber which is the indigestible part of the plant material. This means that much of the raw food passes straight through your digestive system and is not absorbed. These foods act as a cleansing agent to keep the intestines flowing properly. The lack of calories makes them great for people on a diet because it's practically impossible to overeat on veggies. Some vegetables, such as celery, are so low in calories, they contain fewer calories than required to eat them!

Proteins

Proteins are used to fight infections and repair or rebuild damaged tissues within your body. Proteins work side by side, right along with carbs and fats to keep your biological fuel tank filled up at all times, and help produce energy for your physical activities. Proteins in food are broken down into amino acids that are further broken down into other new proteins with very specific functions, such as catalyzing chemical reactions, assisting communication between different cells, or transporting organic molecules throughout your body. When there is a shortage of fats or carbohydrates, proteins can also produce energy.

Good sources of protein are unsalted seeds and nuts, seafood, lean meat and poultry, eggs, soy products, beans and peas. Protein can also be found in many dairy products, although it is much higher in fat than plant-based sources are. Most dieticians agree that your protein intake should be between 10 and 35 percent per day, with an average of 15 percent.

Fats

Fats give you energy and normally curtail or suppress your appetite after you're done eating by making you feel full. Shortening, oils, butter, and margarine are types of fats, and salad dressings, mayonnaise, sour cream, and table cream are high in fat. Some animal-based food sources and certain plant foods like nuts, seeds, nuts, coconut and avocado, also contain fat.

Following are descriptions of the various types of fat.

- **Monounsaturated.** These include olive oil, peanut oil, canola oil and safflower oil. They are found in peanut butter, avocados and some nuts and seeds.
- **Polyunsaturated.** Some are soybean oil, flaxseed oil and corn oil. These are also found in fatty fish, walnuts and some seeds.
- **Saturated.** This type of fat can be found in milk products including butter and red meat, as well as palm and coconut oils. Regular cheese, dairy desserts, pizza and grain-based foods are common sources of saturated fat in our meals.
- *Trans* **fats (*trans* fatty acids).** Processed trans fats are found in vegetable shortening and stick margarine. Trans fats are often used in store-purchased baked goods and many fried foods at some fast food restaurants.

Most dieticians agree that your fat intake should be between 20 and 35 percent of your overall dietary intake per day, with an average of 30 percent.

We'll start combining all of our topics coming up in the next few sections. From there, we'll start reviewing the five most popular nutritional lifestyles. We'll close out this chapter focusing on important fueling strategies.

Nutritional Lifestyles vs. Diet Plans

At this time, I'd like to point out the difference between *nutritional lifestyles* and *diet plans*. A nutritional lifestyle is a personal choice to live your life in a certain way. A diet plan, on the other hand is how you maintain that particular lifestyle, and what you eat within the constraints of the lifestyle choice. For instance, you may select the *vegetarian lifestyle*, but that doesn't define *what* you'll eat. It only states that you'll eat from a plant-based menu. The *diet plan* describes which plant-based items you choose to eat.

As I mentioned in the previous section, I don't want to tell you what you should eat or how you should live your life. And I'm certainly not trying to write a book on diet plans. There are already enough of those! Instead, we'll take a look at each lifestyle and a few of the more popular diet plans. If you have the desire to research it further, feel free to peruse your favorite book store or search the Internet for more information.

> **Motivation**
>
> **"If it is important to you, you will find a way. If not, you'll find an excuse."** – *Unknown*

Vegan Lifestyle

For all intents and purposes, *veganism* is the abstention from the use of animal products, not always from a dietary perspective, but from an overall philosophy towards the treatment of animals. A follower of veganism is known as a *vegan*. There are two basic forms of veganism with *dietary vegans* being the focus of this portion of the book. Dietary vegans refrain from consuming animal products; meat, eggs, dairy products such as milk, cheese, animal-based enzymes and other animal-derived substances. For clarification purposes, *ethical vegans* extend their beliefs into other areas of their lives, and are against the use of *any* animal products. For example, an ethical vegan is opposed to the commercial or personal consumption of leather, silk, feathers and animal based jewelry (pearls), just to name a few. Many avoid by-products of animals, including the honey made from bees. This led to the discussion (or argument) of what makes up a "true" vegan.

With that said, let's now focus on the subject matter at hand – dietary veganism. In this market space, there are many skeptics. For years, many nutritionists felt that good health through veganism was not possible, or at the very least, not sustainable. The so-called experts of the time were convinced that it was only a fad, a temporary lifestyle or diet solution. With modern science on our side, we now know that veganism is not only good for weight loss, but for the most part, is a completely healthy lifestyle.

In general, vegan diets tend to be higher in magnesium, folic acid, dietary fiber, vitamin E, vitamin C, iron and phytochemicals. These diets are also lower in calories, cholesterol, saturated fat, vitamin D, long-chain omega-3 fatty acids, calcium, zinc and vitamin B12. B12 is produced by micro-organisms such as naturally occurring bacteria. Uncontaminated plant foods don't provide vitamin B12, so most researchers agree that vegans should find alternative sources by consuming B12-fortified foods or take some sort of vitamin supplement.

Well-planned vegan diets can reduce the risk of some types of chronic disease, including heart disease, and are considered appropriate for all stages of the life-cycle by the American Dietetic Association, Dietitians of Canada and the Australian National Health and Medical Research Council.

Since 2005 or thereabouts, the vegan lifestyle and diet appeared to become main-stream in the public's eye. Vegan entrees became popular, and restaurants began to mark vegan items on their menus. Many politicians, celebrities and athletes began to adopt vegan diets - some seriously, some part-time. Some of these high profile figures include politician Al Gore, body builder Jim Morris, Olympic sprinter Carl Lewis, actors Alec Baldwin and Beau Bridges, NFL players Arian Foster and Tony Gonzales, and ultramarathon runners Scott Jurek and Damien Stoy.

Motivation

"I've found when all I'm eating is really fresh, healthy foods, I stop craving pizza and burgers." – *Lauren Conrad*

Famous Vegans

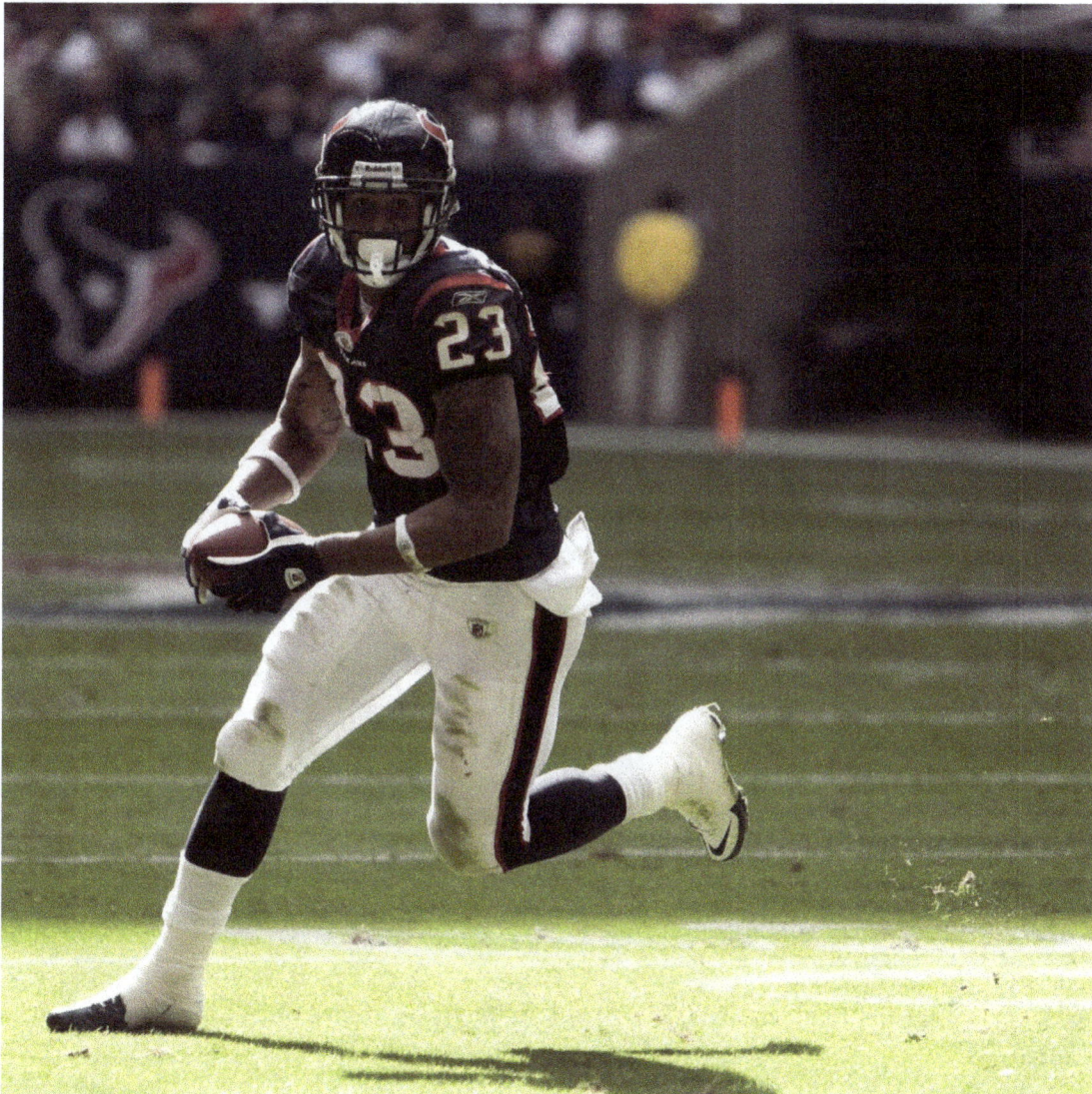

NFL Running Back Arian Foster

From the uninformed consumer perspective, a vegan diet may seem unhealthy. Much of this perception is contrived by people with little exposure or knowledge of veganism, who don't know where to go to get the nutrients they need to maintain a healthy lifestyle. As we saw in the examples of NFL players, body builders and extreme athletes, a vegan diet can be as healthy, if not more healthy than the other nutritional lifestyles.

Personally, I've tried a vegan diet and used it primarily for weight loss. Unfortunately, when it comes to food, my inner cravings usually give way to my eventual lack of commitment.

> **Motivation**
>
> **"Age is no barrier. It's a limitation you put on your mind."** — *Jackie Joyner-Kersee*

One of the most prolific vegan runners is Scott Jurek. Very few athletes have made such an impact on the sport of ultramarathon running as Jurek has made. Based in Colorado, he has elevated veganism into the spotlight as much as, or more than any other professional athlete. Scott has led the sport with some amazing performances, including multiple wins and course records.

On June 25, 2005, Jurek won his seventh consecutive Western States 100 mile ultramarathon event, and then won the Badwater ultramarathon just two weeks later. (See **Badwater** pg. 27 and 32) Not only did he win Badwater, he also set a new course record.

A vegan since 1997, Jurek supports and observes a 100% vegan diet and asserts that this is critical for endurance events, overall recovery and good health.

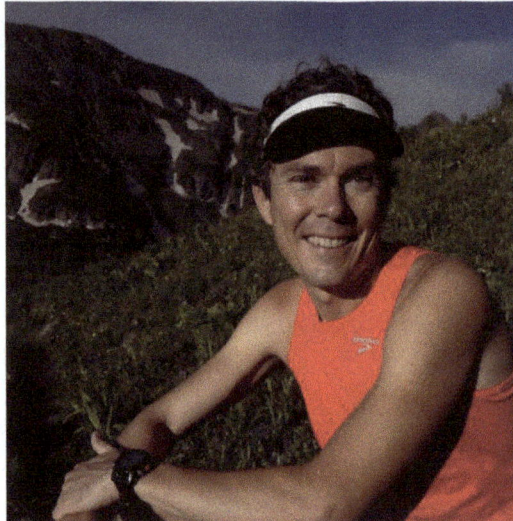

Ultramarathon runner Scott Jurek lives and breathes a vegan lifestyle

Career highlights include:

- Setting the speed record for the 2,200 Appalachian Trail (running and speed walking) in 2015
- Winning at least 24 ultramarathons between 77km and 246km.
- Winning the Western States 100-mile endurance run seven *consecutive* times (1999-2005).
- Winning Millwok 100k three times.
- Winning the Leona Divide 50-mile four times.
- Setting the American 24-hour record with a run of 165.7 miles.
- Becoming the first American to win the Spartathlon (246km), before winning it a second time.
- Setting ten ultramarathon course records.
- Awarded Ultrarunning Magazine's "Ultra Runner of the Year" three times.

As you can see, veganism can be very effective in terms of healthy living and dietary needs. Once scrutinized and deemed as "dangerous," it's proven its worth in recent years, allowing consumers to benefit from this healthy lifestyle.

Be sure to read Scott's Book: **Eat & Run** – *My Unlikely Journey to Ultramarathon Greatness* (www.scottjurek.com)

Vegetarian Lifestyle

By most definitions, a true **vegetarian** does not eat any meat, poultry or fish products and centers the entire diet on fruits, nuts and vegetables. There are also eight different variations of vegetarianism, but to avoid a complete rewrite of diets, I'll focus on the four main varieties.

- **Vegetarian:** consumes no flesh from any animal source
- **Lacto vegetarian:** does not consume eggs, but does consume dairy products
- **Lacto-ovo vegetarian:** consumes no meat, but will consume dairy products (milk, butter, cheese) and eggs
- **Ovo-vegetarian:** consumes eggs, but not meat or dairy products

The other four types of vegetarianism are *pescatarian, flexitarian/semi-vegetarian, raw vegan, macrobiotic*. (Veganism, which we previously covered, can also be considered a vegetarian diet.)

In most cases, vegetarians are usually not as extreme when it comes to cultural, religious, ecological or personal beliefs and therefore are not inclined to use such strict diets that a vegan might commit to. Many of us realize the health benefits of the vegetarian diet, including easier weight loss and maintenance, lower levels of LDL (bad) cholesterol and lower risk of disease linked to eating meat, such as obesity, colon cancer, diabetes and cardiovascular diseases.

Tip

Unless you're facing a critical medical issue, don't just dive into a vegan or vegetarian lifestyle. People who rush into these particular diets often face protein deficiencies from the upstart. Going from an omnivore-type diet directly into a veggie-based diet can leave you weak and hungry. Do your homework and follow common practices to avoid health and dietary problems. Try to make a slow but steady transition into your new plan, network with other vegans or vegetarians, and consult your physician or nutritionist if you have questions. Simply choosing a plant-based diet does not make you healthier!

The four most common mistakes for those who are just beginning a vegan or vegetarian lifestyle:
- Meal Planning - plan your meals well in advance. This is a big change from a mixed diet, so you will be lacking in several areas of nutrition.
- For the first few weeks, take in EXTRA amounts of protein – chickpeas, lentils, and soy products.
- Focus on veggies with a lot of iron. Red meat was one of your best sources of iron, so direct your attention to lentils, spinach, sesame seeds, garbanzo beans, olives, lima beans, navy beans, and kidney beans.
- Be aware of your B12 supplements. Remember, there are NO plant sources for Vitamin B12, so you will need to buy supplements or other foods fortified with B12. Pay more for the good quality supplements - you'll be glad you did.

As with veganism, the downside of this lifestyle is that you need to eat a broad variety of foods to make sure you meet your nutritional requirements. It takes a great deal of effort, research and knowledge to sustain a vegetarian lifestyle. These are a few of the reasons why some people oscillate between vegetarian and omnivore or paleo lifestyles.

Just like the vegan lifestyle, you can be a very healthy person, but you have to know where to obtain all of the nutrients and similar to the vegan lifestyle, B12 deficiencies are common. Make sure you supplement your diet as you plan it out.

Famous Vegetarians

As obesity is on the rise in the United States so is the battle to fight it. Vegetarianism has become a very popular lifestyle with as many as 7.3 million people following a strict fruit, nut and vegetable based diet. More importantly, statistics now show that a whopping 22.8 million people follow a "mostly" vegetarian lifestyle. Even though these numbers were compiled recently, many popular actors, politicians, athletes and scientists led this lifestyle before it became main-stream. Some of the high profile vegetarians, past and present, include scholars and inventors Thomas Edison, Albert Einstein, entertainers Ozzy Osborne and Alicia Silverstone, activist Rosa Parks, writer George Bernard Shaw, and athletes Mike Tyson, Robert Parish and many more.

Refer to the Nutrition Charts on pages 110 through 112 and use them to build your own menu, and don't forget your Vitamin B12 supplements!

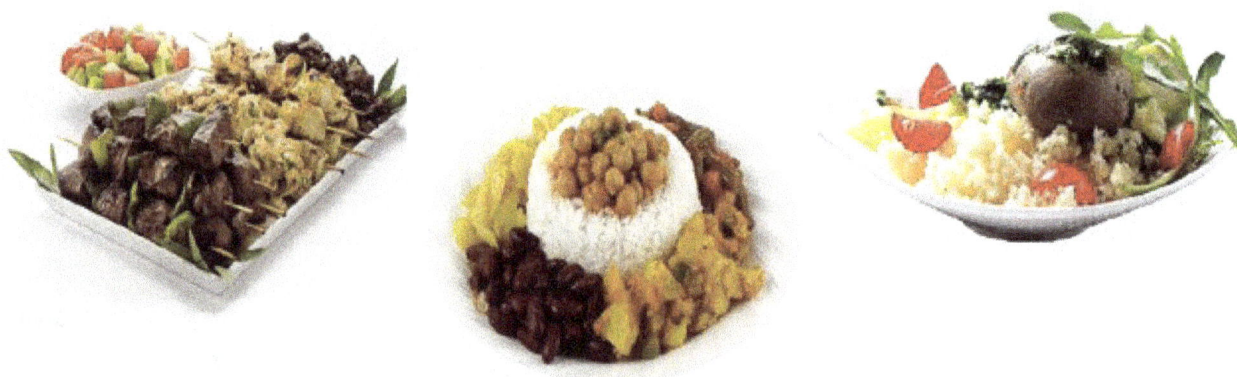

When it comes to vegetarian meals, the choices seem endless

> ### Motivation
>
> **"Some people are willing to pay the price and it's the same with staying healthy or eating healthy. There's some discipline involved. There are some sacrifices."** – *Mike Ditka*

Paleo Lifestyle

Throughout this book, I've tried to offer historical facts, philosophies and stories, and this section is no different. This particular lifestyle choice takes us w-a-a-a-a-y back to that of the caveman. Yes, into the Paleolithic age – a cultural period that lasted from 2.6 million years ago to just over 10,000 years ago. At the time, man used rocks for weaponry, tools, and more, hence the "stone age" moniker.

In the true sense of the word, the **Paleolithic diet,** also known as the **paleo** or **caveman** diet, is very similar to the omnivore diet, because the person still eats fruits, nuts, vegetables AND meat such as fish, poultry, pork and beef. The difference however, is that the Paleolithic diet does not include foods that have been processed.

The human species evolved from Homo habilis to Homo sapiens (modern man) during this period. At this time in history, humans grouped together in packs or bands and survived by gathering plants, hunting or fishing, or simply scavenging for their food. As a point of reference, the paleo diet is based on the food that early humans would have likely eaten, such as meat, nuts and berries, and excludes food they likely wouldn't have had access to, like processed dairy and grain-based products.

Exactly what is processed food? It's normally described as commercially prepared food that is made more portable, has a longer shelf life, is easier to prepare, and is, in many cases, ready to eat. These are also known as **convenience food**, or **tertiary processed food.** This can include foods like frozen foods, prepared cake mixes, dry goods, snacks, or any food that has its useable, consumable life extended by artificial means, such as the use of preservatives. Even modern day staples such as whole wheat bread and homogenized milk are considered to be in this category. And yes, your favorite restaurant – sorry, they're packed with processed foods.

Advocates of the paleo diet state that the metabolic rate of humans hasn't adapted fast enough to process many foods that are available in today's modern world. For this reason, they claim that humans aren't properly adapted to eating dairy products, grains and legumes, in addition to all of the other processed foods available in our society. They assert that the processed food we eat today has contributed heavily to modern day maladies such as obesity, diabetes, cancer and heart disease.

Furthermore, they declare that a Paleolithic lifestyle will allow devotees to enjoy a healthier, longer and more active life.

On the flip side, critics of this specific diet plan indicate a number of flaws in this philosophy, including the fact that early man did indeed eat grains and legumes. Forensic science results from burial excavation sites show digested foods, along with early man's DNA to prove that he ate from these food sources. Because the Paleolithic period lasted several million years, man clearly had plenty of time to adapt to many, many types of diets, and must have been extremely flexible, given the nomadic lifestyle and variations of available food sources. And of course, several studies suggest that Neanderthal and early modern man were almost or completely vegetarian. This theory implies that legumes and grains were most likely in their diet, although the processing method was most likely very different. And some say that they probably ate anything they could find, just to avoid starvation!

The paleo diet seems to be one of controversy, and proponents of the diet assure us that it's safe; there are plenty of fuels – carbs, proteins and fats, but the fuel sources are quite different than most other diets. In theory, I think it would work, but in reality, this diet is too restrictive for people like me because I like my milk, breads and beans - foods that seem very basic to me, but everyone has their own opinions, so I leave it up to you to decide. I just can't imagine life without chili with kidney, pinto or black beans, grated cheese, crackers and a big glass of milk! Surprisingly, almost every type of meat is permissible, including everyone's favorite – bacon. And the favorite protein source for vegans and vegetarians – beans – are not permitted! That includes *all* beans – black, Lima, kidney, red, navy, pinto. If it's a bean, it's not permitted under this diet plan.

Permitted	Not Permitted
Grass-fed, free-range, meats	Cereal Grains
Fish/seafood	Legumes including peanuts, all beans, peas
Fresh fruits	Milk, cheese
Eggs	Refined sugars, candy, junk food
Sweet potatoes, yams	White potatoes
Seeds	Processed Foods
Nuts	Refined vegetable oils
Healthy Oils – olive, flaxseed, avocado, coconut	Soft drinks, fruit juices with fructose
Butter	Beer and other alcohol products

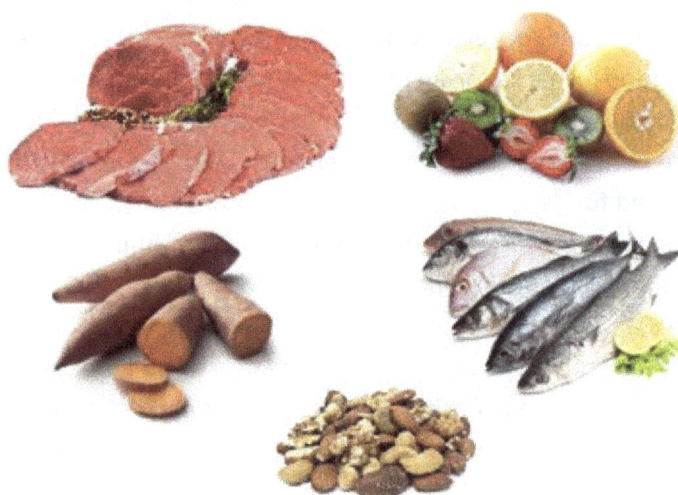

Many running experts, with scientific results supporting their cause, promote this particular diet for long distance runners. There are a number of books and websites that underwrite the Paleo plan, and if you're really interested, I suggest that you look to them for more information.

The Paleo lifestyle has gained popularity in recent years, especially in 2013, but its numbers are still relatively small compared to the other popular lifestyles. In 2015, there were only 1 to 1.5 million people in the United States on this diet plan. It includes singers Miley Cyrus and Tom Jones, actor Matthew McConaughey, actress Gwyneth Paltrow, and NBA star Grant Hill.

Motivation

"It's easy to impress me. I don't need a fancy party to be happy. Just good friends, good food, and good laughs. I'm happy, I'm satisfied, I'm content." – *Maria Sharapova*

Gluten-Free Lifestyle

As runners, we always seek out the top fuel sources for our running program – a solid base of proteins, fats and plenty of carbs from healthy foods such as barley, wheat, rye, farina, many different types of bread, cakes and pies, and many types of pasta. But what happens if we can't tolerate the protein known as **gluten**? *Gluten* is found in all of these and many people suffer from this intolerance, known as **celiac disease**.

Does this mean we can't participate in long distance running because our bodies are allergic or hypersensitive to these proteins? Well, there is good news ahead. Not only can we forgo these protein sources, we can actually excel without them.

In persons with celiac disease, gluten can cause inflammation in the small intestines. Avoidance of foods with gluten helps affected people control the symptoms and prevents complications from the disease. Many find the gluten-free diet frustrating at first, but with patience, research and creativity, you'll find that many substitutes are available for the foods you enjoy. Not all people on a gluten free diet do it for medical reasons, and many folks claim that this particular diet helps in overall weight loss and makes them just "feel better."

Because of its rise in popularity, many food manufacturers and restaurants are now offering gluten-free products – anything from gluten-free spaghetti in your grocery store to gluten free breads, buns and pizzas in your fast foods establishments.

For some, switching to a gluten-free diet is difficult because they feel deprived with all of its restrictions. There are however, many alternatives and there are many books and online resources supporting this particular lifestyle.

On the next page, and as I did in the Paleo section, I'll list a few of the foods that are permitted and not permitted in the gluten-free lifestyle. Of course, this is only a small sample for reference only.

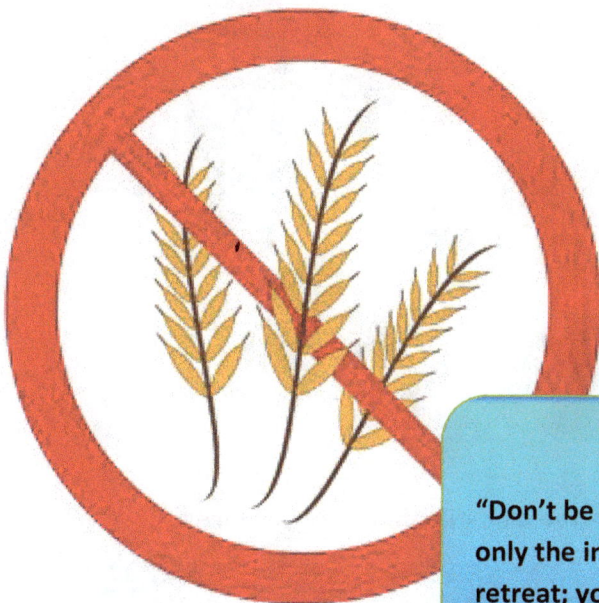

Motivation

"Don't be afraid if things seem difficult in the beginning. That's only the initial impression. The important thing is not to retreat; you have to master yourself." – *Olga Korbut*

Permitted	Not Permitted
Beans, seeds and nuts in their natural, unprocessed form	All food and drink containing barley, rye, wheat, durum flour, Farina, graham flour, kamut, spelt, semolina
Fresh eggs	Triticale – a cross between wheat and rye
Fresh fruits and vegetables	Beer unless labeled as gluten-free
Fresh meats, poultry and fish (not breaded or marinated)	Breads, cakes, pies, candies, cereals, cookies and crackers, croutons, French fries, matzo and pasta unless labeled as gluten-free
Grains and starches such as corn and cornmeal, flax, millet, quinoa, rice, soy, sorghum, tapioca	Processed lunch meats, salad dressings, sauces, snack foods, soups and soup bases, and vegetables in sauce unless labeled as gluten-free
Buckwheat, hominy, gluten-free flours (rice, soy, potato, bean), arrowroot, amaranth	Any processed food such as oats that could be contaminated by gluten during the growing and processing stages

While the benefits of this lifestyle are effective for persons with celiac disease, it should be noted that this diet may lack many key nutrients such as iron, calcium, fiber, thiamin, riboflavin, niacin and folate, and should be supplemented when required.

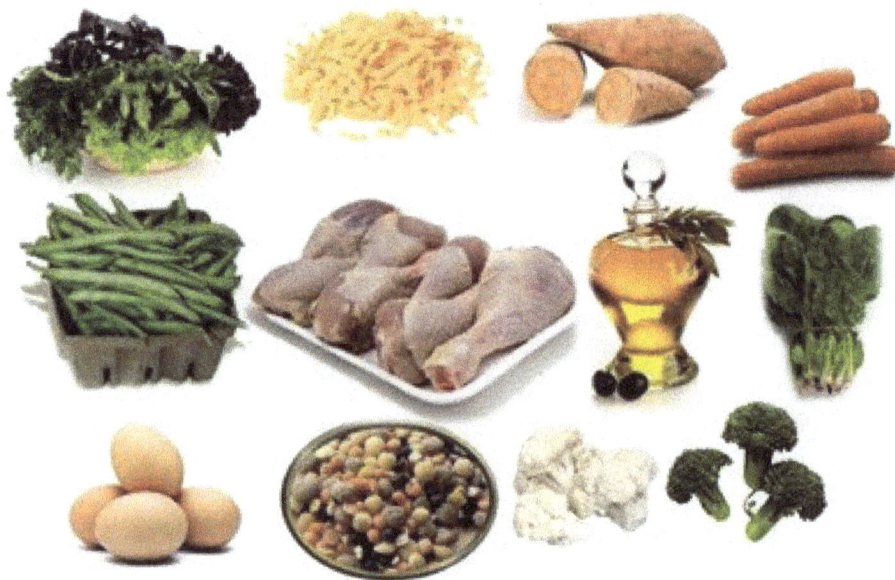

Despite some limitations, the gluten-free diet still offers many choices

Motivation

"Acknowledge all of your small victories. They will eventually add up to something great." – *Kara Goucher*

Omnivore Lifestyle

Up until now, we've talked about diets that only a small percentage of people take part in. By the numbers, about 6% of the people on the planet are vegetarians, with most of them living in India. In the United States, only 2% to 3% of Americans are vegetarians, with .05% of those being pure vegan. That leaves the remaining 97% to 98% of the people living the lifestyle of the **Omnivore.**

Biologically speaking, ALL humans are omnivores by the way our teeth and digestive systems are designed. Philosophically speaking, however, many humans choose to participate in other diet types.

The omnivore lifestyle is comprised of eating both animal and plant-based foods, in stark contrast from the plant-only based diet of the vegan or vegetarian.

As I mentioned earlier, I support the other four nutritional lifestyles (vegan, vegetarian, paleo and gluten-free), but it can be difficult to understand and implement those diets. Some also find that it's more difficult to plan meals, especially if the family is on mixed menus. While there is more and better information available today, some will still struggle to find out where to get the right amounts of nutrients. Finally, the other four lifestyles can be very restrictive and more expensive. Sadly, many will spend a small fortune on inexpensive supplements that are doing little or no good at all.

It's more difficult to balance your daily nutrition with the previous four diets. And that brings us to the omnivore lifestyle, where it's much easier to find your basic nutritional needs because you're getting vitamins, minerals and other nutrients from both animal and plant-based foods. The omnivore diet provides abundant and inexpensive food sources, and we don't have to rely on supplements as often.

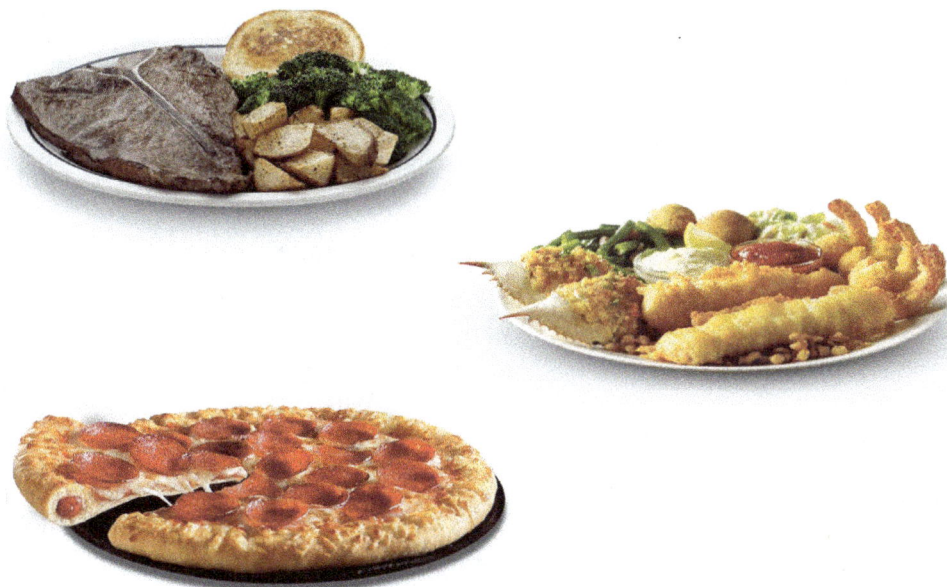

Motivation
"The pain of discipline is far less than the pain of regret." – *Sarah Bombell*

Earlier in this chapter, I pointed out the differences between nutritional lifestyles and diet plans. Now that we've discussed those differences, I'll briefly talk about the popular diet plans. In casual conversation, we usually refer to a *diet plan* as a structured menu with a selection of food to choose from, whereas *dieting* normally refers to a way of losing or maintaining a specific health threshold, usually measured in weight. For instance, we may have an *omnivore lifestyle* and be 20 pounds overweight. In this case a *diet plan* is used to lower the caloric intake in an effort to lose weight. More specifically, a *diet plan* is the *menu* that we use to maintain our particular lifestyle. In this example you'll be eating a lower calorie diet to cause an *offset* or *imbalance* in your caloric intake. As I mentioned earlier in this book, to lose weight, you must burn more calories than you consume – and not just a few hundred here and there. You must burn a whopping 3,500 calories – just to lose a single pound!

With that said, if you've decided on your *nutritional lifestyle*, you can now select a particular *diet plan* to achieve your goals. The diet plan choices are many, but here are the top five and their general highlights. We'll take a brief look at them and their associated strengths and weaknesses. The top five are the **Atkins Diet, Zone Diet, South Beach Diet, Raw Diet** and the **Mediterranean Diet**.

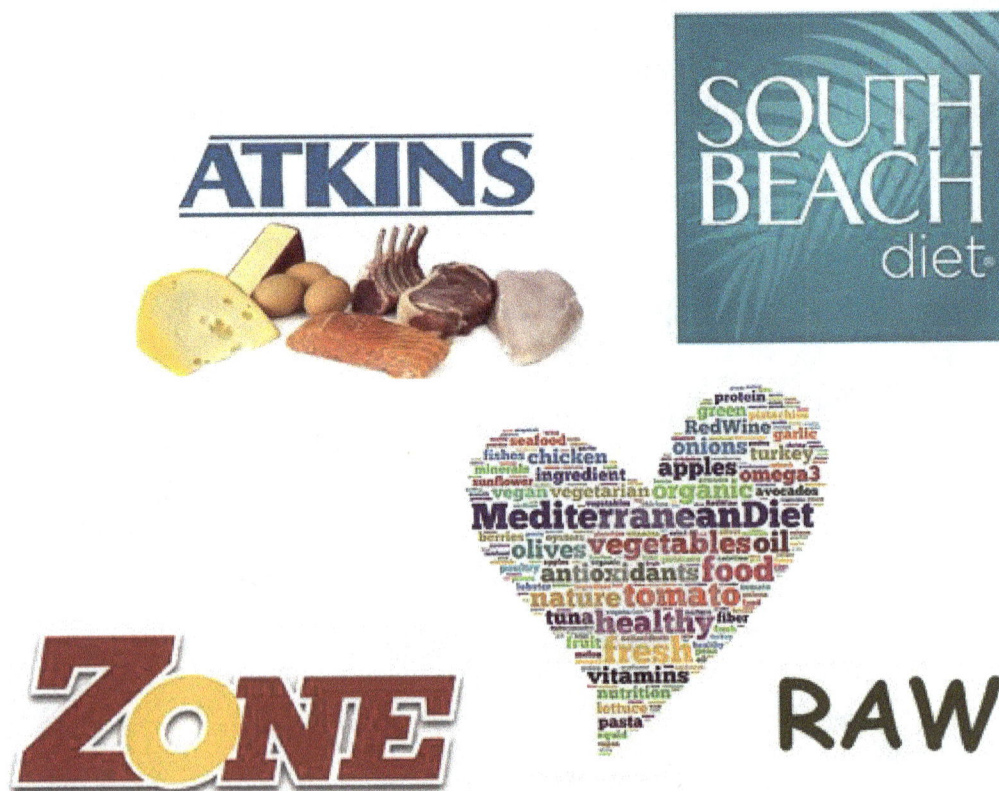

Tip

You can tell monounsaturated and polyunsaturated fats because they are liquid at room temperature. These types of fat seem to lower your chance of heart disease. But you still shouldn't eat more than the dietary guidelines suggest. *Trans* fats and saturated fats are usually solid at room temperature. *Trans* fat and saturated fat can put you at greater risk for heart disease and should be limited.

Popular Diet Plans

As we just learned, a diet plan is simply a menu in which you follow to attain a certain health standard. I'm going to briefly touch on the five most popular diet plans with a one-line description, the obvious pros and cons, and my non-scientific theory about each one. Generally speaking, a diet plan is normally used to lose or maintain a specific weight, but in some circumstances, can be used to *increase* weight, for people such as body builders or professional football players.

Diet Plan: Atkins Diet

Focus: A diet high in protein and fat and low in carbohydrates, prescribed for weight loss.

Pros: This diet can help you lose weight in a short time.

Cons: Lacks sufficient carbohydrate intake for activities such as distance running.

My Analysis: I fully support the Atkins diet for *short term* weight loss programs, and I feel that it is a good diet plan for those of us who were, or are overweight and wanting to get into a running program. Because its fundamental concept is to decrease the amount of carbs, I recommend it on a full-time basis only for non-runners or short distance running. As we saw in earlier chapters, middle and long distance runners rely heavily on diet plans that consist of a caloric intake of at least 55% carbohydrates, 30% fats, and 15% protein.

Diet Plan: Zone Diet

Focus: A diet that balances out the intake of carbs, fat and proteins into nearly equal amounts.

Pros: Targets the burn of fat, not water loss or muscle tissue.

Cons: This diet can be challenging for meal planning as you try to balance the 30% protein, 30% fat, and 40% carb ratio. Because it targets fat, weight loss can be a slow process. Smaller, more frequent meals and snacks are required for the efficiency of this diet.

My Analysis: There have been many surveys regarding the benefits for athletes on this diet. It seems to be a stable diet and can be used long term with few or no side effects for athletes. The actual planning of the meals seems to be the most difficult part – equalizing the fat/protein/carb percentages.

Diet Plan: South Beach Diet

Focus: It emphasizes eating high-fiber, lean protein, unsaturated fats, and low-glycemic carbohydrates, and categorizes carbohydrates and fats as "good" or "bad."

Pros: Rapid weight loss can be achieved in this three step diet program. (13 pounds in 2 weeks)

Cons: Lacks scientific evidence of a "healthy" diet in the first of the three phases, when glycemic blood levels are greatly affected, causing side effects including nausea and constipation, a dry mouth with "bad breath," dizziness, tiredness and insomnia.

My Analysis: While it seems like a good diet program in the second and third phases, I side with the opponents that cite the "brute force" approach in the first phase. I'd like to see more scientific reports and in-depth analysis. For now, I'd have to call this a "fad" diet until more accurate and verifiable information is available, especially in regards to running.

Diet Plan: Raw Diet

Focus: A raw foods diet is made up of fresh, whole, unrefined, living, plant-based foods: fruits, nuts, seeds, and leafy green vegetables, which are consumed in their natural state, without cooking or steaming.

Pros: Moderate to good weight loss because the foods allowed are naturally lower in calories, fat and sodium, and high in fiber. They are normally higher in vitamins, minerals and phytochemicals because cooking decreases the amount of vitamins B and C.

Cons: Can be difficult to consume acceptable amounts of protein, iron and calcium, as well as minerals such as B12. This diet can cause stomach distress for some people.

My Analysis: I am a proponent of this diet plan, as it works for both weight loss and nutritional intake; however, you must enhance this diet with good quality vitamin and mineral supplements, particularly B12.

Diet Name: Mediterranean Diet

Focus: Eating primarily plant-based foods, such as fruits and vegetables, legumes, nuts and whole grains, and replacing butter with healthy fats, such as olive oil. Replace salt by using herbs and spices to flavor your foods; limit red meat to no more than a few times per month.

Pros: A heart-healthy and flavorful diet plan, this diet plan is easy to follow for you and your entire family.

Cons: This diet does not list specific amounts of calories to consume, instead using terms such as 'low' to 'moderate' amounts. Because of this, weight gain can occur if it is not monitored.

My Analysis: I find this to be an excellent diet plan because of the variety of nutrients and flavors and the emphasis on healthy oils, nuts and veggies. All around, this looks like a great diet as long as you don't overdo it with your portions.

As I mentioned earlier, these are the basic overviews of the most popular diet plans. There's a wealth of information on these and more, available in your local book stores or online. Before you make any drastic changes in your diet plan, you should always consult your healthcare professional, clinical dietician or doctor. Do what works best for your health, your goals, your budget and lifestyle.

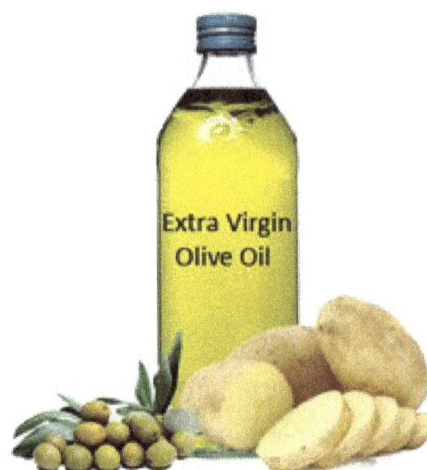

Fueling Up Before You Run

No matter what your nutritional lifestyle is, or what your diet plan is, you still need to approach your running with nutritional foods that will foster good health and results. As we just learned, a healthy diet is comprised of the proper amounts of carbohydrates, proteins and fats, whether you're a runner or not. As far as these three fuels go, carbs are definitely the athlete's main fuel source. Your body metabolizes them into glucose and stores them in your liver and muscles as glycogen. When you're active, your body changes your glycogen into energy – normally enough energy for about 90 minutes of high-intensity activities.

Carbohydrate Strategy – If you're going to exercise for more than 90 minutes at a time you should always:

- Load up on carbohydrates three to four days before your race or long run.
- Focus on a diet that is made up of 55% to 70% of carbohydrates.
- On race day, eat your meal three to four hours before your event to allow enough time for proper digestion and absorption into your system.
- Replenish your simple carbs, electrolytes and water BEFORE and DURING your race or high-intensity workout. This may include sports drinks, gels and other simple sugar carbs.
- Replenish your complex carbs AFTER your race or high-intensity workout, which may include whole-grain bagels or carrots.
- Don't eat sugary or starchy foods within 30 minutes of your race, as this can speed up dehydration.

Protein Strategy – Balance and common sense

- Don't overdo it with the proteins – while they are great maintenance nutrients for your muscles, they don't provide a lot of fuel for intense or lengthy workouts or races. Too much protein can put a strain on your kidneys.
- Ignore protein supplements, and go for the foods that have natural, high-quality proteins, such as lean meats, fish, poultry, nuts, beans, eggs and milk.
- Milk – both white and chocolate, contain whey protein and casein, and is one of the best foods for quick recovery after a strenuous activity. And of course, milk contains a significant amount of calcium to help maintain strong bones.

Fat Strategy – Go easy on fats!

- Be sure to follow the basic dietary guidelines to eat mostly unsaturated fat from foods such as olives, avocados, nuts, vegetable oils, and fatty fish like salmon and tuna.
- For long events such as marathons, your body may turn to fat for energy when carbohydrate sources run low. Keep glycogen stores at high levels prior to race day.
- Avoid fatty foods on race day since they process slowly and can upset your stomach.

> ### Motivation
>
> **"Early to bed and early to rise, makes a man healthy, wealthy and wise."** — *Benjamin Franklin*

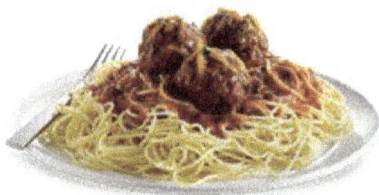

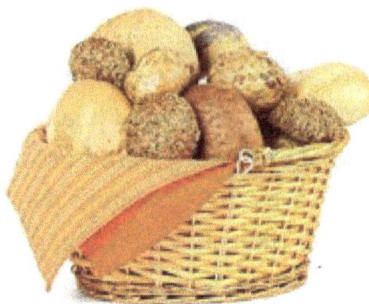

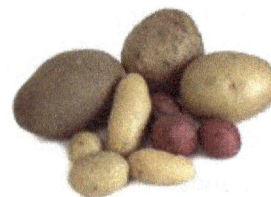

Challenge!

Proper nutrition

In the beginning of this chapter, we heard from Tom and Alice. Proper nutrition during Tom's training program reaped positive results on race day. Alice on the other hand, had a miserable experience. She learned a tough lesson, but she fixed it on her next marathon, finishing better than expected. Alice finished strong because she *took control* of her diet and training. And it didn't matter which diet or lifestyle she was utilizing – she would have been successful with any of them because she became a student of nutrition. She learned how to read food labels and found out where to acquire the right nutrients and supplements.

Instead of finding *excuses*, she found a *way*.

Your challenge: *Become a student of nutrition. Learn how to read labels and understand what it takes to fuel your body properly and **take control** of your nutritional needs. Doing so will also allow you to take control of your personal time and money, by avoiding convenience foods and other stressors in your life. Finally, plan your meals well ahead, so you can focus on other things.*

Motivation

"I've realized that I'm more important than food is. I love a big slice of pizza, but I love myself more. Being thin is about changing the way you think about yourself. It's about saying that you deserve to be healthy." *– Valerie Bertinelli*

Chapter 11 – Equipment and Safety

My Story

When I first began to run, I made just about every mistake a "rookie" can make, when it came to clothing and equipment. I didn't know about the "20-degree" rule, so I was prone to overdressing and subsequent "meltdowns." I didn't understand that each pair of shoes react and wear differently, so I fought through long stages of blister recovery. I was nearly run over early one morning because I didn't have adequate lighting and reflective gear.

Read this chapter carefully, and avoid making these common mistakes!

As I mentioned in earlier chapters, running is relatively simple and inexpensive. However, you'll soon find that as your running activities grow, so will the need for more and better equipment. Of course, this increases your spending, and if you're not careful, you'll soon be over budget – and that can take the fun out of running from the onset. The key is to purchase quality equipment wisely and plan your equipment needs and race entries well in advance. In this chapter, we'll look at the fundamental components to get you out the door. The obvious place to start is with the shoes.

Sole Source

I've read many books, blogs and testimonials telling stories about how the runner would modify their shoes to get them to fit right. Some would cut out the toe box, or remove new inserts to use their old inserts to get them to feel "right." Some would "break in" their shoes for 100 to 200 miles before using them for a race. I've seen others cutting grooves in the soles to make them more flexible. I understand re-lacing shoes in a different way or making little tweaks here and there, but I don't believe in drastic modifications to brand new shoes. I think there are enough shoes out there, that SOMETHING should fit you without reinventing the wheel, so to speak. I also believe that modern shoe technologies put real science into the fit, form and function of today's running shoes. Shoe companies spend millions of dollars to ensure proper fit and performance right out of the box. Break-in periods should be minimal with an average distance of 10 to 20 miles. If you're cutting up brand new shoes in today's marketplace, I urge you to keep looking for the correct shoes instead of butchering new ones. They're out there – you just need to find them. And if you do need to return your shoes, most companies will offer full refunds with no questions asked, even from online sources.

So how do you go about finding the right shoes? What brand should you buy? How much should you spend? There are many questions, and fortunately, there are answers.

If you're new to running or you've been away from the sport for a while, leave the sizing of your shoes to the professionals at the local shoe store. Most modern running stores will be able to video-record you on a treadmill and quickly analyze your stride and gait. They'll be able to see if you pronate normally, overpronate, or supinate. Additionally, they'll be able to see if you're a forefoot, midfoot or heel striker. But that's only the beginning. Once they help you with the basic analysis, you'll need to tell them what your goals are, what type of running you'll be doing, what distances you'll be covering. Alas, once that's done, they'll be able to accurately measure your feet for a correct fit of the shoes and make a recommendation from the information they've collected. Finally, you'll be able to select a color that you like.

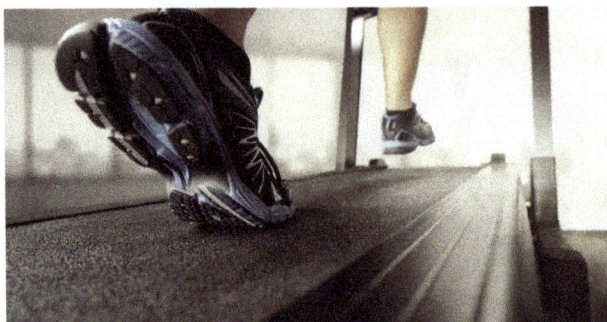

Let the experts at your local running store analyze your running gait

In summary, here are the important decisions to help you with your new shoe purchase:

Pronation determines shoe type – The running store expert should be able to quickly analyze your running style and determine if you pronate normally, overpronate or supinate. This analysis will determine the type of shoe you need. The shoe types are *Neutral, Stability* and *Motion Control*.

Arch Type	Foot Mechanics	Shoe Wear Pattern	Recommended Shoe Type
High Arch	Supination or Underpronation	The shoe has an extreme wear pattern on the outer edges.	Neutral
	Neutral Pronation	The shoe has an even wear pattern throughout the bottom.	Neutral
Medium Arch	Mild Overpronation	The shoe has a minor wear pattern on the inner edges.	Stability
Flat Arch	Severe Overpronation	The shoe has significant wear on the inside of the shoe, front to rear.	Motion Control

- **Running goals** – Tell your shoe expert what type of running you'll be doing. Are you going to be running a 5k or 10k, or will you be running half-marathons, marathons or ultramarathons? Giving this information to the running store shoe expert will allow him to match your new shoes to your running goals.

- **Training or Racing** – Are you looking for a high mileage trainer, or a light weight racing flat? Racing flats are extremely lightweight but are not usually comfortable for multiple long runs and they tend to wear out much faster than trainers. Most good trainers will last 400 to 750 miles if they fit you correctly. Heavier runners should expect shorter life cycles for their shoes.

- **Location –** Will you be running on the streets or heading for the trails? Modern technologies have changed the way shoes are made and each type of shoe has a different purpose. Buy the type of shoes you need and don't try to run on streets with trail shoes and vice versa. If you run on streets and trails, buy both street and trail shoes.

- **Overall health** – Always let the store employee know if you are aware of any kind of health problems that you might have. Known problems with your feet, knees, hips or back should always be relayed to your running expert. Running shoes will not fix biological deficiencies or gait problems – you still need to strengthen and correct your running form to become an efficient runner.

- **Minimalist shoes** – Shoes with a heel drop of 0mm to 4mm are designed for advanced runners who are ready for shoes with a lower heel. Barefoot and "minimalist" runners will often use these for racing or transitioning to barefoot running. Do not try these shoes until you are ready and already have strong feet. Running with this type of shoe when you're not prepared, can cause undue pain, or damage to your plantar fascia, and other tendons of the feet and ankles.

- **First impressions DO matter** – Trust your first instinct – if the shoes are not comfortable in the shoe store, they're not going to get any better when you run. Find a shoe that leaves a good impression as soon as it's laced up. Be sure to try BOTH shoes on in your sporting goods store to check for comfort and fit.

- **Buy wisely** – I can't tell you how many times I bought a pair of shoes at the local running store, found out that I really liked the shoes, and then went online to purchase more of the same shoes for a deeply discounted price.

- **Stock up**! – If you find a make and model that works really well for you, and if your budget allows, stock up, since shoe manufacturers update their models very quickly.

Motivation

"The most important investment you can make is in yourself." – *Warren Buffett*

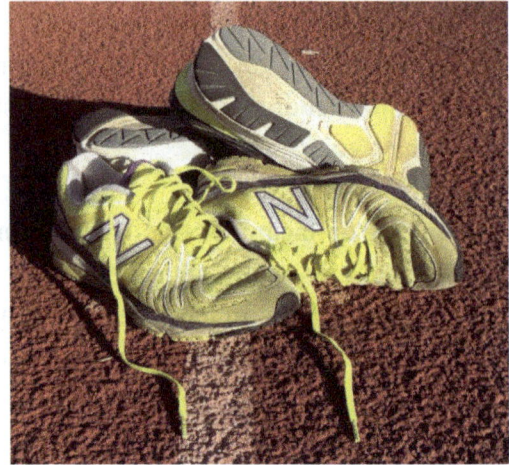

- **Think green** – Finally, once you're done with your old shoes, find a running store that deals with shoe recycling. The old shoe composite materials are ground up at a recycling facility and remanufactured into rubberized material for running tracks and playgrounds. It's a great concept and you can do your share by donating your old shoes! Over the years, Nike has led this initiative and others are catching on quickly.

- **Replacing your shoes** – Your favorite running shoes will eventually wear out and you'll need to replace them with a new pair. Hopefully, you purchased several pairs of the shoes that you like the most. There are a couple different ways to know when your shoes are worn out and are due for replacement. The obvious indicators are normally visible on the bottom of your shoes. Your foot type may play into your shoe wear and clearly show the worn out portions of the shoe. It's not always easy to tell when your shoes wear out because they may have a very subtle and even wear pattern. They may *look* just fine, but if your feet are starting to hurt, it may be another indicator that the shoes are breaking down internally. Over the years, I've had many shoes that appear to last and show little wear on the sole, but when I switch to a new pair, there's a noticeable difference in the comfort of the shoe.

- **Shoe inventory** – Keep track of the distance you're getting from your running shoes. I normally number my shoes, particularly if I purchase several pairs of the same model. Then, I keep track of the distance I get out of the first pair of shoes, and note when visible wear or pain starts to occur. This can help me predict the mileage I can expect out of the next pair and give me an idea of when it's time to order new ones again. This might sound like a lot of work, but if you keep a good running log, it can make a difference of how and when you order your next pair of shoes – and how much you pay. This can also keep you pain-free from worn out shoes.

- **Cost** – On average, good quality shoes should run between $90.00 and $150.00 per pair. As noted above, if you shop around and find a shoe you like, you may be able to find your shoes online at deeply discounted prices, sometimes as much as 60% off. If this is the way you like to shop, it can save you a lot of money. Act quickly, though, because popular sizes sell out fast.

Motivation

"Running has always been a relief and a sanctuary—something that makes me feel good, both physically and mentally. For me it's not so much about the health benefits. Those are great, but I believe that the best thing about running is the joy it brings to life." – *Kara Goucher*

Sock it to me!

An automotive painter once told me that the shiny paint job on the car is only as good as the body work underneath it. We can analogize this expression when it comes to running shoes and socks. Your magnificent new shoes on the outer layer will not provide you with foot comfort unless you have a comfortable layer underneath them.

Good medicine – You would think that socks would be the simplest, most basic item for running. Frankly, it's just the opposite. In this modern era of science and technology, socks have become part of the multi-billion dollar running industry, and with good reason. Socks can easily make a difference in the comfort and health of your running experience. Socks are rarely noticed when the fit is right and they're providing clean, dry conditions for your feet. If they don't fit or react properly, they can complicate what should be a very simple run and invoke misery during your training or race. Just like shoes, socks should be an investment in your *health*, not just another layer of clothing.

Good quality socks are imperative for running, especially if you're going to be out there for extended lengths of time, or running in less-than-ideal conditions. Let's take an in-depth look at sock technologies and options to keep your feet clean, dry and blister-free.

Leave the cotton at home – Cotton socks are soft, warm and comfortable for everyday living and may work just fine for short races, but if you're going to run races longer than 5 kilometers, you need to invest in socks other than 100% cotton materials. Cotton cannot wick away sweat and moisture like synthetic materials do and cotton actually absorbs and retains moisture against your skin. This moisture can cause friction inside of your shoes and encourage the creation of painful and performance limiting blisters.

Say yes to cotton blends, polyester, nylon and Merino wool – Unlike 100% cotton, cotton blends are acceptable because they will allow wicking of moisture away from your skin, much like nylon and polyester materials will do. There are a number of synthetic materials that are excellent for their wicking qualities. Gortex, ClimaCool and CoolMax are all popular synthetic blended materials used for outdoor activities ranging from hunting to cycling to running and all are extremely good at wicking moisture away from your skin. Unlike traditional wool, Merino wool does not make you itch and it easily wicks away moisture and features antimicrobial properties to keep bacteria at bay and prevent odors.

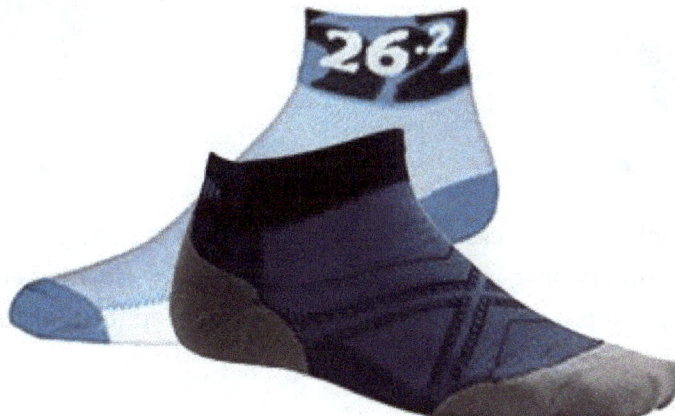

Invest in good moisture wicking socks such as these CoolMax and Merino wool socks

Thick or thin – When it comes to running socks, you have a plethora of styles, colors, sizes and a myriad of thicknesses and varying degrees of cushioning. All of these attributes are of personal choice and only *you* can say if your feet are comfortable or not. Most research indicates that a thin sock provides better wicking qualities; thus they offer better protection from blistering. Thick socks are usually better for trail running where a good degree of cushioning is needed. Thick socks are ideal for people who are prone to foot issues such as bunions and rapid foot fatigue. Additionally, manufacturers of cushioned socks can target specific areas of the foot, adding thicker insulation for problem areas such as the ball of the foot or the back of the heel where blisters can prevail.

Crew cut, low cut, ankle cut – Personal preference will dictate the cut of socks that you select, and they may vary by the type of running you're doing on that day. You might want a very low ankle cut for your road marathon, and a high cut on the trails when you need extra protection from the elements.

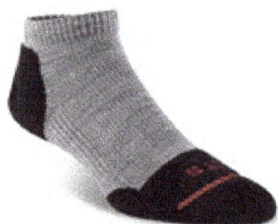
Crew cut

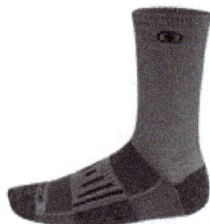
Low cut

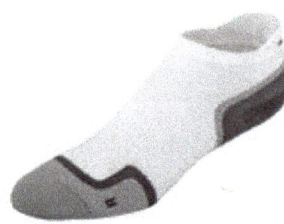
Ankle cut

Specialty socks – There are a number of special purpose socks sold to enhance the health of your feet.

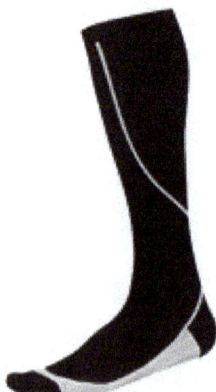
Compression socks

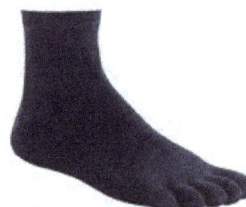
Toe socks

In the medical world, compression socks are designed to keep blood from pooling in your legs but the results are unproven in the running world. Some runners swear by them, stating that their legs feel fresher during and after a run. However, some say they can be uncomfortable on hot days.

Toe socks are designed to keep your toes from blistering by isolating each toe away from the next, to keep the moisture and friction away.

"Smart Socks" – It was bound to happen – In this world of technological advances, there are even "smart socks" that can track your stride, pace, distance, and calories. This modern technology can determine how and where your feet land, and measure the distance of your stride. This can offer a form of analysis that can help to prevent injuries. These types of devices typically use blue-tooth connectivity to your smart phone.

Colors galore! – Running socks can be found in just about any color imaginable and some companies will even print custom logos and designs for those who are willing to pay a little extra.

Test drive your socks, too! – As you do with the rest of your running wardrobe, test fit your socks. A well cushioned sock may feel just right on your hardwood floors, but may be very uncomfortable inside your shoe. An overly snug fit from a cushioned sock may end up causing blisters rather than deterring them. Likewise, overly thin socks that leave extra room in your shoe are dangerous as they may allow blisters to form because of the extra slack in your shoe.

As with shoes, your socks should give you a good first impression. If they feel hot and restrictive when you first try them on, or if they feel to thin or loose, use your intuition and keep shopping until you find the right ones.

No socks – Of course, there will be a number of runners out there who prefer no sock at all. Some people can tolerate the absence of socks and it's neither right nor wrong – do what works best for you.

> **Motivation**
>
> **"You have brains in your head;**
> **You have feet in your shoes.**
> **You can steer yourself any direction you choose!"** – *Dr. Seuss*

Under Where?

Basics – Perhaps the most overlooked items that a runner might need are the undergarments. The same rules that apply to socks should apply to running underwear. Avoid 100% cotton and buy good quality wicking materials that move the moisture away from your skin. The longer your run is, the more you'll appreciate clothing that keeps you dry.

For men, underwear should be made of a cotton and synthetic blend of materials. They should keep parts of the male anatomy in their proper places without too much restriction to make them uncomfortable. Seams and stiches should be minimal or well placed and should not rub in those sensitive areas. Some men still prefer an athletic supporter (jock) but the straps may be irritating on long runs, particularly in hot or humid weather.

For women, a good wicking material is imperative, not only for comfort, but for the health of the woman athlete. Thongs should also be avoided as they can become bunchy and cause all kinds of issues during long runs. Again, smooth seams are important.

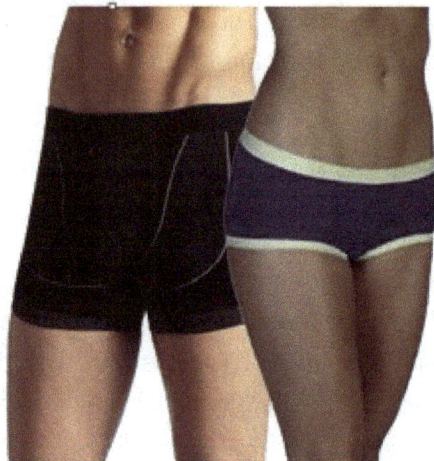

Other hints for comfort – Both genders should get used to applying moisturizing creams or other healing creams to avoid chafing in sensitive areas. This may sound silly, but always launder your new undergarments before using them, as they may still contain manufacturing chemicals that can irritate the skin, particularly when you sweat.

Specialty wear – Beyond the basics, there are other pieces of clothing that can keep you supported, dry and comfortable. Compression shorts are normally worn by sprinters or short distance runners and can be worn underneath regular running shorts, or can be used as the outer layer. There are several theories that suggest compression shorts may improve performance, but there is no definitive proof of that.

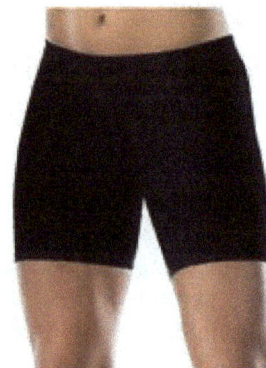

Athleisure wear – As with other layers of clothing, women's running bras should be constructed of a good quality wicking material, and offer good support. Proper fit is essential to the comfort of the runner, and there should be very little movement of the breasts when exercising. Again, seams should be minimal to avoid irritations of the skin. Some sports bras even have sewn-in pockets for small items such as MP3 players or keys. Be sure to shop around for the best value.

In recent years, there has been a movement in women's fashion known as "athleisure wear," which basically refers to women wearing athletic wear (like sports bras and yoga pants) for non-athletic activities such as running errands. Because of this rise in demand for athletic apparel, many non-specialty stores are now carrying sports bras, running shorts, yoga pants, etc. A good sports bra used to cost $25-$40, but now you can get them for under $10!

Motivation

"In the end, it's extra effort that separates a winner from second place. It takes desire, determination, discipline, and self-sacrifice. Put all these together, and even if you don't win, how can you lose?" – *Jesse Owens*

Running Apparel

If you're starting to sense a general theme with clothing, you should be noticing that it focuses on lightweight, synthetic wicking materials with an emphasis on minimal seams. Running shorts, tights, tanks and tees – should also fit this criteria to keep you warm, dry and happy.

The Bottom End – Wild prints, loud colors, skorts for women, split leg, compression, short, medium, long, fitted, 2-in1, full length stretch tights, warmups. You name it, the styles and varities seem endless into today's marketplace. While there are some very catchy designs out there, your primary focus should still be comfort. Each style may be dictated by the type of running you're doing on that particular day. For example, if you're running a marathon in warm weather, you might consider split leg shorts that provide minimal coverage so you don't overheat. If you're out on a winter run, you would most likely be comfortable in a pair of long, stretchy running tights.

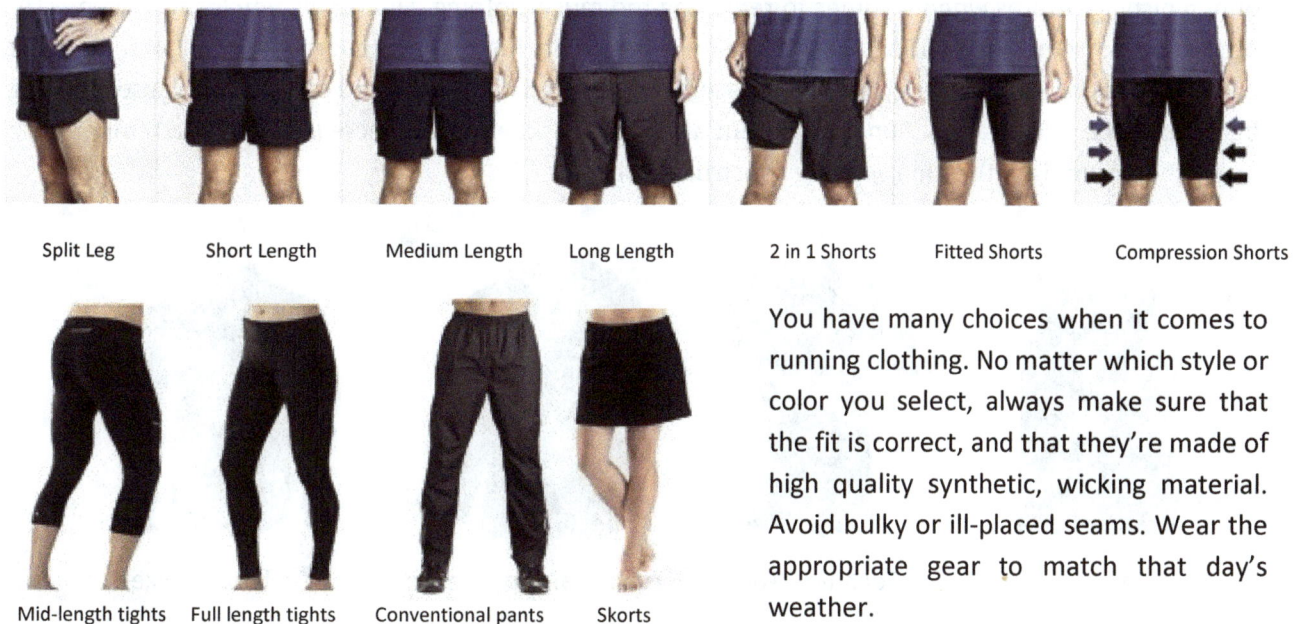

Split Leg   Short Length   Medium Length   Long Length   2 in 1 Shorts   Fitted Shorts   Compression Shorts

Mid-length tights   Full length tights   Conventional pants   Skorts

You have many choices when it comes to running clothing. No matter which style or color you select, always make sure that the fit is correct, and that they're made of high quality synthetic, wicking material. Avoid bulky or ill-placed seams. Wear the appropriate gear to match that day's weather.

Tip

The 20-degree rule - If you don't take any other tips from this book, at least take this one. I can't tell you how many times I've seen people who are midway through their race and they're stifled by the amount of clothing that they're wearing. Inexperienced runners tend to over-dress. They have good intentions to "be prepared for anything," but when they're out there and very active, their body temperatures rise and they simply overheat, they slow down, have a poor performance and a bad overall experience. The easiest fix for overdressing is to not do it! Instead, use the *20-degree rule*, and you'll be fine almost every time. So, here it is: If the start temperature is 40 degrees, add 20 so you'll be dressing for 60 degrees. If it's 70 degrees, dress for 90. If it's 30 degrees, dress for 50. I've done this for years, and it's never failed me yet! This applies to the bottom and top half of your body.

The Top Side

When it comes to clothing for the top half of your body, most of the same rules apply. Once again, 100% cotton can be your enemy when it comes to running. First of all, it tends to collect moisture rather than wicking it away from your body. This, of course, can you leave you very hot, wet and uncomfortable. The bigger threat, however, is the lack of ultra-violet (UV) protection that cotton material gives you. Because cotton is a natural material, it lacks the filtering components that most synthetic materials offer. The lighter the color, the less filtering ability it has. Morever, when it gets wet from rain or sweat, it loses even more of its UV protection ability. If you insist on wearing cotton, make sure you still apply your normal sunscreen under your clothes. And, of course, long sleeves are better than short sleeves when it comes to protection from the dangerous rays of our sun.

As mentioned in my "Tip" on the previous page, use the 20 degree rule to avoid overheating. Guys, I know the temptation is there to go shirtless in very hot weather, but try to avoid it. There is a point of diminishing returns when it comes to removing too much clothing. First of all, you lose all of your UV protection by removing your shirt completely. In extremely hot, sunny conditions, you'll actually start baking your skin. The salt from your sweat becomes encrusted in the skin, and can actually cause bleeding because of the skin irriation. Running without a shirt in hot weather can increase your core temperature faster than running with a thin, wicking constructed shirt.

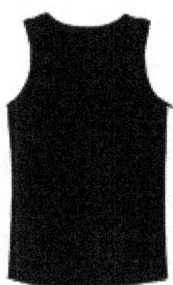

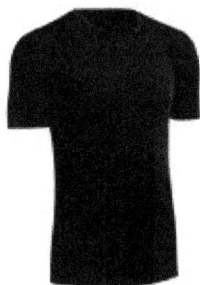

| Singlet | Technical Tee | Technical Long Sleeve | Technical Jacket |

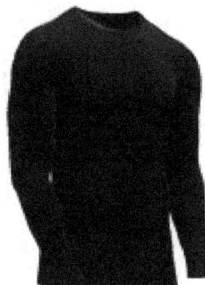

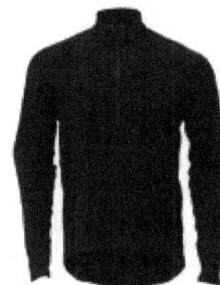

What to wear, when to wear it

For the top half of your body, the 20 degree rule is particularly important. You have choices from short tops, singlets, sleeveless, short sleeve and long sleeve shirts, and each has its proper place with respect to weather conditions. Below, I've added my recommendation for basic weather conditions, with considerations of the 20 degree rule.

Negative 10 to 10 degrees – Wear three to four layers, which should include an effective wicking layer, a thermal layer such as a lightweight sweatshirt, a very warm layer (coat or insulated running jacket) and a protection layer. This protection layer may be made of water- or wind-proof materials, depending on the conditions. Head, facial protection and quality gloves are a must. A wicking layer is *always* essential, no matter what the temperature is, especially in cold weather. If you don't wick the moisture away in these cold temperatures, you could end up with a miserable experience, a nasty cold or maybe even hypothermia. Stay dry in very cold conditions!

10 to 20 degrees – Wear two to three layers which include a wicking shirt, an insulated running jacket and protection layer for water and wind. Lighter weight gloves are possible, and you might be able to shed the facial protection, but keep the hat and make sure it covers your ears!

20 to 30 degrees – As the temperatures rise, overdressing becomes easier and easier, and this temperature range is one of the most difficult to manage. Remember, with the 20 degree rule, this range is like running in 40 to 50 degree temperatures. In this range, wear your wicking layer, a thermal layer and bring along that running jacket. You may be able to drop it off later or tie it around your waist once you get going. You may feel a little chilled at the beginning, but you'll warm up quickly. Bring a hat, good gloves and a protection layer.

30 to 40 degrees – The perceived temperature of this range will be 50 to 60 degrees. At this point, dress for comfort, starting with a good wicking layer. Multiple lightweight layers are optimal for these conditions. Long sleeves can be rolled up if you get too warm, or you might use your arm warmers. Tie a light jacket around your waist in case you do get chilled. Lightweight gloves are still recommended.

40 to 50 degrees – You can be quite comfortable running in shorts and long-sleeved, lightweight technical shirts. Again, sleeves can be rolled up or traded for short sleeves. Lightweight gloves and arm warmers are optional.

50 to 60 degrees – Multiple layers are no longer required, and you can probably get away with a short sleeve shirt, but you should still be prepared to tie a lightweight longsleeve tech shirt around your waist – just in case.

60 to 70 degrees – Think comfort. Add the 20 degrees to calculate the perceived temperature. You shouldn't need additional layers at this temperature range. Just go out and have fun!

70 degrees and higher – Again, you can wear with confidence anything that you're comfortable in, but don't forget the 20 degree rule! If you're running in this temperature range, you'll most likely need a hat with a bill for additional shade.

In any condition – As long as the sun is shining, you need to wear a quality sunscreen to avoid skin problems down the road. Always match your socks with the current weather conditions! Warm socks are imperitave in cold running conditions. Be sure to bring layers that will protect you.

Tip

Stowaway vs. Throwaway –To keep the chills away on race day, you have several options: 1) At the start line, remove your extra clothing to send to the finish area in a clothing bag if the race offers this service. 2) Wear extra, OLD clothing for the first few miles and shed it to the side of the road as needed. Don't expect to get these clothes back as most race directors give them to charities. 3) Bring a large trash bag and cut holes for your arms and head. Use it to repel wind and moisture. It's amazing how warm you'll stay until the start of the race! Be sure to discard properly.

Inclement Weather Gear

There are a few times when you'll need additional protection from the elements. If you're running in wet or windy conditions, you'll need an outer layer that keeps you warm and dry. If you're up for a run in the desert, you'll need extra protection from the sun and arid conditions. Let's look briefly at some of the options for each.

Cold Weather Options

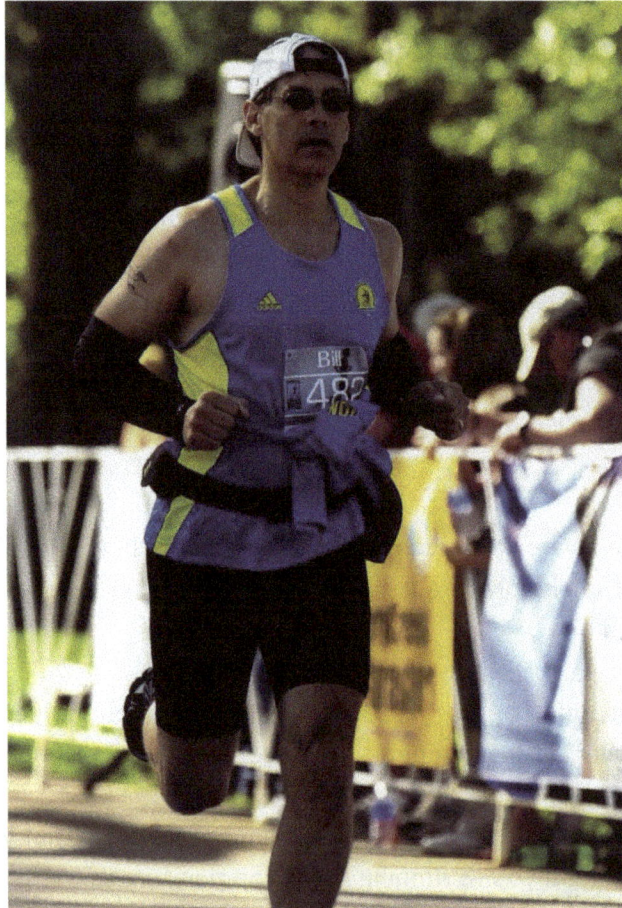

Arm warmers are great for those cool spring or fall marathons!

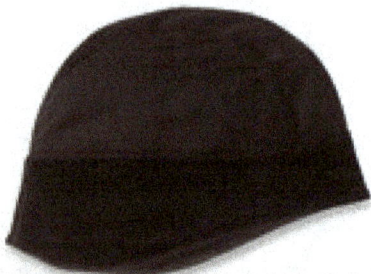

Check out this Merino wool hat!

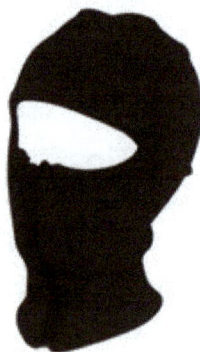

Full facial protection

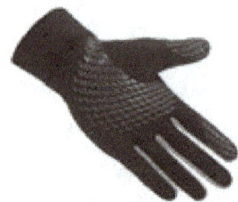

Invest in quality gloves

Hot Weather Options

There are a number of companies that sell "desert" wear for runners. If you plan on a desert run, be sure to buy the right gear. LONG sleeve technical shirts are a must to keep your skin from baking under the hot desert sun. Don't be tempted to remove your shirt in dangerous hot weather conditions. Protection for your head and neck should come from a quality hat with a built-in neck drape.

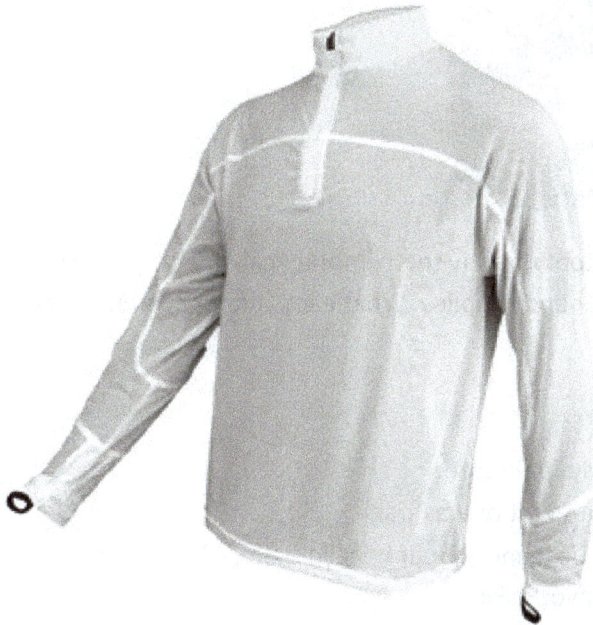

Desert running top   **Hat with neck drape**

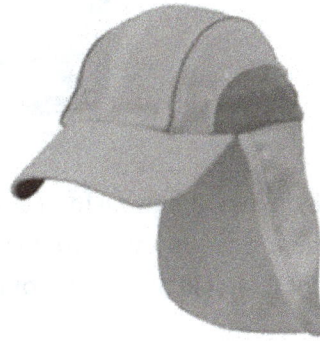

Additional Equipment

Now that we've covered the essentials for clothing, let's take a look at optional, but no less important items that you should have in your running "toolbox." We'll start with the basics and work our way up to the cool technical gadgets! Over the years, I've accumulated quite a list of "must haves" and optional equipment and supplies, and while I don't always need them, it's been nice to know that I'm stocked up when I really do need them. Be prepared!

We'll break it down into groups:

- **The toolbox**
- **First aid**
- **Safety**
- **Hydration and nutrition**
- **Technical gear**
- **Recovery gear**

> **Motivation**
>
> **"A winning effort begins with preparation."** — *Joe Gibbs*

The Toolbox

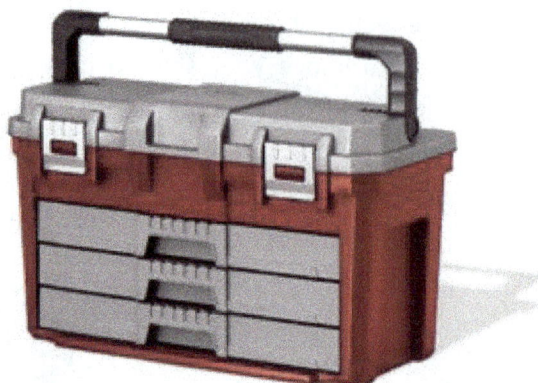

For beginners, the thought of a runner's kit or toolbox may seem impractical, but it actually makes pretty good sense once you start your collection of gear and supplies. What each runner puts in their own kit will vary, but it should have some of these basics:

First Aid Supplies

- Band-aids – for minor lacerations, blisters, and nipple care
- Bandana – get a large one that can double as a splint or washrag
- Lubes and balms – items such as Bodyglide, Vaseline, Aquaphor, lip balm, Blistex, sunscreen – basically anything that you can take to protect your skin
- Antibiotic wipes, antiseptic wipes, hydrocortisone cream, Preparation H
- Travel size shampoo and bar soap
- Cold compress
- Sterile guaze pads (4 x 4)
- Adhesive cloth tape 10 yards x 1 inch
- Anti-diarrheal medicine
- Tylenol, Ibuprofen, Aspirin, Benedryl
- Scissors, tweezers, oral digital thermometer (not glass)
- Snake bite kit
- Iodine tablets for water purification
- Mosquito repellent
- Foil "Space blanket"
- Basic first aid guide, CPR guide
- Safety pins
- Toothpicks, toothbrush
- Cotton swabs
- Toenail clippers
- Rubbing alcohol, hydrogen peroxide or iodine

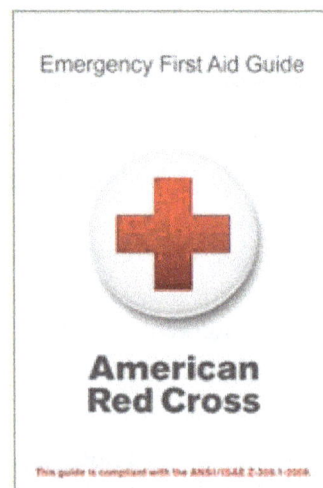

Emergency First Aid Guide

American Red Cross

This guide is compliant with the ANSI/ISA2 Z-308.1-2009.

While it sounds like a lot of "stuff," most of it is small and it should be very easy to stow in your toolbox. Some of it might be specific to trail running, but as they say, it's better to have it and not need it, than to need it and not have it! See, the top deck or drawer of your toolbox is already full, and we've only just begun!

Safety Equipment

- LED headlamp or flashlight (or both)
- Reflective wrist and ankle bands
- Reflective safety vest
- Insurance cards, emergency contact information

- Mace or pepper spray
- Spare car key
- Safety whistle
- Road ID (see below)

Market Leaders

While I try not to spotlight any particular brands in this book, there is one company that deals with awesome and innovative safety products for runners. **Road ID** is one of the vendors that just can't be ignored. Their flagship product is, of course, their ID bands. The Road ID band or tag is designed to let first responders know who you are, if you have any health issues, emergency contact information and even leaves a place for special instructions such as "Never give up." Other examples might be "Diabetic" or you can list any medical allergies that you might have. You can even get a matching ID band for your canine companion. Several different styles are available, including wrist and ankle bands, or military "dog tag" styles. Alternatively, you can buy shoe IDs. They also have a line of reflective gear and LED lighting for running in the dark.

Visibility Products

All runners should have some type of LED light and additional reflective gear for those early morning or evening runs. Increase your visibility by having multiple points of light, such as reflective wrist and ankle bands or clothing, a quality headlamp and/or a flashight.

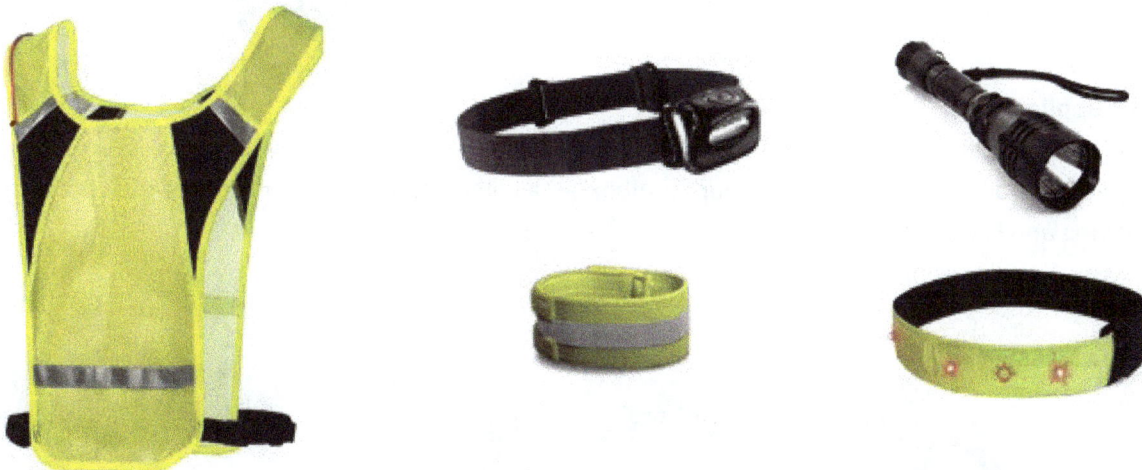

Full reflective safety vest, LED headlamp and flashlight, reflective wrist band and LED arm band

---

Motivation

"The door to safety swings on the hinges of common sense." — *Author Unknown*

Miscellaneous Toolbox Items

Sunglasses with UV protection are a must for runners. Also, if you wear glasses, make sure you have a good lens cleaner with a soft rag designed to wipe plastic lenses. An eyeglass repair kit will fit neatly into your tool box. If you wear contact lenses, make sure you have contact cleaner solution and a lens case.

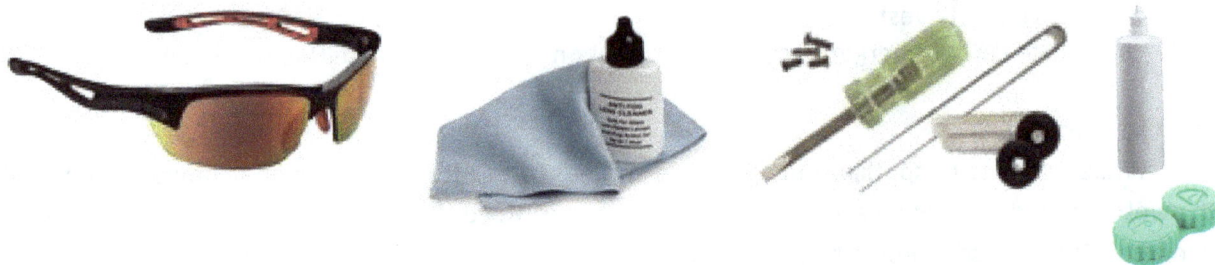

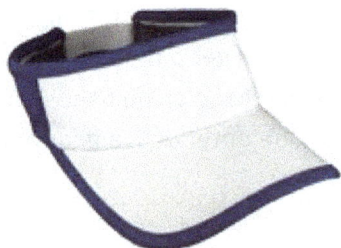

Keep a lightweight visor or hat in your tool box at all times. Also, place a couple of trash bags in your toolbox – one for trash, and one that you can convert into a windbreaker at the start line.

You never know when you might need to make an emergency repair while on the road. Pack a travel size sewing kit in your tool box.

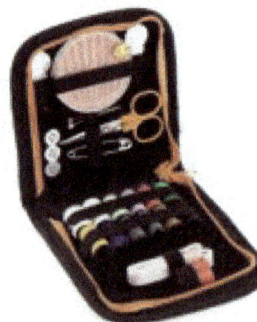

Hydration Supplies

We've talked about the importance of hydration and nutrition in the previous sections of the book. Let's add a hydration ensemble for your "toolbox" – a collection of necessary tools and supplies to get you moving and keep you moving.

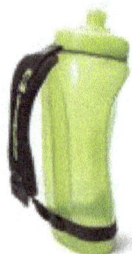

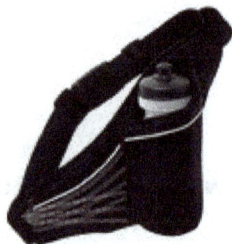

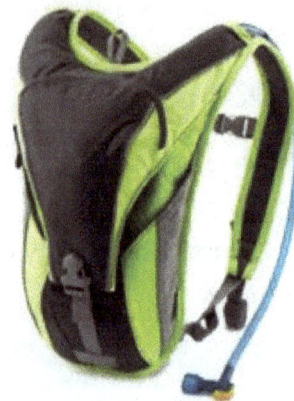

| **Hand-Held** | **Waist Band Bottle** | **Fuel Belt** | **Over-the-Shoulder Hydration Pack** |

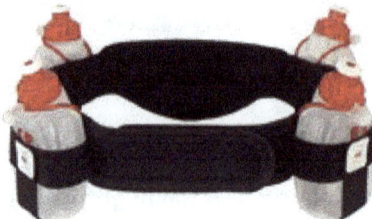

Nutritional Items for Your Toolbox

- Electrolyte tablets, salt tablets
- Gels, Gummy Bears or other simple sugars
- Pre-race hydration and post-race recovery drinks, bars and gels. Look for brands such as Hammer, CLIF, PowerBar, Cytomax, Vega, and GU.

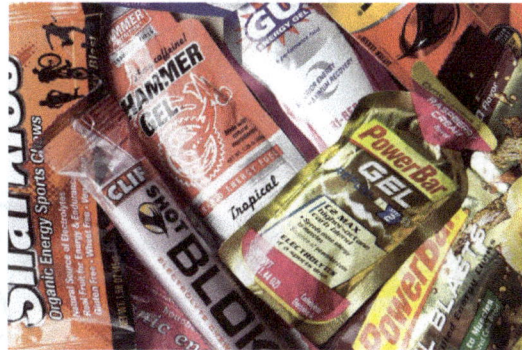

Technology gear, apps, websites and more

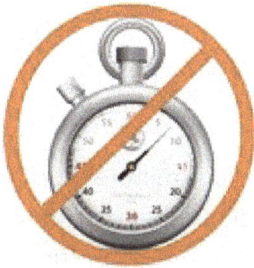

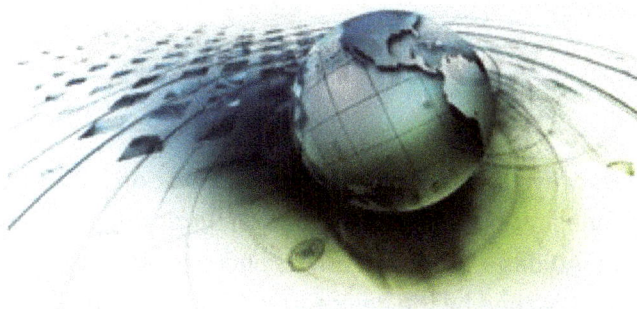

Gone are the days of the analog stopwatch and manual mileage estimates. Over the past couple of years, technology has caught up, and in some ways overtaken the running, biking and swimming industries. It has ferried them under one umbrella of concepts and unimaginable amounts of data in graphs, charts and tables. Technology has pushed the envelope and allowed the athletes to be coached by devices and driven even further by instant and accurate results that can be presented worldwide.

In this section, we'll take a look at the rising technological advances with respect to running, and how they can help you with your goals.

- Music
- Monitoring gadgets - watches, heart monitors, and pacing devices
- Running websites
- Smart phones and running apps
- Live cameras

Motivation

"Safety is something that happens between your ears, not something you hold in your hands." – *Jeff Cooper*

Tuning In

Most of us enjoy music, and why not? It allows us to shut out the world and listen to what we want to hear as individuals. It can motivate and inspire, and it can help keep us on pace.

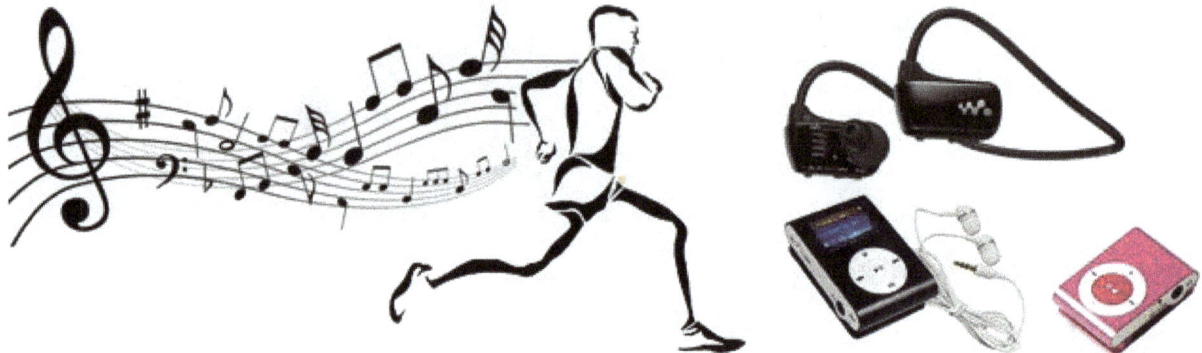

Tip

Earlier in this book, I mentioned that you should try to run a pace of 90 footsteps per minute. Try to match music that has 90 beats per minute, and it will help you keep your pace. Remember to turn down your music or remove one ear piece in high traffic areas. Search the internet for "music for 90 steps per minute," and you'll get a ton of great music web sites!

Monitoring

Modern technology has introduced countless ways of tracking your pace, elevation, distance, heart rate, stride and much more. And, nothing provides monitoring better than GPS tracking watches. Manufacturers such as Garmin, Timex, Polar, TomTom, Adidas and several others have paved the way for accurate measurements and allow the consumers to be coached by the device as it collects real-time data for graphs and charts, trending and goal-setting.

When you shop for a GPS watch, ALWAYS look at consumer reviews as you would if you were buying a car. Features, accessories, battery life, device life expectancy, and warranty should all play a part in your decision making.

A good GPS watch should have a minimum of the following accessories or features:

- Real-time GPS data collection for pace, altitude, distance
- Pace monitor for steps per minute (built in to the watch or a foot pod)
- Heart rate monitor (built in to the watch or a chest strap)
- Wireless upload and synchronization to your PC or support website
- USB or compatible charger
- Electronic compass
- Personal data entry for age, weight, heart rate zones, etc.
- Optional soft straps

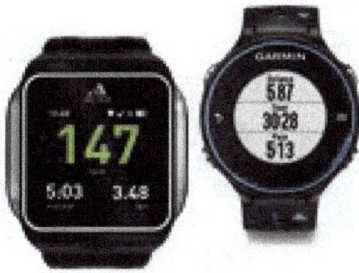

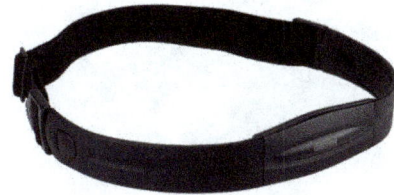

Leading brand GPS watches **Foot pod** **Heart rate monitor**

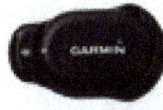

Additional features found on the high-end models should include:

- Vertical Oscillation detection
- Virtual Trainer with pace alerts
- Notification from other smart devices such as phones
- Touchscreen
- Ground contact time
- Ambient temperature

A decent GPS watch system will have a suitable website and support system behind it, complete with Smart phone apps available. Uploads from your GPS device should be seamless and available immediately.

Athlete Websites

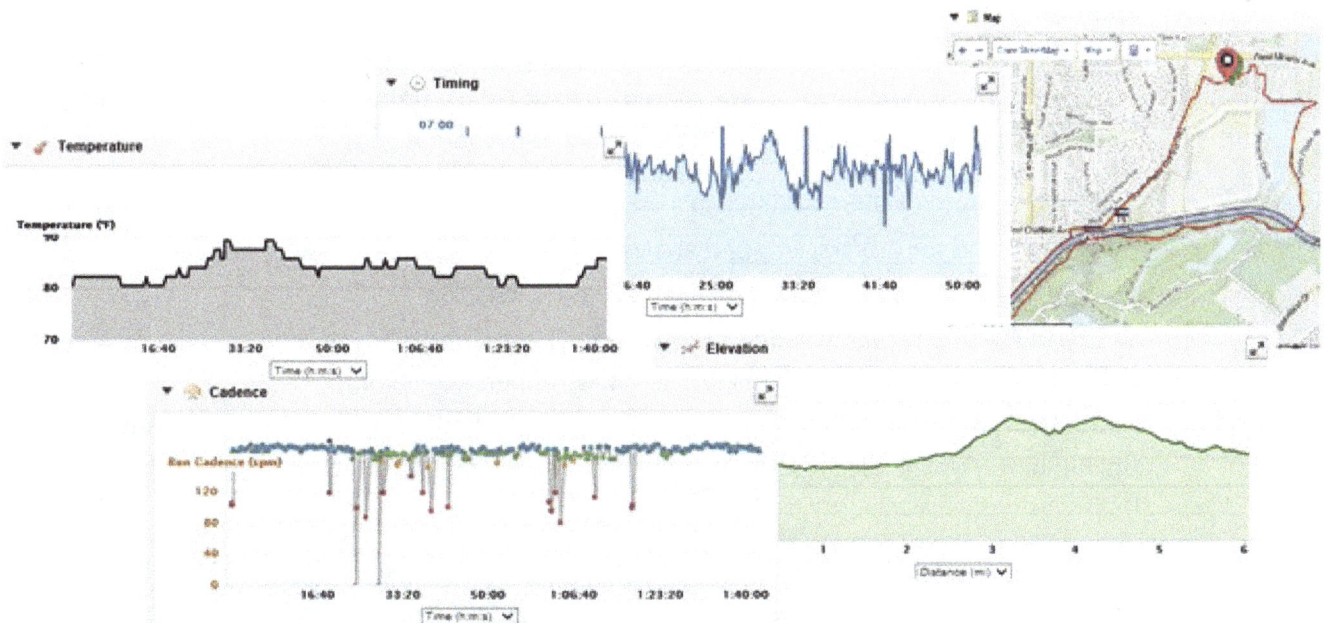

Popular websites like Garmin and Strava display important information for your run, such as pace, elevation, ambient temperature, cadence, oscillation, foot contact and more. Most will allow you to set custom goals and review past performances.

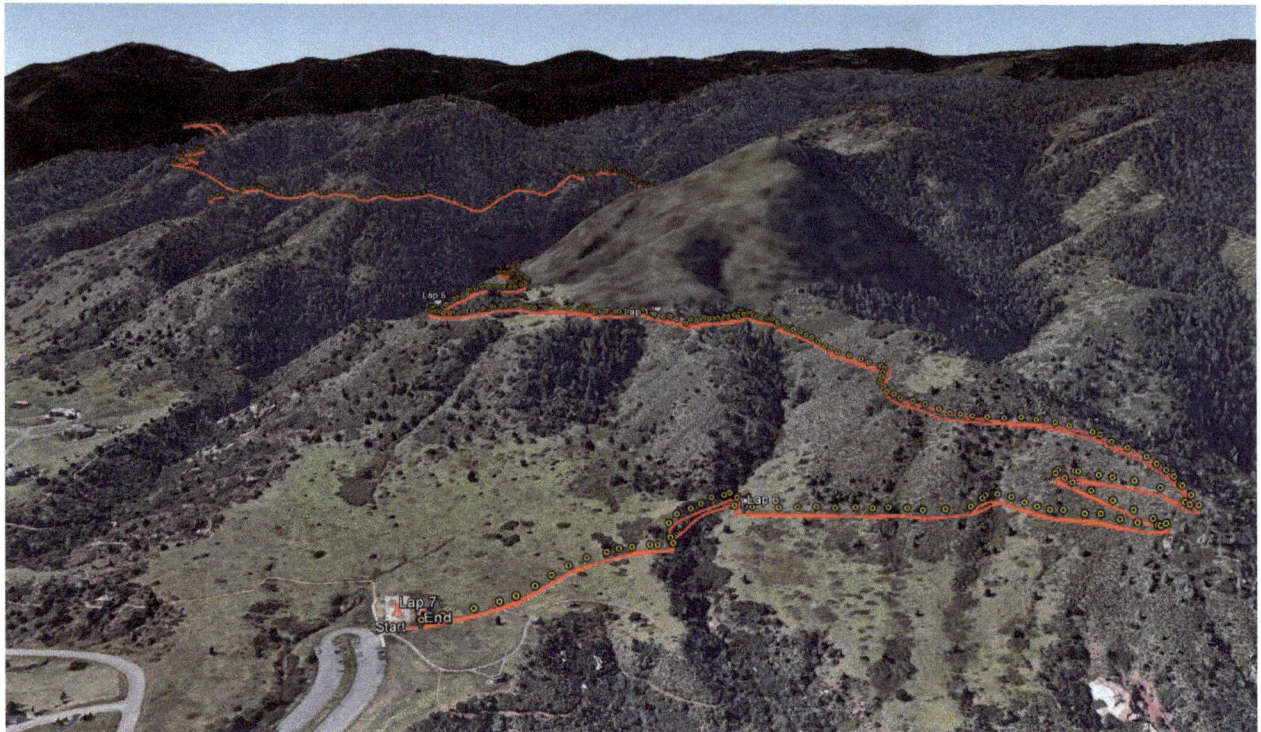

Data can be exported as .GPX or .TCX file types for mapping programs, or directly into topographical programs such as Google Earth ®, MapSource ® or EasyGPS ®, and show your run in 3D animation.

Running Websites

There are a number of websites dedicated to running technology, statistics, races, facts and trends. Some of the more popular sites are geared toward GPS tracking, reporting and trending, and others are used to advertise upcoming races. Here are a few of them:

- Garmin ® – Used for GPS tracking and analysis of Garmin branded devices (www.garmin.com)
- Strava ® – Used for GPS tracking and analysis of popular devices (www.strava.com)
- Athlinks ® – Tracks athlete performance (www.athlinks.com)
- RunningUSA – Online race schedules (www.runningusa.com)
- Runner's World – Online runner magazine (www.runnersworld.com)
- MarathonGuide – Online marathon resource and race schedules (www.marathonguide.com)
- Cool Running – Online race resources, information, and tools (www.coolrunning.com)

> **Motivation**
>
> **"You can't put a limit on anything. The more you dream, the farther you get."** — *Michael Phelps*

Bill Watts

M - 57 Littleton, CO, USA

Facebook G+ Share Tweet Email

	Marathon 67 Race Results	1/2 Mara 27 Race Results	10K 19 Race Results
Total Races **220**	2:59:01 Personal Best	1:26:04 Personal Best	38:32 Personal Best
Total Race Miles **3,939**	Top **35.8%** Athlinks Rank	Top **14.8%** Athlinks Rank	Top **11.1%** Athlinks Rank

Bill is a Runner, Trail Runner, Triathlete.

ATHLINKS — Search by Event or Athlete Name — Events & Results Athletes Bill ▼

2009

Event	Pace	Age	Gender	Overall	Final Time
St. George Marathon — St. George, UT, US • Oct 3rd	6:49 /Mi	5	133	151	2:59:01
Aetna Park To Park 10 Miler 2009 — Denver, CO, US • Sep 7th	6:58 /Mi	5	61	77	1:09:42
Georgetown To Idaho Springs Half Marathon 2009 — Georgetown, CO, US • Aug 8th	6:34 /Mi	4	50	62	1:26:04
Stadium Stampede - St. Joseph's Hospital 2009 — Denver, CO, US • Jun 21st	7:24 /Mi	9	82	98	23:01
Steamboat Marathon 2009 — Steamboat Springs, CO, US • Jun 7th	6:52 /Mi	1	7	7	3:00:09
The Denver Post Colfax Marathon 2009 — Denver, CO, US • May 17th	7:24 /Mi	2	17	18	3:14:06
Cottonwood Classic 2009 — Thornton, CO, US • May 16th	7:13 /Mi	14	47	56	22:26
Sierra's Race Against Meningitis 5K Run-Walk 2009 — Loveland, CO, US • Apr 25th	6:56 /Mi	4	51	62	21:34
Hrca Heritage/Adventure 5/10K Run/Walk — Highlands Ranch, CO, US • Apr 11th	7:08 /Mi	1	11	13	44:22
Platte River Half Marathon — , CO, US • Apr 5th	6:46 /Mi	4	55	59	1:28:50

Use a website like Athlinks to track your races

There are thousands of running-related websites and blogs available on the Internet today and a quick online search will retrieve answers for most of your questions. Use these sites to accurately track your accomplishments!

> **Motivation**
>
> **"You can't achieve what you don't believe."** — *Bill Watts*

Smart Phones and Running Apps

There are literally hundreds of smart phone apps available for download. Some are free and some charge a nominal fee, but all are geared to benefit you, as a runner, to keep you informed and on track. There are pace calculators, statistics apps, heart rate and health apps, as well as tons of social networking apps to keep friendly competition between you and your running companions.

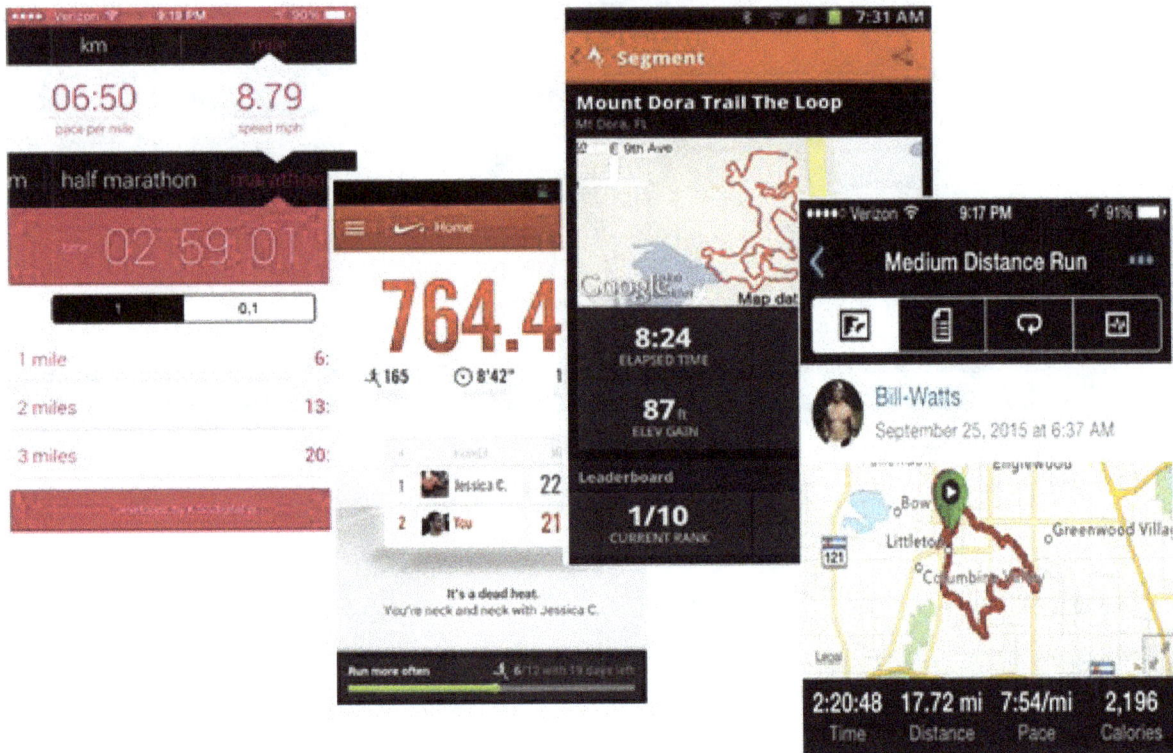

Let's take a look at a couple of them:

- Garmin ® – much like their website, this app is geared for runner history and analysis and has several social networking tools built in. You can track your own performance or anyone in your group.

- Endomondo ® – A new player in the running tech gear that talks to most of the popular smart phones and devices, including iPhone, Windows Phone, Blackberry, Polar and Garmin devices.

- Strava ® – Similar to the Garmin app, this one is designed for runner tracking and statistics but the social networking features have a leg up on the competition.

- Nike+ ® – Another great tracking and statistical app with a very user friendly interface.

- Road ID ® – This little app is aimed mostly at runner safety. It adds an emergency contact list to the lock screen of your phone and allows you to send "eBread-crumbs" to your family or friends so they can track you on your hike or run.

- Runne – This is one of the best pace calculators and allows you to estimate your time or distance in miles or kilometers, and has one of the easiest interfaces to use.

- MapMyRun – Obviously, this great little app tracks your run, along with the distance, pace, calories, elevation and nutrition for the day.

Live Cameras

High definition video cameras have been around for a while, used for anything from underwater scuba diving to helmet cams on Mount Everest. Race car drivers, motorcyclists, surfers, skiers and bicyclists have adopted their use over the past few years. Well, they've finally arrived on the running scene and their impact is already being felt, offering views of long trail runs, road marathons and full speed sprints. Until now, these spectacular views were only available to the runner, but now they can be stored and shared!

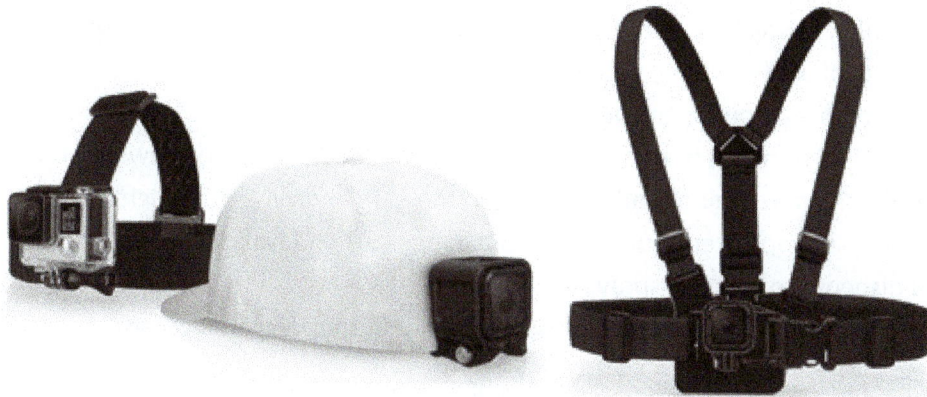

Hat, head and torso mounted cameras

Recovery Gear

Massage accessories such as foam rollers or massage sticks are great for post-race aches and pains. Of course, if your race includes a free massage afterwards, you should always try to take advantage of it. Most of the massages are done by professional therapists or their apprentices, and they do a wonderful job of massaging those aching leg muscles.

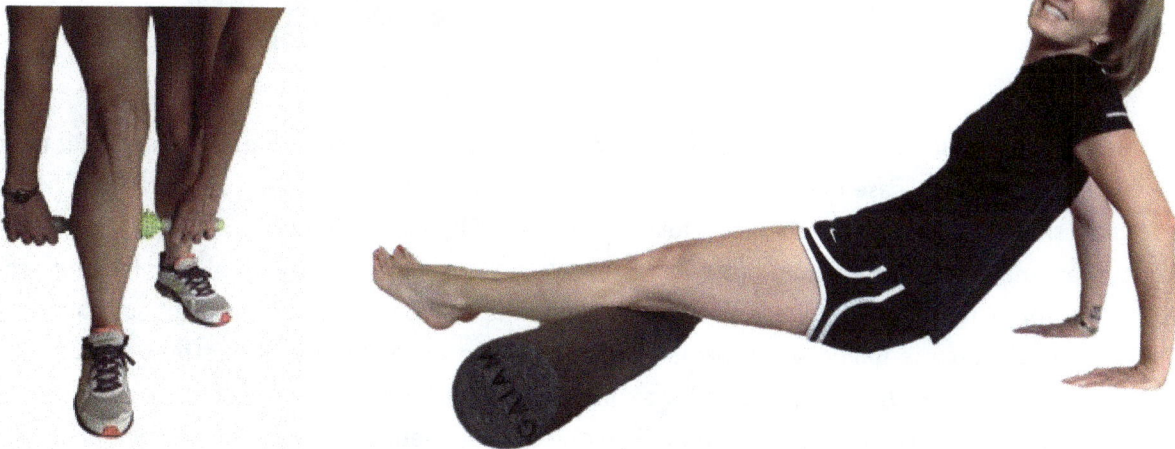

Massage sticks and rollers work wonders after your race

Safe Running

So now you have an idea of the equipment you'll need for your running, but none of it does any good unless you practice safe running technique. When it comes to running or most other outdoor activities, safety comes down to little more than common sense. Be safe by following these pieces of advice, and add them as a safety checklist for your run.

- Get a physical before you start your running program.
- Have a current identification card with you at all times.
- Avoid running during the hottest part of the day in summer.
- Drink plenty of water before, during and after your run.
- Take your mobile phone with you.
- If using an iPod or headset, don't play the music too loud – stay alert, aware and alive.
- Wear reflective materials if you're running in the early morning or at night.
- Choose well-lit, populated routes and avoid dangerous and isolated areas.
- Carry a dispenser of pepper spray.
- If you injure yourself while running, stop immediately and seek medical advice. Call 911 for serious injuries.

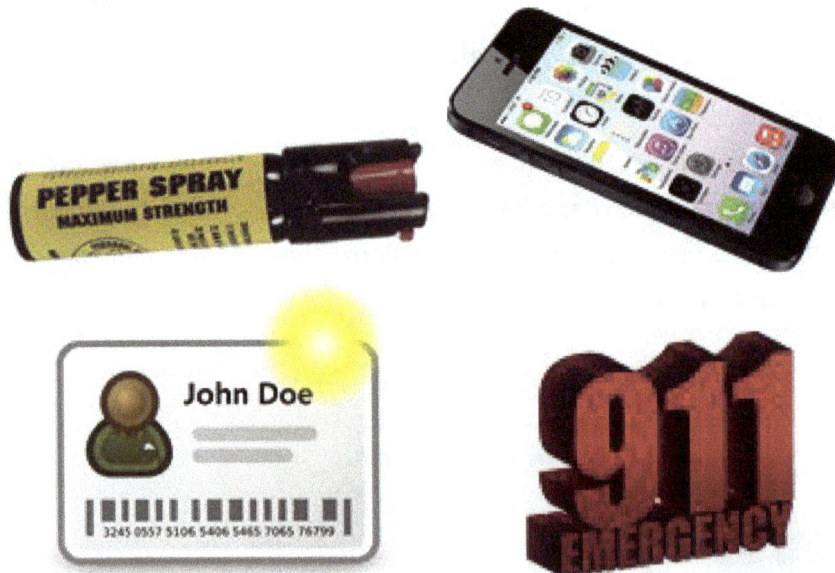

- **Be prepared** – Be prepared for any emergency by toting your smart phone. You can use it to call first responders in case of an emergency, or simply use your GPS to find your location. Always carry small amounts of cash and carefully plan out your hydration needs.
- **Pay attention to your surroundings** – It seems like a no-brainer, but things always look different when you're running the opposite direction. From time to time during your run, glance backwards and try to make mental notes of special landmarks, geographical features or street signs.
- **Share your plan** – Whenever you go for a run, someone should know where you're going and the time you expect to return. If you don't talk to one of your friends or family, at the very least, leave a note.

- **Know the Route** – Make sure you know where you've been and where you're going. In a group setting, try to run with someone if you can. There truly is safety in numbers. If others at your pace are also concerned about running alone, you can agree to stay together, even if one or more of you needs to slow down. As always, safety is paramount. If you're running by yourself, make sure you study your route before you go out. If you don't have a GPS device, you can always sketch out a map to carry with you.

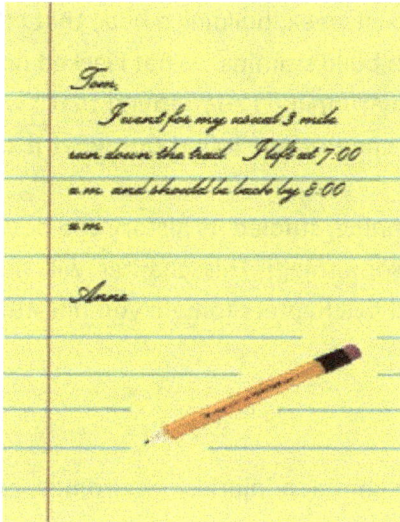

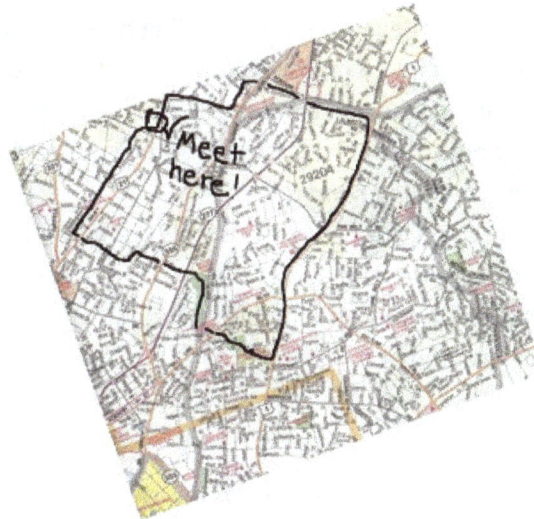

Leave a note and know where you're going!

Challenge!

Gear Up and Stay Safe

In this chapter, we had glimpses of a lot of equipment to help us overcome many challenges that running can present to us. We now know how the "20-degree rule" works and why it's important to dress properly when we go outside to run. We examined advanced technologies that can supplement and enhance our running lives.

Your challenge: *Build your very own "tool box" and stock it up with an inventory that's useful and efficient. Keep first aid supplies clean and in good condition, and always replace expired medicines and ointments. Leave nothing to chance – always expect the unexpected.*

In summary, be smart about the equipment you buy and the way you use it. You never know when it could save a life – maybe even your own.

Chapter 12 – Strength and Conditioning

My Story

Early in my running career, I thought it might be possible to run a full marathon, but when I'd run five or six miles at a time, my endurance would fade quickly. I didn't understand why this was happening because I was spending hours at the gym each week, building a body that I thought would hold up for 26 miles. I was also running frequently to build stamina. What I lacked however, was a training plan to *combine* my weight training with my running. I soon found that I wouldn't ever be able to reach my goal if I didn't do *both!* In this chapter, we'll find out what it takes to become *strong and conditioned!*

In the first 11 chapters of this book, we defined running, studied its history and dove into a cache of science and facts. But, now it's time to DO something! This chapter will build the foundation for your running program, and will be followed by chapters to help you fine-tune your running program.

In **Chapter 7 – Dealing with Injuries,** we exposed the common injuries, syndromes, conditions and symptoms that runners can experience. Statistics show that nearly 50 percent of all runners will encounter some type of injury in any given year, and more than 80 percent will experience a running-related injury in their lifetime. Many runners will simply quit after being injured because they assume they were injured *because* of running. Clearly, I can say that running in itself is not dangerous, unless you have some kind of pre-existing condition or illness, such as an enlarged heart. Lack of physical preparation is normally the cause of injury.

A pilot would not fly a plane without carefully studying the flight manual, practicing hundreds of hours of flight training, and weighing the risks involved in flying an aircraft. He would make sure that his plane was properly maintained and that it would pass regularly scheduled safety inspections. He would make sure that all of the electrical and hydraulic systems work as they should and that the plane was fueled up before each flight.

We could use this same analogy for a runner. He would study and research books and manuals to gain information about running. He would train for many miles before a race, and know what the risks are for each type of injury. He would make sure that he maintains a healthy body by consuming nutritious food and drink. He would submit to an annual physical examination from his doctor. He would make sure that all of his systems were in working condition, such as his cardiovascular system, digestive system and musculoskeletal system, ensuring that each were strong and capable of the trip ahead.

Drawing from these two examples, we can deduce a common thread, even though flying an airplane is much different than running a marathon. The mutual connection between each is that we must *study, develop, prepare, focus, engage and execute* for the intended results. As in flying, we must treat running as a *skill* rather than just an *activity*.

Similar to any other skill, we must learn how to adopt best practices, and adapt to other ways of thinking so we can continue to improve. The best way to improve is to increase our *strength* and *conditioning*, relevant to running. Some sports professionals will argue that strength and conditioning are one and the same. In this book I'm going to break them into individual topics to make it simpler for me to explain and easier for you to understand.

Strength – What is it?

Strength can be defined in a number of different ways:

- *Physical* strength, such as a physical capacity to employ power and mobility; to resist strain or stress; to be durable.
- *Mental* strength, such as a capacity to deal with issues, situations or to maintain a moral or intellectual position.
- *Resource* strength, such as a numerical capacity or quantity.
- *Attribute* strength, such as a characteristic or asset of yours.
- *Situational* strength, the ability to adapt to different conditions, plans or situations.

Generally speaking, strength can most easily be described as "the state or quality of being strong," whether it's one of the strengths listed above or all of them together. Granted, physical strength may be the only one you need to run a mile, for example. But what happens if you're going to run a marathon?

Obviously, you will need a great deal of *physical* strength just to complete the marathon, but late in the race, you may need to depend on your *mental* strength to push you through to the finish line. One of your *attributes* or characteristics is that people say you always finish what you start. You may also rely on *resource* strengths, such as a fellow runner, a pacer, an assistant, or even the fans along the course to encourage you to the finish line. Finally, you may need *situational* strength, if you need to *adapt* while you're on the course. *Strength* is the capacity to create energy from a power source, such as human muscle, thoughts, resources, attributes or situations.

In this chapter, we'll deal primarily with *physical* strength. We touched on *mental* strength in **Chapter 5 – Running Psychology** and we'll examine *resource* and *situational* strengths in **Chapter 16 – Training Plans**.

Physical Strength – To become a successful athlete, you must strengthen and enhance your body's musculoskeletal system for the activities in which you plan on doing. For runners, the obvious and primary strengths must originate from the legs. I'm not sure why some runners shy away from the gym and weights, but from what I've experienced, weight training will enhance your running in many ways. There are a few myths that I'd like to address before we go any further.

Running and Weight Room Myths

MYTH: Runners need more VO2 max (a measure of the maximum volume of oxygen an athlete can use), not more strength or muscle mass. VO2 max is simply a measure of the maximum volume of oxygen that an athlete can use. It is measured in milliliters per kilogram of body weight per minute (ml/kg/min). See page 50 for an easy-to-understand description of VO2 max.

MYTH-BUSTER: As we saw in **Chapter 6 – Running Physiology**, we learned the importance of VO2 max for elite and high efficiency runners, and ways they can improve it. We also took note of the fact that "average Joe" runners may not need to be concerned with VO2 max. According to most Sports and Exercise Physiologists, about 80% of VO2 max is related to genetic design. A well-conditioned "average Joe" has a VO2 max of 45ml/kg-/min and may be able to increase to 52 ml/kg-/min through hard work.

To keep things in perspective, pro cyclist and triathlete Lance Armstrong has a VO2 max of about 80ml/kg-/min, nearly the highest rating a person can possess. If this is true, what are the alternatives to having a low or average VO2 max? How can a runner who is predisposed with a low VO2 max become a better athlete? Well, I'm happy to tell you that there are alternatives for VO2 max when it comes to endurance sports. Proper strength and conditioning, even without increasing your VO2 max, can lead to better running economy.

MYTH: Strength training makes you heavier, slower, inflexible and "muscle-bound."

MYTH-BUSTER: While it is true you can actually gain weight by increasing your muscle mass, this is usually balanced by a loss of fatty tissue because of an increased caloric burn. The advantages of a complete and comprehensive strength training program far outweigh the benefits of a sedentary or one dimensional "running only" curriculum. Another benefit of strength training is the increase of muscle group coordination (neurological adaptations) that allows the different parts of your body to work together in harmony. For example, many runners perform two leg squats to increase the strength in their quadriceps. But what are the real advantages of two leg squats when running is defined as: "to go quickly by moving the legs more rapidly than at a walk and in such a manner that for an instant in each step, both feet are off the ground"?

Two-leg squats would be great if you were going to hop through your next race like a kangaroo. Instead of two-leg squats, why not *one-leg* squats? Not only would one-leg squats increase your strength because you would be supporting your entire body on one leg, but it would also improve your balance and coordination. This is the kind of logical thinking I'd like you to embrace in this chapter. While conventional weight lifting may be fine for body builders, we need to adapt their beliefs into a running philosophy. When doing your gym work, try to think "outside the box," and keep the focus on running.

MYTH: High running volume should dictate your running plan.

MYTH BUSTER: In **Chapter 7 – Dealing with Injuries**, I told you "My Story," citing examples of how I called myself the "king of junk miles." I learned the hard way that the *quality* of your running mileage is much more important than the *quantity*. Therefore, every mile of every training session should have a purpose. I can't stress this enough, so I'll simply repeat it – "*every* mile of *every* training session should have a purpose!" Admittedly, at some point, you'll have to run the distance it takes to meet your eventual goal. If you're planning a 10k, you'll need to practice that distance at least one time before your race. If you run a marathon, you should run the distance, (or close to it) at least once before you race it. We'll take a deep-dive in the next chapter – **Chapter 13 – Training Basics,** and again in **Chapter 16 – Training Plans.** With all of this in mind, please keep your focus on *quality mileage*. Quality mileage will improve your overall *running efficiency* and *decrease your propensity for injury*, and those, my friends, are the main objectives.

On the previous page, we looked at the myth that conveys the message that high volume should dictate your running plan. One running camp may say that you have to work up a solid strengthening program before you ever start your running program, while another says to start your running program and build into your strengthening program. Why does it have to be one way or the other? Why can't we allow the two disciplines to co-exist and work on both at the same time? After struggling with my own array of injuries over the years, I found that you really shouldn't do one without the other. By focusing on "run-only" or "strength-only" training, you condition your body to do just one at a time. If you *strengthen* AND *condition* your body to do both, you won't limit your body's potential. Instead, you'll allow different muscle groups to work together in a coordinated effort.

As I'll state many times in this book, you need to start with a goal. Once you define your goal, work on your plan. Is your plan based on a certain event such as a 5k or marathon? Do you know how many days you should run each week? How many days should you cross-train or work with weights? How long will it take you to reach your goal? How do you stay on track if you have a set-back or injury?

This chapter and the next one will help you plan and achieve your goals. In this book, I'm going to assume that you have just made your decision to take up running and will tag you as a "beginner." With this in mind, let's define each of the categories, so you can make your own decisions on where you stand:

- **Beginning Runner:**
    - I feel overweight or unhealthy and need a place to start
    - I consider myself healthy but have never run regularly
    - I haven't run in a long time
    - I'm a jogger/runner but my mileage is limited to 1 to 5 miles per week
- **Intermediate Runner:**
    - I feel healthy and can run a 5k or 10k
    - I'm an average runner, but I want to raise my level of intensity or duration
    - I'm a jogger/runner but my mileage is limited to 5 to 25 miles per week
- **Advanced Runner:**
    - I've been running for quite some time
    - I can run 15 miles without stopping
    - I can run, or do run more than 25 miles per week without injury
    - I want to run competitively

Motivation

"You can wish as hard as you like but all that really matters is the shape you're in on the day of the race. I've always felt these really big races aren't necessarily won by whoever is the fastest. They're won by the athlete who is the smartest and in the best shape on the day." – *Paula Radcliffe*

Earlier in this chapter, I said that we'd define *strength* and *conditioning* as two separate topics, even though in reality they are intertwined with respect to running. I mention this because a person can possess a tremendous amount of *strength* because he can squat 400 pounds or bench press 200 pounds. However, having this strength doesn't necessarily mean he can effectively run 5 miles down the road.

Likewise, just because he may be able to run a marathon, it doesn't mean he can do 30 pushups or 50 sit-ups. While an athlete may have an incredible amount of *strength*, it doesn't mean he can run an entire marathon, and vice versa – a person *conditioned* to run a marathon, may not possess a great deal of weight lifting strength.

Ultimately, our goal should be a *combination* of strength and conditioning - to allow us to run that marathon with plenty of *strength* and be *conditioned* to go the entire distance. So what do we call this *combination* of *strength* and *conditioning?* At this point, I'd like to propose another equation or formula:

Strength + Conditioning = Fitness

While it's fairly easy to measure strength with the amount of weight an individual can push, pull or lift, and we can measure conditioning with a defined limit on endurance, it becomes much more difficult to measure fitness. What *is* fitness? How can you tell when you have become "fit?" Are you "fit" when a 10 mile run suddenly becomes easy?

What is the definition of "fitness?" What specific characteristics make us fit?

According to the United States Department of Health and Human Services, physical fitness is defined as "a set of attributes that people have or achieve that relates to the ability to perform physical activity." The study goes on to state that "fitness" is made of 5 distinct categories:

- Muscular Strength – Defined as the ability of muscle to exert force during an activity
- Muscular Endurance – The ability of a muscle to continue exerting force without tiring out
- Cardiorespiratory endurance - How efficiently your heart and lungs deliver oxygen to your body and how efficiently your body creates the energy your muscles need in order to contract
- Body Composition – The relative amounts of fat, bone and muscles that make up your body composition
- Flexibility – Defined as the range of movement across a joint. In this chapter and the next, we'll take a look at how we can increase our strength, improve our conditioning and achieve our preferred level of fitness.

Tip
Don't forget that proper nutrition is paramount to your strengthening program. Read **Chapter 10 – Nutrition** to help customize your nutritional needs.

Motivation

"The will to win is important, but the will to prepare is vital." – *Joe Paterno*

Where Are You in Your Training Program?

On the previous page, we took a look at current fitness descriptions. Take the time to evaluate your own personal fitness level and calculate the time to your next (or first) event. Be realistic in your approach and allow "slack" time for unforeseen injuries. Make sure you include enough time to rest or "taper" before your race. We'll take a closer look at these topics in **Chapter 16 – Training Plans.**

Let's Begin!

After you've made an honest assessment of your fitness level, start with building your foundation several months in advance. Don't be too aggressive in your program, or you may become injured or miss your "peak" training period if you don't plan accordingly.

Strength training is typically made up of:

- Repetitions (reps) – the number of time you repeat the exercise, lift, etc.
- Sets – how many sets of reps you do, with a rest period or alternate activity in between
- Resistance used – how much weight or resistance is used in the activity
- Rest periods between sets

In the upcoming pages, we'll take a look at various strengthening exercises and activities that are specific to running. Most of these activities will not use free weights or weight machines, although you can certainly benefit from the use of these devices.

In the following example, we'll assume that you're just starting out as a "beginner." Based on this assumption, I'll give you my recommended schedule for a one to six month strengthening program. Remember, do your strength training in conjunction *with* the customized running schedule that you'll build in **Chapter 16 – Training Plans.**

Month 1: One to two strength training sessions per week using all exercises shown in the next section; two sets of each exercise with 8 to 10 reps and a 90 second rest between each set.

Month 2: Two strength training sessions per week using all exercises shown in the next section; three sets of each exercise with 8 to 10 reps and a 75 second rest between each set.

Months 3 to 5 ½: Two to three strength training sessions per week using all exercises shown in the next section; four sets of 8 to 10 reps and a 60 second rest between each set.

Month 5 ½ to Race Day: Two strength training sessions per week using all exercises shown in the next section, one set of each exercise, 8 to 10 reps and a 90 to 120 second rest between each set. In this example, the volume of resistance training gradually increases until you peak at around 5 ½ months. At this point, your strengthening volume should taper in parallel with your running taper. You do not need to be concerned about losing your "fitness" level and at this point. Besides, your body will appreciate the down time!

Which exercises should I use?

All strengthening exercises can be beneficial to anyone, but as a runner, you should focus on anything that will allow the different parts of your body to *work together*, especially if you're going to engage in long distance running such as half-marathons, marathons or ultramarathons.

The mainstays of your program should focus on:

- Balance
- Stability
- Multiple-joint exercises
- Core strengthening
- Emphasis on quality over quantity
- Upright exercises (bench presses don't help much with running – stay vertical)
- Single-leg strengthening instead of two-leg exercises
- Work muscle *groups* not individual muscles

Specific to Distance Runners

If you plan on running long distances, please note that you should not sacrifice weight training for miles on the road. In fact, you should emphasize and maximize your strengthening program. Muscle tissue weighs more than fat and it's easy to be concerned when you start to gain weight through an effective strength and conditioning program. Too many of us worry that the additional weight gained in the weight room due to increased muscle mass will somehow hamper our running ability.

As an "average Joe," I've experienced almost all of the running-related injuries and in the final analysis, I firmly believe that if I had spent more time in the weight room, I probably wouldn't have had so many injuries. Running puts an incredible amount of stress and strain on the human body, and if you don't prepare accordingly, you'll increase your probability for injury. The bottom line – don't shy away from the weight room! Go ahead and build up those muscles, joints and connective tissues so your body can handle the load. Get strong and stay strong – finish your race feeling fit!

Finally, consider the following when you go through your program:

- One workout per week can help you *develop* during your program.
- Two workouts per week can help you *maintain* that fitness.
- Three workouts per week can help you *advance or improve* your fitness level.

Motivation

"I would rather be ashes than dust! I would rather my sparks should burn out in a blaze than they should be stifled by dry rot. I would rather be a superb meteor, every atom of me in magnificent glow, than asleep and permanent as a planet. The proper function of man is to live, not to exist. I shall not waste my days trying to prolong them. I shall use my time." *– Marshall Ulrich*

Weight Training for Runners

Up to this point, we've looked at many aspects of running and the components that make up some of the reasons why we might take up running, yet we've not lifted a single weight or run a single mile. As if we were about to build a house, we need to implement a few basics.

- **Goals** – We need to set our goals of *when* we want to accomplish this. Stick to the timelines you've agreed to and make sure those timelines are sensible and achievable.

- **Concept** – We need to get an idea of *what* we want to achieve. You have an idea of what you're going to accomplish, but you must be willing to adapt and think "outside the box" when the ideas have to change for one reason or another.

- **Blueprint** - We need to decide *how* we are going to achieve our goal. You can be the designer of your own running program. Use sound design techniques and best practices and apply them accordingly.

- **Foundation** – We need to build a *strong foundation* to support our goals. Be sure to build a strong foundation so you can keep your injuries to a minimum and stay healthy for years to come.

- **Framework** – We need to build our body in this phase. Proper strength and conditioning should correspond to your original blueprints, but don't be afraid to modify when necessary. Remember, the finished product is only as good as what lies underneath!

- **Fit and Finish** – We need to apply the finishing touches to our project. Tune as you go, and customize to make it fit *your* plans. While this book can provide the basic architecture, it's really up to you to modify to fit your needs.

To be effective, runners need four critical attributes:

- Postural alignment
- Specific stabilization
- High strength
- Ability to produce this strength quickly

Postural alignment can be best achieved by hard work and practice. As humans, we spend much of our time in a sitting position, which shortens our anterior hip muscles (a group of muscles that attach to the pelvis – namely the hip-flexors, quadriceps and iliopsoas). In turn, this pulls the pelvis forward into a tilted position to the front, and can eventually lead to back pain and poor posture because it creates an exaggeration to the curve of our lumbar spine. Good posture is required for overall musculoskeletal health and is something that we should all strive for, whether we are running in a marathon, or simply walking in the park. While core exercises don't require additional weights or equipment, the use of an exercise ball can help with stability, strengthening and balance.

First, we'll look at exercises that can aid in good posture focusing primarily on the back muscles. Then we'll examine the core and the legs, and finally we'll analyze the arms, shoulders and neck, all of which are important for running efficiently. Most of the techniques can be done without the use of hand weights or gym equipment. A yoga mat and elastic band can be helpful, and you can always choose to enhance your workouts with the use of weights.

Lower Back Strengthening Exercises Without Weights:

- Diagonal Back Extensions

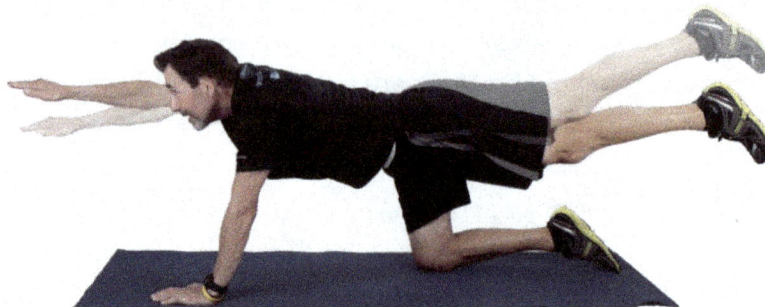

MUSCLE TARGET:
Erector spinae, gluteus maximus, back thigh muscles
HOW TO DO THIS EXERCISE:
With both hands and both knees on the floor, lift and extend your right leg and left arm in line with your torso. Hold this position and then extend the opposite arm and leg. Make slow and controlled diagonal torso extensions until you reach the leg and arm position above the horizontal torso line. Switch sides and repeat.
HELPFUL HINTS:
During the exercise, try to keep your hips in a horizontal position; this way you prevent undesired lifting of the hips and rotation of the spine. Allow the head to be an extension of the spine and never cover your head. Inhale while lifting arm and leg and exhale when returning to the start position

- Floor Back Extensions

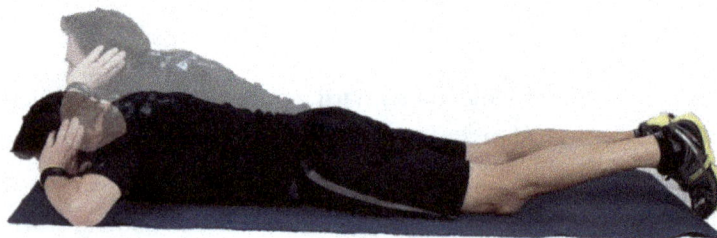

MUSCLE TARGET:
Erector spinae, intrinsic muscles of the back
HOW TO DO THIS EXERCISE:
From the prone position, place your feet in line with your hips. Look downwards and put the hands behind your ears. Make slow and controlled torso extensions until you slightly lift the torso off the floor.
HELPFUL HINTS:
During the exercise, don't let your head fall back or forward, keeping your head in a straight line with your spine. Don't lift your torso too high because it increases the pressure on the lumbar spine. Keep your legs on the floor. Inhale while lifting the torso upwards and exhale when returning to the start position.

- Superman Back Extensions

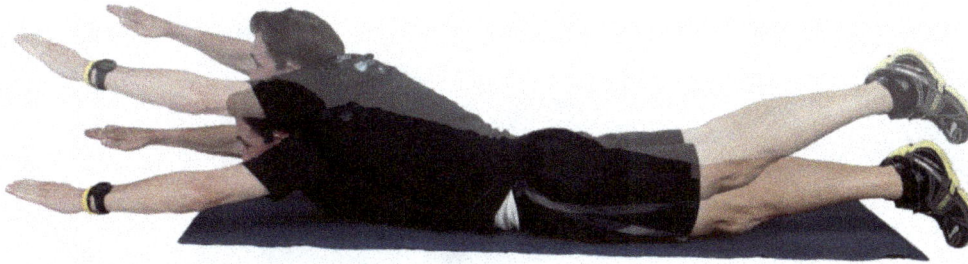

MUSCLE TARGET:
Gluteus maximus, erector spinae, intrinsic muscles of the back

HOW TO DO THIS EXERCISE:
In the prone position, extend your arms in front of your head, and at the same time extend the legs and place them in line with the hips. Look downwards. Make slow and controlled "Superman" back extensions until you extend your legs and arms as high as possible without causing pain.

HELPFUL HINTS:
During this exercise, the head again acts as an extension of the spine. In the extended position, keep your arms in line with your upper back. Don't lift your torso too high because it increases the pressure on your lumbar spine. Inhale when lifting to the extended position and exhale when returning to the start position.

- Reverse Back Extensions with Leg Lifts

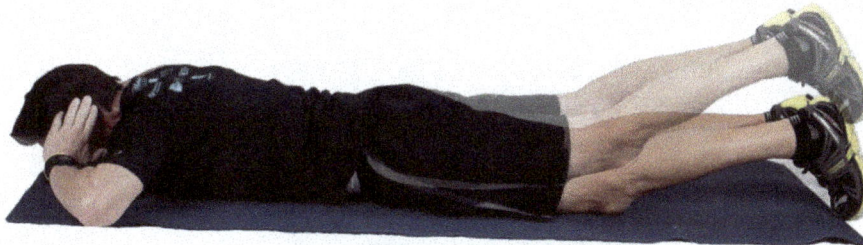

MUSCLE TARGET:
Gluteus maximus, erector spinae, intrinsic muscles of the back

HOW TO DO THIS EXERCISE:
From the prone position, place your feet in line with your hips. Look downwards, and allow the head to be an extension of the spine. Make slow and controlled leg lifts so that the toes are raised to the height of the buttocks.

HELPFUL HINTS:
Perform this exercise in a slow and smooth technique so you don't put too much pressure on your lumbar spine. To make the exercise more challenging, hold your heels together when lifting your legs. Inhale when lifting the legs upwards, and exhale when returning to the start position.

Motivation

"Push yourself again and again. Don't give an inch until the final buzzer sounds." – *Larry Bird*

Abdominal Strengthening Exercises Without Weights:

- Conventional Crunches

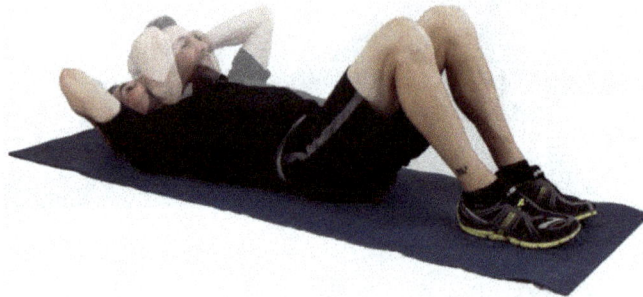

MUSCLE TARGET:
Rectus abdominis, obliquus externus, obliquus internus
HOW TO DO THIS EXERCISE:
Lie on your back and bend your knees at a 90-degree angle. Place the feet flat on the floor, in line with your hips. Look upwards and put your hands behind the ears. Make slow and controlled lateral torso flexions and bring the chest as near as is possible to the hips.
HELPFUL HINTS:
During this exercise, keep the natural arch of the lumbar spine. Allow the head to act as an extension of the spine. Keep the chin at least a fist's length away from the chest. For easier control over the lumbar spine, place your heels (not the entire foot) on the floor. To make the exercise more challenging, don't allow your shoulders to return to the floor. Exhale when lifting yourself forward and upwards and inhale when returning in the start position.

- Conventional Crunches With Rotation

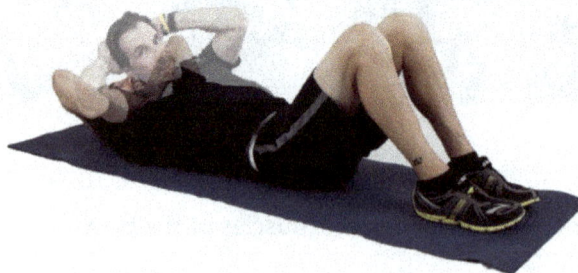

MUSCLE TARGET:
Rectus abdominis, obliquus externus, obliquus internus
HOW TO DO THIS EXERCISE:
Lie on your back and bend your knees at a 90-degree angle. Place the feet flat on the floor, in line with your hips. Look upwards and put your hands behind the ears. Make slow and controlled lateral torso flexions and bring your elbow as near as possible to the opposite knee without taking the other elbow off the floor. Switch sides and repeat.
HELPFUL HINTS:
During the exercise, keep the natural arch of the lumbar spine. Allow the head to act as an extension of the spine. Keep the chin away from the chest. Focus on using your obliques (side torso muscles). Exhale when lifting and twisting your torso and inhale while returning in the start position.

- Conventional Crunches With a Crossed Leg and Rotation

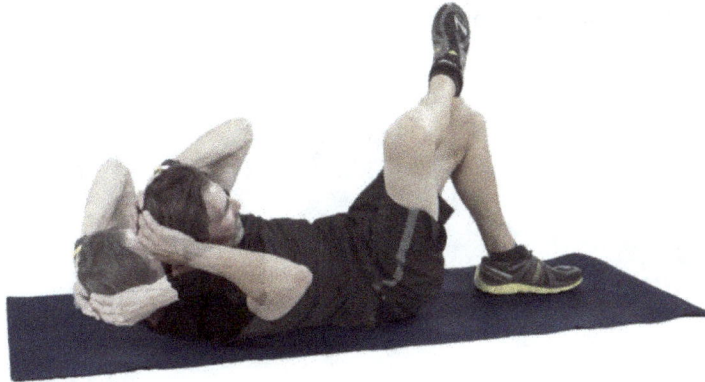

MUSCLE TARGET:
Rectus abdominis, obliquus externus, obliquus internus

HOW TO DO THIS EXERCISE:
Lie on your back and bend your knees at a 90-degree angle. Cross one leg over the knee of the other. Keep your hands placed behind your ears and look upwards. Make slow and controlled lateral torso flexions and bring your elbow as close to the knee as possible. Switch sides and repeat.

HELPFUL HINTS:
During this exercise, you will primarily use your side abdominal muscles, keeping one elbow on the floor at all times. Exhale when lifting and twisting your torso, and inhale while returning to the start position.

- Conventional Sit-ups

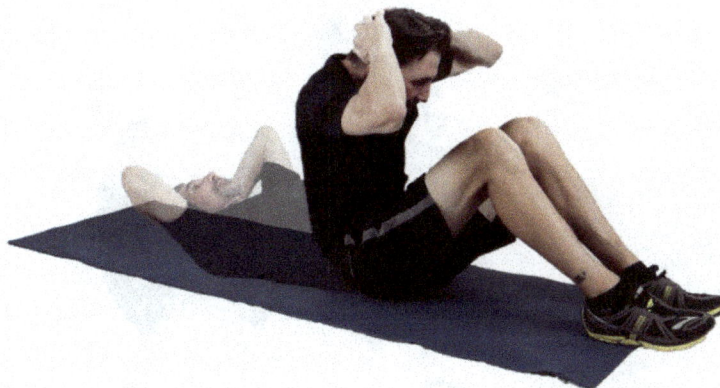

MUSCLE TARGET:
Abdominal muscles, hip flexors

HOW TO DO THIS EXERCISE:
Lie on your back and bend your knees at a 90-degree angle. Place the feet flat on the floor, in line with your hips. Look upwards and put your hands behind the ears. Make slow and controlled lateral torso flexions and bring the chest as near as possible to the hips.

HELPFUL HINTS:
During this exercise, keep the natural arch of the lumbar spine. Keep your head aligned with your spine. Keep the chin a fist away from the chest. Make this exercise easier by crossing your arms over your chest. Exhale and lift yourself upwards and inhale when returning to the start position.

Upper Leg Strengthening Exercises Without Weights:

- Two Leg Squats with Three Variations

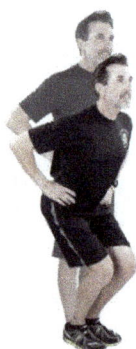

| Legs Together | Legs Parallel | Legs Apart |

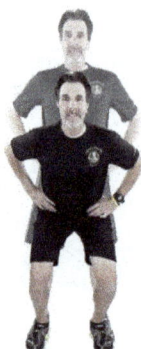

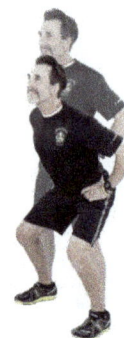

MUSCLE TARGET:
Quadriceps femoris, gluteus maximus, back thigh muscles

HOW TO DO THIS EXERCISE:
Stand upright and place your feet together, parallel or apart, and your hands resting on your hips. Look straight and keep your back straight. Make slow and controlled squats until you reach a 90-degree angle position of your knees. Return to the start position.

HELPFUL HINTS:
Keep the natural spine curvature and your knees pointing in the direction of your feet. Your knees should not extend over your toes. Inhale while squatting and exhale while returning in the start position.

- One-Leg Squats

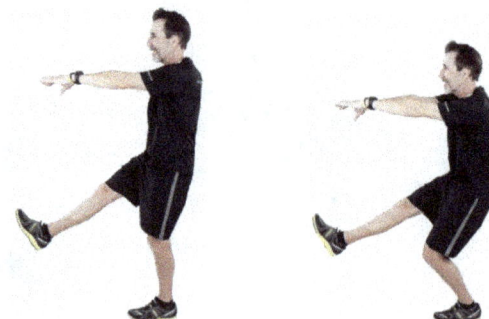

MUSCLE TARGET:
Abdominal muscles, gluteus maximus, lower back, shoulders

HOW TO DO THIS EXERCISE:
Balance on one foot and squat down, bending the knee at a 90- to 110-degree angle. Keeping your balance on one foot, return to the start position. Make slow and controlled squats until you reach a 90-degree angle position of your knees.

HELPFUL HINTS:
Keep the natural spine curvature and knees pointing in the direction of your feet. Your knees should not extend over your toes. Inhale while squatting and exhale while returning to the start position.

- Lying Leg Abduction With Elastic Band

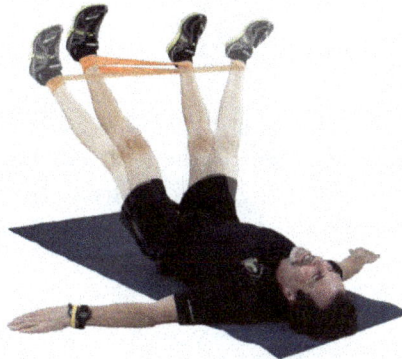

MUSCLE TARGET:
Gluteus medius, gluteus minimus, tensor fasciae latae
HOW TO DO THIS EXERCISE:
Place the elastic band around your ankles and lie down on your back. Lift your legs, bending them at a 45- to 90-degree angle from the hips, with your feet extended skyward. Use your hands for support on the floor. Make slow and controlled pushes of your legs. Do not reach the point where it causes pain.
HELPFUL HINTS:
Keep your effort balanced between each leg, as symmetrical as possible. It should be more difficult as you spread your legs apart. Keep your torso firm and stable with your lower back on the floor, if possible. Exhale while spreading your legs, inhale while returning to the start position.

- Lying Leg Adduction

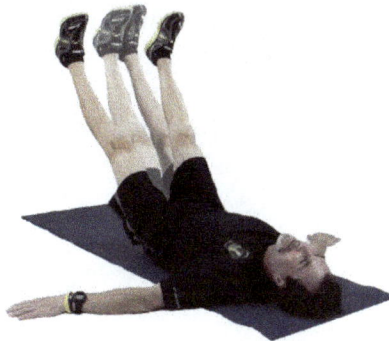

MUSCLE TARGET:
Adductor, gracilis, pectineus
HOW TO DO THIS EXERCISE:
Lift your legs, bending them at a 45- to 90-degree angle from the hips, with your feet extended skyward. Use your hands for support on the floor. Maintain natural curvature of the back. Make slow and controlled movement to spread your feet and touch your feet together.
HELPFUL HINTS:
Keep your effort balanced between each leg, as symmetrical as possible. It should be more difficult as you spread your legs apart. Keep your torso firm and stable with your lower back on the floor, if possible. Exhale while spreading your legs, inhale while returning to the start position.

- Standing Hip Extension With Optional Sandbag

MUSCLE TARGET:
Gluteus maximus, back thigh muscles
HOW TO DO THIS EXERCISE:
Drape the sandbag over your shoulders, gripping it with both hands in an upright position. Place your feet in the width of your hips, with your knees locked. Make slow and controlled hip extension movements while bending forward with your back straight.
HELPFUL HINTS:
Keep your back straight all the time, and keep your head aligned with your spine. Hold the weight or the sandbag so that it cannot slip from your grip. Exhale in the upright position, inhale when bending forward.

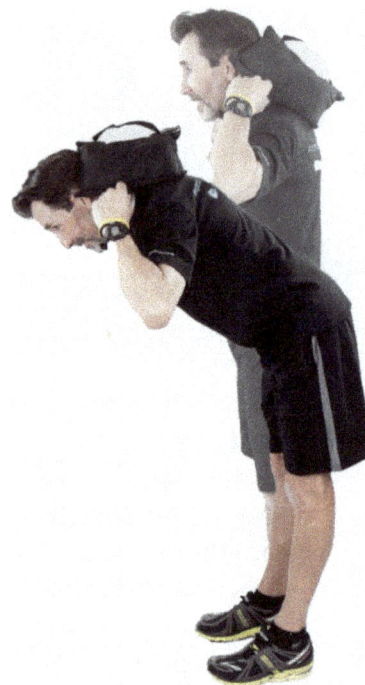

- Hip Flexion With Optional Elastic Bands

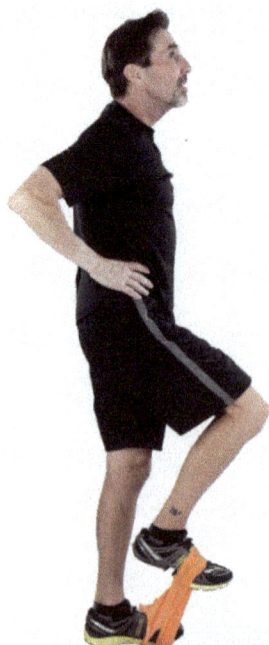

MUSCLE TARGET:
Iliopsoas, rectus femoris
HOW TO DO THIS EXERCISE:
Place your feet shoulder width apart and slide the elastic band under around each foot. Lift one leg in a slow and controlled motion to a 90-degree angle and then alternate the other leg.
HELPFUL HINTS:
Inhale while lifting your leg, exhale while returning to the start position.

Motivation

"Most people give up just when they're about to achieve success. They quit on the one-yard line. They give up at the last minute of the game one foot from a winning touchdown." – *Ross Perot*

172

- Side Lunge Squat

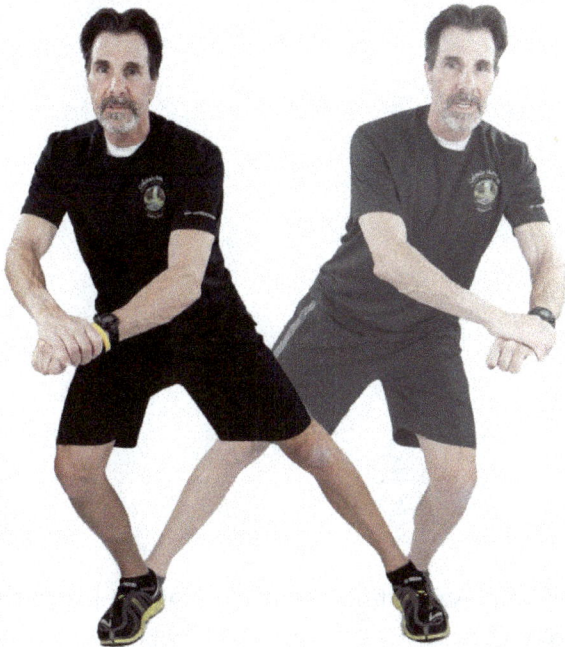

MUSCLE TARGET:

Quadriceps femoris, gluteus maximus, back thigh muscles, adductors

HOW TO DO THIS EXERCISE:

Stand upright and place your feet wide apart, arms extended in front of you. Look straight ahead and keep your back straight. Make slow and controlled side-step squats until you reach a 90-degree angle in the knee of the active leg. (The active leg is the one that is supporting the majority of your weight.

HELPFUL HINTS:

Your knees should never go over the imaginary line of your toes. Inhale while squatting and exhale when you are in the upright start position.

- Forward/Backward Lunge

MUSCLE TARGET:

Quadriceps femoris, gluteus maximus, back thigh muscles

HOW TO DO THIS EXERCISE:

Stand upright and place your feet at shoulder width with your hands resting on your hips. Look straight ahead and keep your back straight. Make slow and controlled backward steps until you reach a 90-degree angle position in the knee joint of the front leg. Return to the start position and alternate the other leg.

HELPFUL HINTS:

Keep your back straight, with your knee and foot directly in front of you. Inhale while squatting and exhale when returning to the start position.

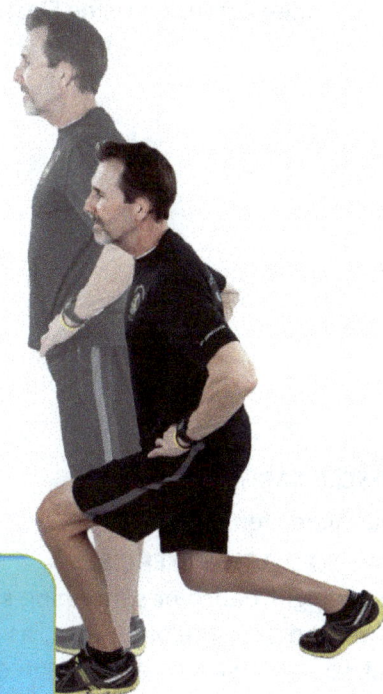

> **Motivation**
>
> **"Obstacles are those frightening things that become visible when we take our eyes off our goals."** – *Henry Ford*

Lower Leg Strengthening Exercises Without Weights:

- Standing Knee Extension

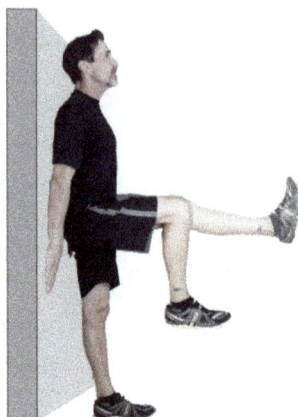

MUSCLE TARGET:
Quadriceps femoris
HOW TO DO THIS EXERCISE:
Stand with your back to the wall and heels touching the wall. Raise the knee of your active leg to the height of the hip. Return to the start position and alternate legs. Keep your back as straight as possible and lift with a slow and controlled motion.
HELPFUL HINTS:
Exhale while extending the knee, and inhale when returning to the start position.

- Knee Extension Using Elastic Band

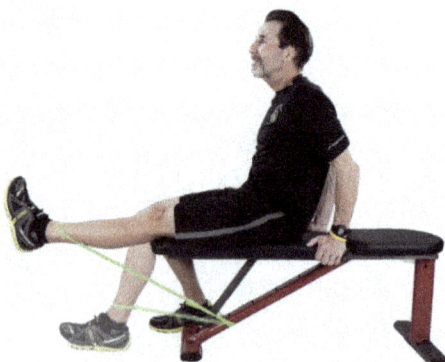

MUSCLE TARGET:

Quadriceps femoris

HOW TO DO THIS EXERCISE:

On a weight bench or something similar, place the elastic band around one foot, through the leg of the bench and over the other foot, as shown in the picture. Support yourself with your arms, keeping your back straight. Straighten your knee with slow and controlled movements, return to the start position and alternate legs.

HELPFUL HINTS:

Inhale while extending the knee, and exhale when returning to the start position.

174

- Standing Calf Extension with Three Variations

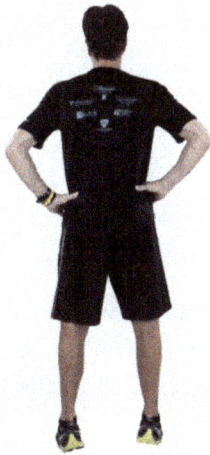 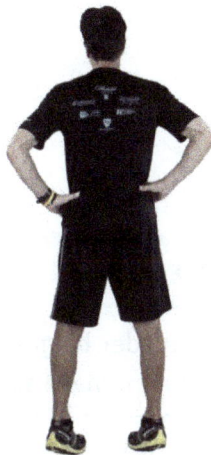 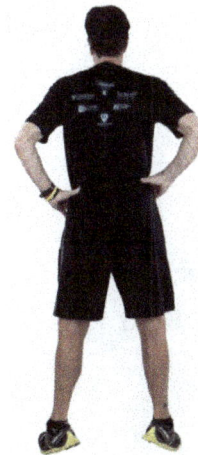

Feet Parallel   **Feet Inward**   **Feet Outward**

MUSCLE TARGET:
Gastrocnemius, soleus, plantaris
HOW TO DO THIS EXERCISE:
Place your feet in line with the width of the hips for better balance, hands resting on the waist, with your feet parallel, pointing inward or outward as shown in the pictures. Make slow and controlled toe lift movement to ankle extension.
HELPFUL HINTS:
Inhale while lifting, exhale while returning to the start position.

- Bench Step

MUSCLE TARGET:
Quadriceps femoris, gluteus maximus, back thigh muscles
HOW TO DO THIS EXERCISE:
Stand upright and place your feet in line with the shoulders. Place the foot of the active leg on the edge of the bench, hands resting on the hips. Make slow and controlled upwards step and stand on the bench. Step down to the start position and alternate legs.
HELPFUL HINTS:
Keep your back straight and try to lift yourself instead of lunging upwards. Inhale while lifting; exhale while returning to the start position.

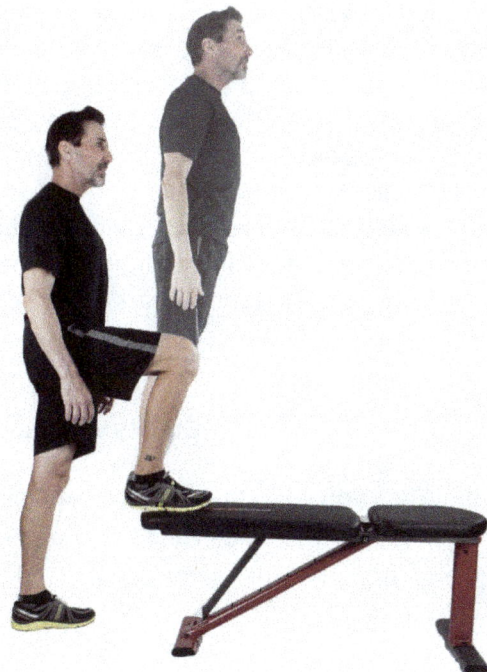

Arms, Neck and Shoulder Strengthening Exercises:

- Alternating Dumbbell Biceps Curl

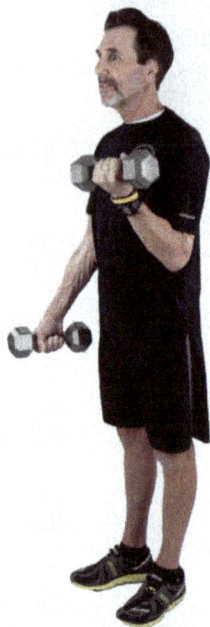

MUSCLE TARGET:
Biceps brachii, brachialis, brachioradialis
HOW TO DO THIS EXERCISE:
Stand upright, keeping the dumbbell at shoulder width while you lift to shoulder height. Alternate arms and alternate normal and inverted grip. Make slow and controlled biceps curl to the highest possible position of forearms.
HELPFUL HINTS:
Keep the elbows locked against your body for better stability. Keep weights light and use more repetitions. Inhale while curling and exhale when returning your hands down to the extended start position.

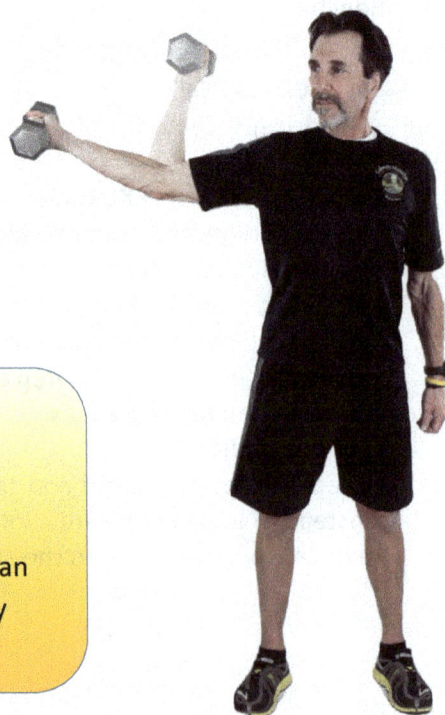

- One-hand Side Dumbbell Biceps Curl

MUSCLE TARGET:
Biceps brachii, brachialis, brachioradialis
HOW TO DO THIS EXERCISE:
Stand upright with feet in the width of your shoulders; hold the dumbbell with your hand, bending slightly at the elbows. Position your elbows to the height of your head. Make slow and controlled side bicep curls until you reach a 90 degree bend of the elbow.
HELPFUL HINTS:
For increased stability hold another dumbbell in the inactive hand. Inhale while curling and exhale when returning your hands down to the extended start position.

> **Tip**
>
> **Quality vs. Quantity**
>
> When you go to the weight room, plan your activities for that day in advance. Just like running "junk miles," you can overdo it in your weight training. Always focus on quality not, quantity.

- Overhead Dumbbell Triceps Extension

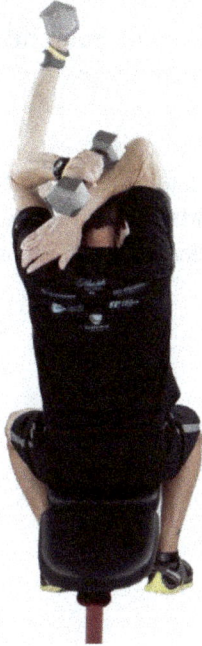

MUSCLE TARGET:

Triceps brachii

HOW TO DO THIS EXERCISE:

Sit on a weight bench or chair and with your free hand, hold your upper part of the active arm. Hold the dumbbell with a prone grip behind your head and then place your elbow in an extended position with the weight towards the sky. Repeat five to 10 times. Return to the start position and alternate hands. Make slow and controlled elbow extensions until you reach full extension.

HELPFUL HINTS:

Use your inactive arm as support for the active arm. Inhale while extending your arm and exhale while returning to the start position.

- Close-Grip Pushups

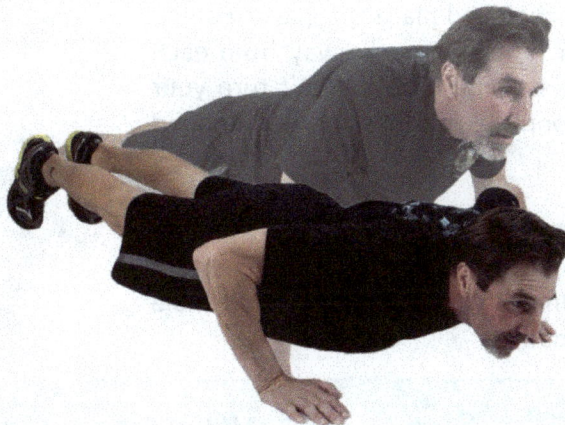

MUSCLE TARGET:

Triceps brachii, deltoideus, pectoralis major

HOW TO DO THIS EXERCISE:

With your toes and palms of your hands on the floor, extend your arms, lifting your body. Keep your back straight. Make slow and controlled motions while lifting and returning to the start position.

HELPFUL HINTS:

Don't allow your chest to rest on the floor and keep your hands at shoulder width. Keep your elbows close to your body. Inhale while lifting and exhale while returning to the start position.

- Neck Extension with Resistance

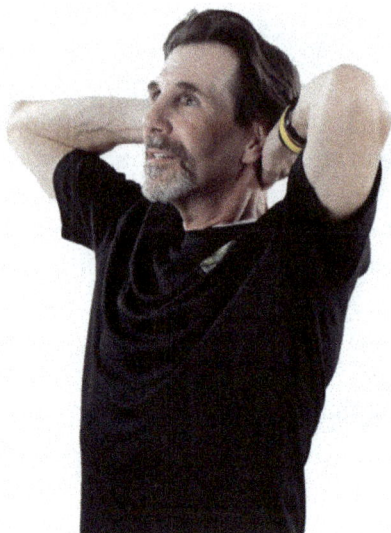

MUSCLE TARGET:
Erector spinae, trapezius, intrinsic muscles of the back
HOW TO DO THIS EXERCISE:
Stand or sit straight and place your hands behind your head, straightening the back. Make slow and controlled neck extensions keeping your head aligned with your spine.
HELPFUL HINTS:
Contract the shoulder and forearm muscles so that your arms are firm and stable during the exercise. Do not rotate your head, look forward at all times. Inhale while moving backwards and exhale while pushing forward.

- Neck Extension Using an Elastic Band

MUSCLE TARGET:
Erector spinae, trapezius, intrinsic muscles of the back
HOW TO DO THIS EXERCISE:
Sit on a weight bench or chair and place the elastic behind your head. Extend your arms and neck away from each other and return to the start position. Don't turn your head, and use slow and controlled motions for the extended and contracted motion.
HELPFUL HINTS:
Spread the elastic wide to ensure safe and equal pressure during the exercise so the elastic doesn't slip. Never overextend your neck. Inhale while extending and exhale while contracting the band.

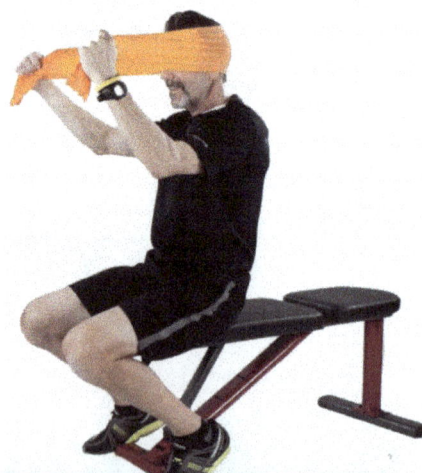

Motivation

"During my 18 years I came to bat almost 10,000 times. I struck out about 1,700 times and walked maybe 1,800 times. You figure a ballplayer will average about 500 at bats a season. That means I played seven years without ever hitting the ball." — *Mickey Mantle*

Stretching: Focus on Flexibility

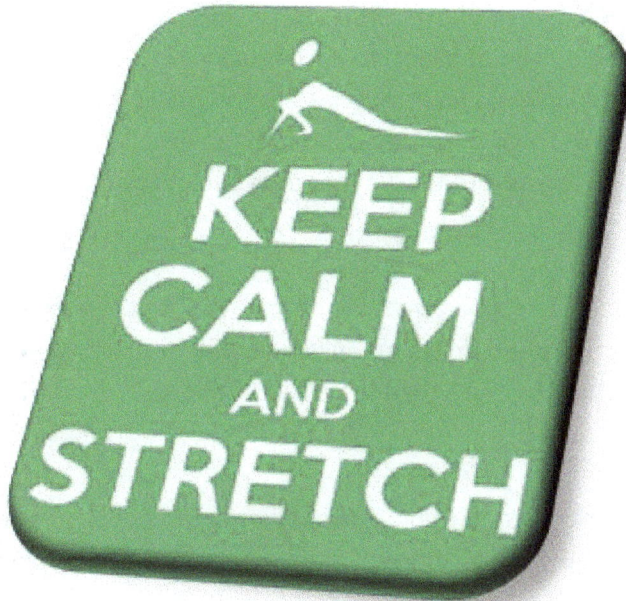

Stretching may not seem like a priority in your normal exercise routine because it takes extra time —time that you might not want to take away from your primary exercise. But beware! Avoiding this part of your routine could result in more frequent injuries.

Studies suggest that stretching may help your overall range of motion, which could help produce better results on race day.

Benefits of Stretching

When stretching properly, athletes seem to improve their overall performance, while decreasing the risk of injury.

Other benefits of stretching include better blood flow to the muscles, which warms the muscles up before a race, and aids in healing after a race. Don't short-change yourself by missing the stretch portion of your workout.

Finally, stretching can help with the mental aspects of your workout, giving you time to focus before a big performance. Make it part of your routine!

Stretching Essentials

Before you begin your stretching strategy, take the time to learn safe and effective ways to do it. One of the side benefits of stretching is that you can do it just about anywhere and you don't need any equipment.

Know When to Exercise Caution

Use caution when stretching muscles that are already injured, as this may cause additional damage. Finally, don't think that because you stretch, you can't get injured. Always consult a doctor or physical therapist if you are unsure about a particular stretch. While stretching does return the blood supply and seem to help limber the muscles and joints before a performance, it does little or nothing to help with soreness after a performance. As a matter of fact, overstretching can cause more tearing and pain and hinder short term performance. And therein lies the problem for many people – they tend to overstretch and cause muscle damage in the process.

Use These Tips to Keep Stretching Safe:

- **Don't Substitute Stretching in Place of a Warm-up** – Never stretch with cold muscles. Before stretching, warm up with a brisk walk, jog or a bit of biking at low intensity for five to ten minutes. Better yet, stretch lightly after you exercise, when your muscles are completely warmed up. Be wary of stretching before an intense activity, such as sprinting or track and field activities, as some researchers suggest that pre-event stretching before these types of events may actually decrease performance.

- **Strive for Symmetry** – Not all of us are as flexible as we'd like to be. You don't have to stretch like a rubber band or bend like a pretzel. Instead, focus on building equal flexibility from side to side, particularly if you injure or favor one side more than the other. Make sure that you stretch both sides equally.

- **Focus on Major Muscle Groups** – Rather than stretching individual muscles, focus on stretching entire muscle groups, such as upper leg (all of the quadriceps muscles), lower leg, hips, back, neck and shoulders.

- **Hold Your Stretch, Don't Bounce** – Stretch using smooth movements and without bouncing. Bouncing can cause injury to your muscle. Hold each stretch for about 30 seconds; in problem areas, you may need to hold for approximately 60 seconds.

- **Don't Aim for Pain** – Expect to feel tension while you're stretching but not pain. If you feel pain when you stretch, you're pushing it too far. Back off to the point where there is no pain, and then hold the stretch for 30 to 60 seconds.

- **Make Stretches Sport-specific** – If you participate in triathlons, stretch your lower body parts specific to the run and bike, and the upper body parts to the swim and always stretch your core muscles.

- **Keep Up with Your Stretching** – Stretching seems like it may take quality time from your workout, but you'll receive the most benefits if you keep a regular schedule of two to three times per week. If you don't stretch regularly, you risk losing any benefits that stretching offers in the first place.

- **Bring Movement into Your Stretching** – Gentle motion can help you be more flexible in specific areas. The gentle motions of yoga or t'ai chi may be a good way to stretch and build strength at the same time. Make sure you're stretching the muscles you're going to use for your athletic performance that day.

> **Motivation**
>
> **"By failing to prepare, you are preparing to fail."** – *Benjamin Franklin*

Isometrics, Plyometrics and Powerlifting

Much of the previous section focused on weight training, using little or no actual weights. We looked at a couple of lifts that used dumbbells, but for the most part, our routine was based on lifting only our own body weight, very light hand weights or the use of elastic bands. But, what about powerlifting? Can a routine with heavy weights help us with our running? Yes, it can! While weights are not required for your running program, they can certainly add to your core strength, balance and agility. From the previous chapters, we know that strengthening the core can result in improved running economy. It allows us to maintain better posture late in a race. This framework keeps you upright and allows better function of the diaphragm, which results in better oxygen distribution and less fatigue.

You can definitely realize benefits from powerlifting, but as a runner, you need to keep the two types of training balanced. Too much powerlifting can add bulk to your muscles and unneeded weight. Yes, you will be stronger, but your performance may suffer from the additional weight. The trick is to keep both activities in balance and allow one to benefit the other.

To begin, you need to have a balanced program, such as powerlifting two days a week and running three days a week. Try to weight train at least two days per week and base all of your training around your long run. If you're a marathon runner, try to schedule your powerlifting two days after your long run, in conjunction with a very short run. Add another powerlifting session two days after that. For instance, if your long run is scheduled for Sunday, do a short run and powerlift session on Monday and Wednesday. Use the remaining days – Tuesday, Thursday and Friday for short training runs (fartleks, strides, etc.,) and/or cross-training, depending on where you're at in your training plan. Always leave at least one day for rest. We'll get into the basic training plans in the next chapter – **Chapter 13 – Training Basics.**

Most powerlifting programs revolve around squats, deadlifts and bench presses. Your lifting days should be difficult, but manageable and relatively pain free from the effects of your long run.

Keep in mind that if you're getting close to your race date, or finding it difficult to schedule weightlifting and running on the same day, mix it up. It might be to your advantage to do "two-a-day" workouts. For example, you might do your heavy weight lifting on a Wednesday morning, followed by a quick weight "refresher," using moderate weights on Wednesday evening. Likewise, you can run a bit longer in the morning and still be fresh enough for a second run that same evening. Remember to *adapt* to your work and home schedule. Be flexible in your planning and schedule a contingency session if the first one doesn't work out. Think outside the box! We're not all the same and we don't all share the same timetables. Create a plan that works for YOU!

Motivation

"**Racing teaches us to challenge ourselves. It teaches us to push beyond where we thought we could go. It helps us to find out what we are made of. This is what we do. This is what it's all about.**" – *PattiSue Plumer*

Plyometrics

A number of studies have shown that training with plyometrics (bounding and jumping exercises involving repeated rapid eccentric and concentric muscle contractions) improves running economy by increasing muscle power. This power is the combination of speed and force, and can be enhanced by heavy weight training to improve overall strength and plyometric training to improve the speed at which muscular force is applied.

Isometrics can also be used as a form of resistance strength exercises. Isometrics are exercises in which the muscles do not expand or contract, such as pushing your fist into the palm of your other hand, and pressing hard. While you feel the tension and resistance in your arms, you're neither contracting nor expanding the length of your muscles.

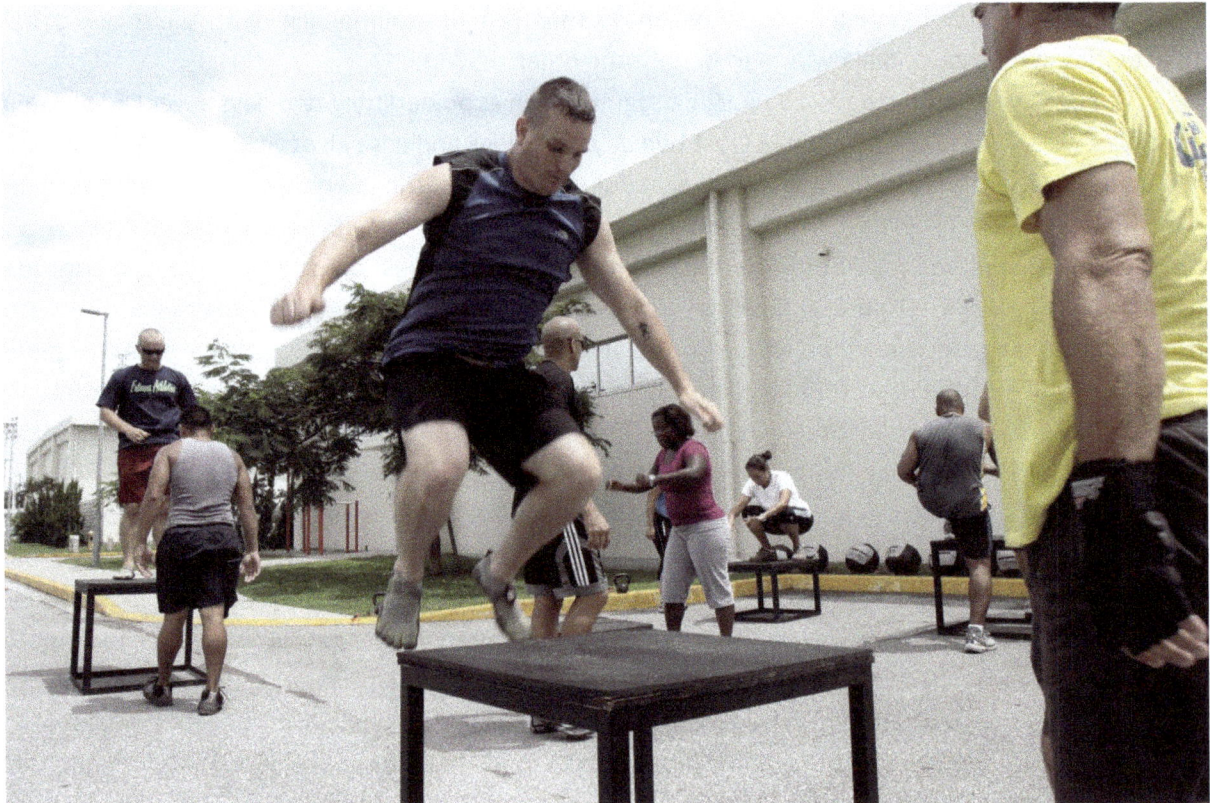

Working out on plyometric equipment

Yoga - Beyond Common Exercises and Stretches

Obviously, this book is about running, but I also submit to you a recommendation: bring yoga into your life. Men, put your ego aside and take a good look at the benefits of yoga. Yoga is not a religion and it's not just for women. It's a way of elevating the life force within you, through a series of physical and mental exercises. The various postures in yoga can help you develop flexibility, stamina, balance, and strength for your physical being, while the mental techniques include breathing exercises or meditation to discipline the mind. Both of these can help you as you prepare for your race, especially before the start when your mind is doing the racing! Ultimately, the goal of yoga is to help the individual to "transcend the self and attain enlightenment."

Importance of Yoga

Yoga is designed to bring the physical, mental and spiritual aspects together to promote a well-balanced individual. Yoga is said to increase your self-awareness, enhance personal power, promote self-healing and attain equilibrium and harmony from within. This helps you deal with everyday stressors in your life, and allows you to be healthier – mentally, physically and spiritually.

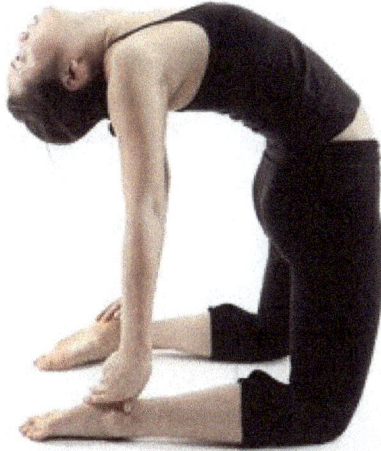

Challenge!

Stay Strong

In this chapter, we learned about the combination of *strength* and *conditioning,* to build *fitness.* The level of fitness you gain from this chapter will directly impact your success in the upcoming chapters, which deal with training basics, cross-training and the creation of your goals and training plans. We are now at a juncture in this book that can define success or failure.

Your challenge: From now to the end of this book, take detailed notes of your gym workouts, and alternate your upper and lower body reps. Stretch properly before and after each workout to increase flexibility. Seek balance and symmetry with every workout, and focus on major muscle groups, rather than individual muscles.

Are you ready to run? Turn to the next chapter, and let's do what we came for!

Motivation

"It's not the will to win that matters—everyone has that. It's the will to prepare to win that matters." *– Paul "Bear" Bryant*

Chapter 13 – Training Basics

My Story

When I first started running, I asked Keith, my friend and mentor, about proper breathing techniques. I said I was struggling to create a rhythm between my foot strikes and my breathing pattern. Keith immediately told me that I was overthinking my breathing – that I shouldn't really be thinking about my breathing; it should just happen naturally. At first it didn't work, but eventually, breathing while running became as natural as breathing while sleeping. Most of my concerns took care of themselves as my fitness increased – most of the breathing problems I had were directly related to shortness of breath. In other words, I was running too hard for my current physical condition. As my fitness level increased, my problems with breathing decreased.

This chapter will reveal things that should be simple, but sometimes get over-complicated – things like posture and breathing. This chapter deals with basics and tells us how to get in running shape within six weeks, even if you've never run before. This chapter gives us a *starting point*.

We've examined everything from the history of running all the way to modern technology for running – and everything in between. I shared some of my personal experiences with you to help you prepare for your very own journey ahead. But now it's time to put the rubber to the road. Let's rewind all the way to the beginning and review the basics.

As I mentioned at the beginning of this book, I wasn't able to run a single lap around the local track when I first started running. Desire, perseverance, willpower, and a healthy dose of stubbornness drove me down the path to a long, happy, and healthy running livelihood. If you've made it this far in this book, you're also showing that same drive.

If you're feeling a bit apprehensive, nervous, or intimidated by running, take heart – you're not alone. Most of us felt the same way when we first began our running program, and some of us still feel that same way before a race, even though we might have done it several hundred times. Embrace that energy and funnel it internally to maximize your potential.

First Things First – See Your Doctor – To begin your running program, start with medical clearance from your doctor. This should be your number one priority, well ahead of the purchase of your running shoes. Make sure your doctor knows what your goals are, what your health issues are, and what your risks are. A doctor visit is even more important if:

- You are a former smoker.
- You are over the age of 40, where most medical issues begin to emerge.
- You've lived a sedentary lifestyle for a year or more.
- You are overweight or obese.

- You have high blood pressure.
- Your family has a history of health issues, including heart problems or high blood pressure.
- You're pregnant.
- You have diabetes.
- You have dizzy or fainting spells.
- You have other health-related concerns.

When you consult your doctor, make sure he or she completes a full health assessment and analysis of existing conditions and make sure to follow your doctor's recommendations. Also, let your doctor know if you are trying to lose weight along with your running program, as he may offer other suggestions pertaining to diet and medication.

A full health assessment should include a stress test on a treadmill to rule out any latent cardiovascular problems that might surface under intense exercise. Benchmarks should be started so you can compare your overall health the next time you go to the doctor. Most doctors now recommend having a physical every five years if you're under the age of 40 and every one to three years over 40 years of age. Of course, you should always contact your doctor if you incur an injury or have other health concerns.

Focus on Form – As I mentioned in **Chapter 3 – What is Running?**, correct running form is vital to a long and healthy way of life. To reiterate, let's look at a few ways to help you run faster and more efficiently, reduce the stress on your body and the likelihood of injury.

- **Look Ahead** – Scan your path 10 to 20 feet ahead, looking for obstacles. If you're running trails, you may have to shorten this distance, as there are plenty of things that can trip you up.
- **Center Up** – Try to land on your midfoot. Research shows that running on your toes can cause tightness in your calves, pain in your shins and early fatigue. Striking your heels first causes a braking effect which wastes precious energy and can cause injury.
- **Point Your Toes Forward** – Keep your toes pointed straight ahead. Pointing your feet too far inward or outward can cause injury.
- **Run Efficiently** – Don't over-stride! By keeping your stride short and your feet close to the ground, you'll increase your running efficiency. Shoot for a pace of 90 steps per minute (each foot, for a total of 180 steps), and focus on this turnover rate whether you're running uphill, downhill, or on a flat surface. Don't bounce when you run.
- **Relax**! – Keep your hands relaxed, at your sides, and at waist level. Keep your arms swinging in a front to back motion, without your crossing your hands in front of your chest. Don't clench your fists or tighten your neck and shoulders. Your hands should be loose enough to grasp an egg without breaking it.
- **Monitor Your Posture** – Due to fatigue, your posture can deteriorate the longer you run, unless you keep assessing it as you go. Keep your head up, your shoulders level, and your back straight. Maintaining your posture is just as important as your target of 90 steps per minute.

Motivation

"I walk slowly, but I never walk backwards." – *Abraham Lincoln*

Warm Up, Cool Down – Before you start your run, you should always stretch or warm up your muscles to avoid injury. A good warmup will dilate your blood vessels to make sure your muscles are getting the proper amount of oxygen. It also raises your body's temperature to allow optimal efficiency and flexibility. Finally, your heart will be happier because it doesn't have such an abrupt increase in pulse rate, which can stress your cardiovascular system.

Likewise, you should finish an intense workout with a cool down that allows your heart rate and blood pressure to stabilize. Stopping suddenly can cause lightheadedness or fainting. (See postural hypotension in **Chapter 6 – Running Physiology**).

Proper warmups and cool down methods are crucial for maintaining a good run. Here's how you should do them:

- As we saw earlier in this chapter, it's not a good idea to stretch cold muscles. Before you begin your stretching, do about five to ten minutes of light aerobic exercise to limber up your muscles and warm you up for your run. A brisk walk, slow jog or a short warmup on a stationary bike will properly warm up your legs.
- When you begin your run, start with a jog or slow run, and gradually build to your target pace. Unless you're racing, your breathing should be easy and if you feel too winded, slow down. Of course, if you're racing, you should complete a good warmup before you start your run.
- When you finish your run, cool down by walking or slowly jogging for five to 10 minutes.
- Stretch fully after your cool down. Your body should be adequately warmed up and stretching should feel easy.
- Stretch your lower back, neck, calves, quadriceps, hamstrings and groin area. Hold each stretch for 15 to 30 seconds.

Breathe Easy

MYTH: You should inhale through your nose and exhale through your mouth when running.

MYTH BUSTER: Your cardiovascular and muscular systems need a lot of oxygen delivered to them. Inhaling only through your nose will simply starve your body. You need to use both your nose and mouth for taking in precious oxygen.

MYTH: You should only breathe using your chest, and avoid "deep belly breathing," in which you let your stomach expand, instead of your lungs above the diaphragm.

MYTH BUSTER: Deep belly breathing allows you to take in more air, and research indicates it may help to prevent side stitches. Make sure you're breathing more from your diaphragm, or belly, not from your chest – that's too shallow. When you breathe, make sure that you exhale completely to remove carbon dioxide.

> **Motivation**
>
> **"Do a little more each day than you think you possibly can."** – *Lowell Thomas*

Walk Before You Run

We've all heard the terms, "crawl before you walk" and "walk before you run." There's nothing more accurate or important than "walk before you run." When you begin your running program, it's best to start it based on a walk/run routine. You started this journey because you felt the need to better your health and lifestyle. You made the choice and commitment to better health, just as I did when I started my running program. Let's look at ten different types of workouts. We'll start with the run/walk program and later in this chapter we'll look at the other nine cardio workouts.

So what is the walk/run routine? How can you transition into a run-only program? How can you convert a sedentary lifestyle into an active one? How much time do you need to commit?

These are common questions that beg to be answered. Well, my friends, these questions are very easy to answer if you don't try to overthink them, or overestimate your potential. One of the biggest mistakes beginners make is to try to put their running goals into mile increments. Because they're thinking purely in terms of miles, their goals are jeopardized from the start. Instead of thinking in mileage, plan your goals in terms of time – minutes, not hours. This will help you build up from a normal-paced walk, to a brisk walk, to walk/jog combination and finally into a full jog or run routine. If this is your first time in a running program, or if it's been a while since you were in one – start slowly. This will help you develop your muscular and skeletal systems, as well as your cardiovascular system. Starting slowly will help you avoid common injuries and give you confidence as you build up.

Let's break it down into four different categories:

- Walking
- Brisk walking
- Walking and jogging
- Jogging and running

Walking Program

At first, set aside ten minutes per day, three to five days per week. It doesn't sound like much in terms of mileage, but the health benefits should begin within two weeks. Gradually work up to 30 minutes per day, four to five days per week. Even if you're overweight, you should be able establish a routine in three to four weeks.

Brisk Walking

When you're comfortable with walking 30 minutes per day, incorporate *brisk* walking into your program. A brisk walk should raise your heart rate and cause you to breathe fairly heavily. You won't be able to get enough oxygen through your nose, so you'll need to use both your nose and mouth for breathing. You will most likely work up a sweat after 10 to 12 minutes of brisk walking. Try to get to the point where you are brisk walking for 30 minutes per workout, four to five times per week. Once you're comfortable with that, you're ready to mix jogging into your program.

Walking and Jogging

Once you've accomplished the brisk walk phase, you're ready to add light running into your regimen. Again, don't think about mileage! Think only in terms of time on your feet, and what you're doing with that time. In the following tables, I've put together a starter program. You may need to adjust it according to your age, fitness level and capabilities. The schedule for the first three weeks is based on seven minute cycles. Of course, you still need to add a few minutes for warmup and cool down periods, before and after your run. If you follow this schedule, you should be able to run the full seven minutes beginning at week four!

Week 1	Brisk Walk Duration	Jog or Run Duration
Sunday	6 minutes	1 minute
Monday	5 ½ minutes	1 ½ minutes
Tuesday	Rest or cross-train	Rest or cross-train
Wednesday	5 minutes	2 minutes
Thursday	4 ½ minutes	2 ½ minutes
Friday	4 minutes	3 minutes
Saturday	Rest	Rest

Week 2	Brisk Walk Duration	Jog or Run Duration
Sunday	4 minutes	3 minutes
Monday	3 ½ minutes	3 ½ minutes
Tuesday	Rest or cross-train	Rest or cross-train
Wednesday	3 minutes	4 minutes
Thursday	2 ½ minutes	4 ½ minutes
Friday	2 minutes	5 minutes
Saturday	Rest	Rest

Week 3	Brisk Walk Duration	Jog or Run Duration
Sunday	3 minutes	4 minute
Monday	2 ½ minutes	4 minutes
Tuesday	Rest or cross-train	Rest or cross-train
Wednesday	2 minutes	5 minutes
Thursday	1 ½ minutes	5 ½ minutes
Friday	1 minutes	6 minutes
Saturday	Rest	Rest

Week 4	Brisk Walk Duration	Jog or Run Duration
Sunday	1 minute	7 minutes
Monday	1 minute	8 minutes
Tuesday	Rest or cross-train	Rest or cross-train
Wednesday	1 minute	9 minutes
Thursday	30 seconds	10 minutes
Friday	0 minutes	10 minutes
Saturday	Rest	Rest

Week 4 begins your transition to a "runner." Your walk duration is minimized to zero minutes and your run time moves into a full 10-minute jog or run.

Week 5	Brisk Walk Duration	Jog or Run Duration
Sunday	0 minutes	10 minutes
Monday	0 minutes	15 minutes
Tuesday	Rest or cross-train	Rest or cross-train
Wednesday	0 minutes	12 minutes
Thursday	0 minutes	17 minutes
Friday	0 minutes	20 minutes
Saturday	Rest	Rest

Week five is where you begin to run with no walk breaks (if you choose to). From there, extend your running time to match your goals. You'll notice that on some occasions, your run duration drops instead of increasing, but the overall trend is to add minutes during the week, with at least one day of rest.

Run/Walk Methodology

Don't be intimidated by the running schedule that I recommend. You can change it to fit your own needs. For example, if you're really struggling with the program, repeat one of the weekly schedules until you get comfortable. Likewise, if you feel you can run for 10 minutes when you're only scheduled to go eight minutes – *go for it!* There are three important elements to the run/walk method:

- Make it YOUR schedule – customize to fit your busy life and your running goals
- Honor the rest days – overtraining is easy to do, especially when you're starting out
- Set an upward trend – even if you run fewer minutes on Wednesday than you did on Monday, make sure that it's an upward trend for the entire week. Again, don't worry about how many miles you cover – focus on time.

Tip

As a beginner, try to run at a pace at which you can breathe easily. Use the "talk test" to figure out if your pace matches your current fitness level. You should be able to speak in full sentences, without gasping for air. Slow down or walk if you're short of breath. If you relax and slow the pace, breathing problems usually take care of themselves.

Motivation

"Be of good cheer. Do not think of today's failures, but of the success that may come tomorrow. You have set yourselves a difficult task, but you will succeed if you persevere and you will find a joy in overcoming obstacles. Remember, no effort that we make to attain something beautiful is ever lost." – *Helen Keller*

Tips

- Before you start your session for the day, warm up with a normal five-minute walk.
- Keep repeating your run/walk pattern until you've covered your goal time. For example, if you want to run/walk for 14 minutes, you can run/walk at a 1:6 ratio for two cycles.
- Make sure that you're using the proper form with your entire body.
- Start your brisk walk cycle *before* your run cycle to properly warm up your body and avoid early fatigue or injury. A brisk start will elevate your heart rate to prepare for the run cycle.
- Use a running watch than can track multiple timers: one for your walk cycle and one for your run cycle. Get a watch that beeps at the beginning and end of each cycle.
- During your run/walk program, try to extend the amount of time you're running and reduce your walking time. Don't increase your run time by more than a couple of minutes when you first start your program.
- After your run/walk session, take an additional five minutes to "cool down" by using a slower walk and good stretching exercises.

History of the Run/Walk Method

The run/walk method has been around for a long time, but in 1974, elite runner and Olympian, Jeff Galloway made it very popular. Jeff led a group of former non-runners by introducing them into his program that featured a run/walk combination. After 10 weeks of training, all of his "students" successfully ran (and walked) a 5k – without injury.

Studies showed continued successes with seasoned runners at longer distances. Jeff's research showed that even average marathon runners, could run a *faster* marathon by using the run/walk combination, than by trying to run the entire 26.2 miles. Further studies showed that his pupils experienced fewer injuries with quicker recovery times, and less stress on the entire body. It also kept the athletes' bodies from overheating and reduced overall fatigue.

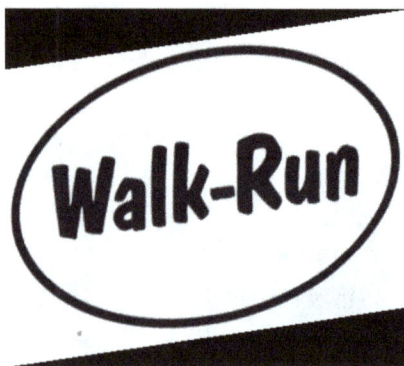

I can personally vouch for Jeff's training method. I have never done it myself, but I've been passed late in a marathon by several, if not many, run/walk participants. The important part of the technique is that you *must* take a walk break at scheduled times for the entire race. If you run a complete marathon, that's 25 one-minute walk breaks. On average, people who use the run/walk routine, finish a marathon 13 minutes faster than they would have if they had run the entire distance!

While it may not be for everyone, at least give it a try if you're struggling to run an entire race, no matter what the distance is.

Workout Types

On the previous pages, I described ways to get you off the couch and begin your new running lifestyle with the run/walk method. Or maybe you're starting over from days gone by. Either way, you should look for other training methods besides the run/walk program to see what works best for you. In this section, we'll look at nine more cardio-focused runs to really get your blood flowing!

- Base run
- Interval run
- Fartlek
- Tempo run
- Progression run
- Hill running
- Hill repeats
- Long run
- Recovery run

Of course, when we're done with this, we'll dive right into the next section: **Chapter 14 – Cross-training.** This will extend your capabilities and increase your physical capacity more than you can imagine! Let's now take the time to see the nine other ways to train and after I describe them, I'll try to cite examples of each type of run.

Base Run

Once you're able to sustain a basic run of 20 minutes or more, the next logical step is to establish your *base run.* A base run is a fairly short to moderate length run at a runner's natural gait and pace. This run does not need to be particularly challenging, but it should be done frequently, and should be the foundation of your aerobic capacity, endurance, and running economy. Base runs will make up the majority of your weekly training mileage.

On a personal level, I try to allow for about 60% of my weekly mileage on the base run, 25% on my long run and 15% on one of the other types, such as hill repeats, tempo runs or intervals.

Example: Run six to eight miles at a natural pace that doesn't completely exhaust you. Focus on 90 steps per minute, as outlined earlier in this book. Enjoy your run!

Interval Run

Interval workouts are exactly as they are labeled. They consist of repeated segments of moderate to fast-paced running separated by slow running or walking for a brief recovery. This allows the runner to avoid complete exhaustion and still be able to focus on a great cardio workout. Intervals are usually categorized as short or long intervals and are generally run on a track or flat trail. Short intervals are generally 400 to 800 meters in length, with a few quick recovery jogs between segments. Long intervals are 800 to 1,200-meter segments run faster than your normal 5K race pace with easy jogging recoveries between them. Effective interval workouts should be very intense and push you hard. You'll be "red-lining" during the interval and just waiting for that segment to end! During your recovery segment, be sure to allow enough time to run the next hard section as well as you ran the first one. Most seasoned runners will try to make each running segment a bit faster than the previous one, allowing just a little more time between each recovery period. The following examples are intended to be done at your local track.

Example #1 – The Short Interval: Warm up with two laps consisting of an easy jog, well below your normal training pace. Next, run 400 to 800 meters (one to two laps) at a 5K race pace or faster, followed by a 400 meter recovery jog. Depending on your current fitness level and your expected goals for the week, do this four to eight times. The mileage won't necessarily add up very quickly, but you'll reap the benefits of a fast-paced workout!

Example #2 – The Long Interval: Warm up with two laps consisting of an easy jog, well below your normal training pace. Next, run 800 to 1200 meters (two to three laps) at 10K race pace or faster, followed by a 400 meter recovery jog. Depending on your current fitness level and your expected goals for the week, do this four to eight times.

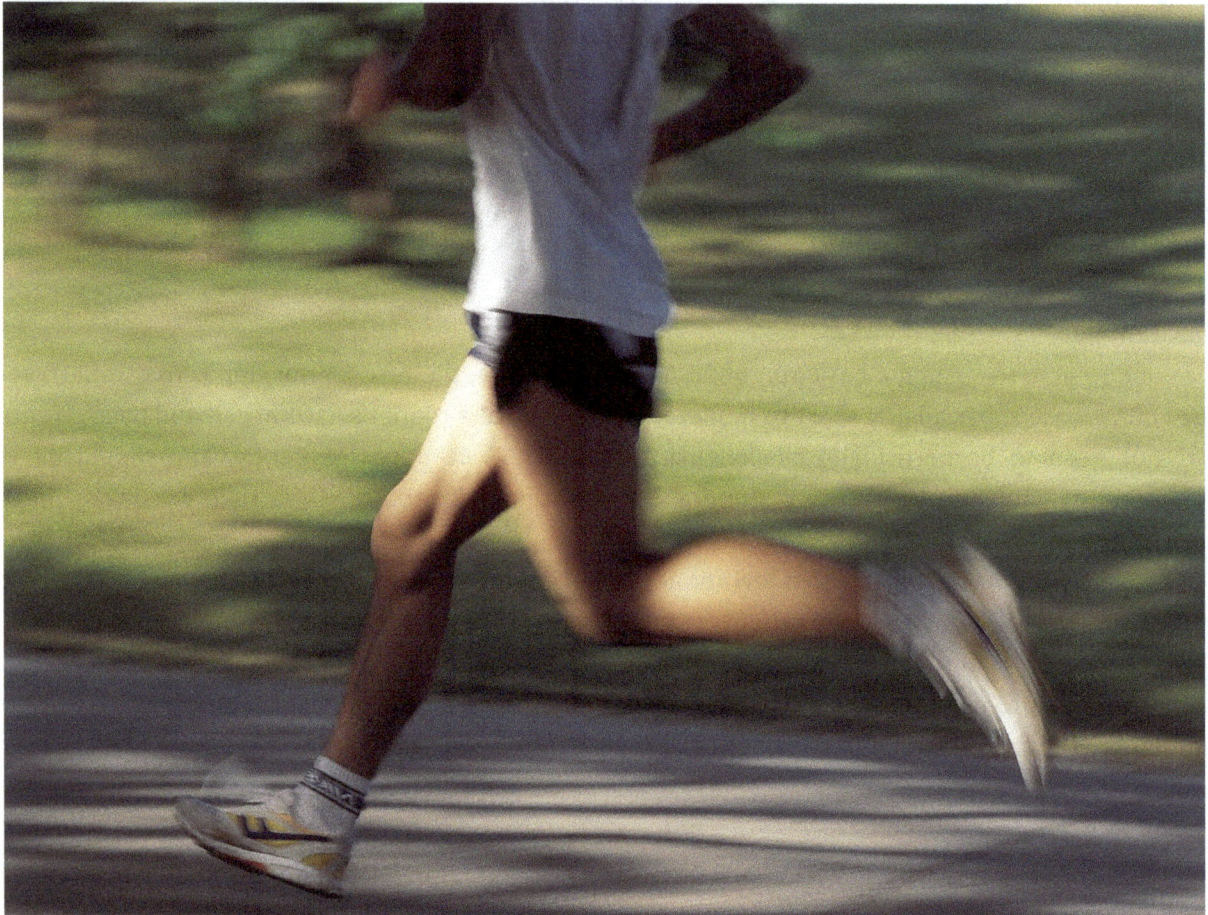

Pick up the pace with intervals, tempo runs and fartleks

Fartlek Run – Combining the Base Run with the Intervals
The term fartlek comes from Swedish origin, and essentially translates to "speed play." Unlike the formal structure of intervals or tempo runs, the fartlek combines the base run with the interval, at a pace and distance that you dictate. If you're feeling good, you simply speed up for as long as you can, and if you start to fatigue, you simply slow down. How neat is that? Just pick a road sign or landmark and pick up your pace until you reach it. For beginners, the fartlek workout is one of the best ways to increase your running efficiency and make the transition from the base run to race pace. Even for experienced runners, fartleks are an important training method to increase endurance with limited "pickups" that can help emulate real race conditions.

Example #1: Start with a quarter- to half-mile warmup run, slower than your normal pace. Run three to eight miles at a natural pace with 10 one-minute pickups at a 5k pace and one-minute recoveries during your run. Try not to walk or slow jog in fartlek exercises – attempt to maintain sustained pickups followed by cycles at a moderate pace. Take advantage of a lengthy cool-down run afterwards.

Example #2: For a stimulating outing, run with friends and take turns leading the group. This promotes teamwork as well as a little friendly competition. It keeps everyone mentally and physically sharp by pushing the entire group.

Tempo Run – Turning It Up a Notch

Back in **Chapter 6 – Running Physiology,** we discussed lactate threshold. In a nutshell, lactate threshold is defined as the fastest pace that can be sustained for one hour by a very fit individual. More or less, it's the fastest pace that can be sustained for 20 minutes in less fit runners. That definition provides the basis for the tempo run – "a sustained effort at lactate threshold intensity." Tempo or threshold runs serve to increase the speed you can sustain for a prolonged period of time and to increase the time you can sustain that relatively fast pace.

Example #1: Start with a half-mile warmup at slower than your normal pace. Start your first mile at your normal training pace, followed by one to four miles (depending on your current fitness level) at lactate threshold pace. Finish your run by slowing to your normal training pace for one mile. Always finish with an adequate cool-down run.

Experienced marathoners can enhance their training by a specific "marathon-pace" training run. Our next example shows how a prolonged run at marathon pace is a perfect way to fine tune your pace and endurance in the final weeks of preparation leading up to marathon race day.

Example #2: Start with your normal warmup of a quarter to half a mile. Start your run with two miles at your natural pace, followed by 13 to 15 miles at threshold pace. Finish your training segment with another two miles at your natural pace. Close out with an adequate cool-down jog.

A note about long tempo runs. Not every day is a good day for a long tempo run. Extreme weather, wind, fatigue, terrain and current energy levels can all be cause for a good day to go bad. If you're just not "feeling it" on your planned day, reschedule it. I know several people who over-trained and ultimately injured themselves because they were inflexible with their schedules. As always, listen to your body.

Motivation

"That's what a comeback is. You have a starting point and you build strength and momentum from there. Stay the course... remain patient. Focus on small steps that are constantly forward."
– *Kara Goucher*

Progression Run

Of all the different training runs, I find the progression one to be my favorite and probably the most beneficial, especially during the later stages of my training, just before a race. The concept is to start out slower than your natural pace, and gradually build to a strong finish. These runs are designed to be moderately challenging, but not to the extent of a tempo run. It should, however, be more difficult than your base run. My progression mantra is "Slow and steady with a strong finish." For years, this run was known as the "Kenyan's Secret," because it was, and still is a large portion of the elite athlete's training program. It teaches mental patience and allows you to "push" when you want to, and extends your base training by allowing your body to warm up completely during your run. The biggest benefit of this run is the way that it builds aerobic capacity and allows you to finish strong on race day!

The primary differences between intervals and the progression run are that the progression run has no break and it allows you to accelerate without strain – simply build up slowly into your finishing pace.

Finally, this is one of the best training runs for you and a running friend or a group of runners. It allows a little friendly competition, without all-out racing.

If I go for a six-mile run, for instance, I like to increase my pace by 15 seconds faster than the previous mile. During marathon distance training runs, I like to trim five seconds per mile faster than the previous mile. Whenever I do this, I always go much SLOWER than my natural pace for the first few miles – it gives me plenty of energy to finish strong, and allows my body temperature and heart rate to build up slowly.

A warmup isn't really necessary for progression runs, since you start out slowly anyway.

Example #1 – 10k Trainer: Mile 1 – 8:45, mile 2 – 8:30, mile 3 – 8:15, mile 4 – 8:00, mile 5, 7:45, mile 6 – 7:30.

Example #2 – 20 Mile Marathon Trainer: Mile 1 - 9:15; mile 2 – 9:10; mile 3 – 9:05; mile 4 – 9:00; mile 5 – 8:55; mile 6 – 8:50; mile 7 – 8:45; mile 8 – 8:40; mile 9 – 8:35; mile 10 – 8:30; mile 11 – 8:25; mile 12 – 8:20; mile 13 – 8:15; mile 14 – 8:10; mile 15 – 8:05; mile 16 – 8:00; mile 17 – 7:55; mile 18 – 7:50; mile 19 – 7:45; mile 20 – 7:40

Hill Running

The benefits of hill running are proven and well documented. Fact: If you want to gain strength and get in shape quickly, science shows that running hills will get you there faster. There are a number of ways that you can benefit from hill running, but we'll just take a look at "basic hill running" and "hill repeats."

Basic Hill Running is comprised of a combination of up and down hill running of various grades and distances. This is the "free-form" of hill running, with no set structure. The idea is to use different muscle groups to build strength in the muscular and connective tissues of your body. When you run hills, focus on form.

Don't forget about your 90 steps (per foot) of turnover. Strive to keep that pace on up and downhill sections, even if you have to shorten the stride dramatically. Remember – a quick turnover will beat length of stride almost every time – no matter the grade or distance.

Example: Run six to eight miles on a moderately hilly route. Combine intervals, tempo runs or progression runs for maximum training benefits. Try to maintain 90 steps per minute and practice good running form throughout. This is the least structured of all the training plans, but the most beneficial for gaining valuable strength in a short time.

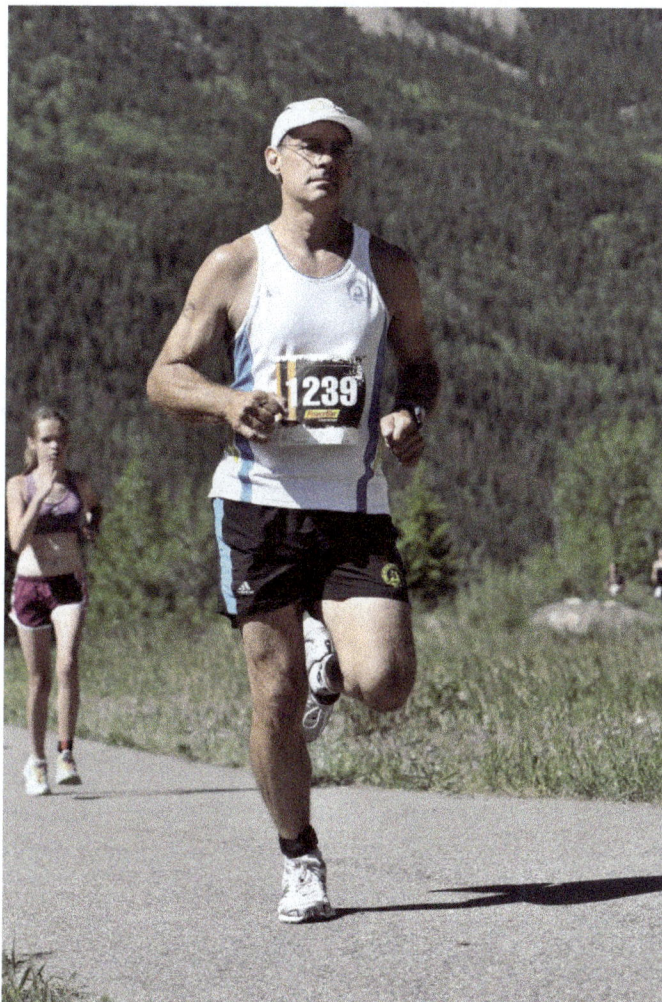

Run hills to boost your strength quickly

Hill Repeats

Hill repeats can help you build stamina and pain tolerance and quickly increase aerobic power. Hill repeats can also cause injury if you're not fully prepared to run them. Make sure you have established your base-building training before you begin hill repeats. The idea of hill repeats is to choose a moderately steep hill (4-6% grade) with 30 to 45 second speed bursts, from bottom to top. A thorough warmup is highly recommended before hill repeats are started. I like to run one to two miles at a slow to moderate pace before beginning my hill repeats.

Example: Begin with a one to two-mile warmup. Run ten 45-second hill repeats at a hard effort with a recovery of one to two minutes, which may include a slow jog back down the hill. You should always run a one to two-mile cool down after any intense run such as tempo runs or hill repeats.

Long Run – Simply put, the "long run" is an extended base run. I normally consider a "long run" as a run that leaves you moderately to severely fatigued and exposes you to "the wall" – the point at which your glycogen stores are nearly or completely depleted. "Hitting the wall" gives you the experience you'll need to finish a marathon and it normally hits around mile 18 or 30 kilometers for most runners. If you plan on running a marathon, be sure to read "My Story – the Marathon Owns You" in **Chapter 16 – Training Plans.**

As a point of reference, I usually consider the following distances to classify my training distances:

- **Short Distance Run** – 1 to 9.99 miles
- **Medium Distance Run** – 10 to 17.99 miles
- **Long Distance Run** – 18 to 26.2 miles
- **Ultra-Distance Run** – more than 26.2 miles

The Long Run should extend your base run and build stamina and endurance to run a given distance without stopping. This run should give you confidence to finish your race. If you're training for a marathon, I recommend going the full distance at least one time in your race preparation. Once you get comfortable with the long run, feel free to mix in tempo runs, fartleks and progression runs to fully boost your stamina – and your confidence!

Example: Run 19 miles at your natural pace. Ease into your run, and you won't need a warmup. Your first mile should be your slowest, and the remaining 18 should be fairly consistent, depending on the weather and terrain.

Recovery Run – The recovery run should be treated as a very easy run or jog. Recovery runs are used to maintain current fitness levels without taking away from performance. They're usually done right after or right before a strenuous training session. Recovery runs should not create additional fatigue and should be done as slowly as necessary to feel comfortable despite lingering pain or fatigue from your previous run.

Example: Without a warmup, run four miles at a pace that is comfortable and does not cause pain or additional fatigue.

Where to Run – Pick a location that matches your training plan for the day. If you're going to run hills, try to find a soft trail or road in a rural location. If you plan on running tempo runs, fartleks or intervals, you can go to your local track. For a long run, try to find a soft trail that's not interrupted by local motorized traffic. Each time you have to stop at an intersection, it becomes harder to restart. Avoid hard surfaces such as concrete or asphalt, if possible.

> **Motivation**
>
> **"The difference between the impossible and the possible lies in a person's determination."**
> – *Tommy Lasorda*

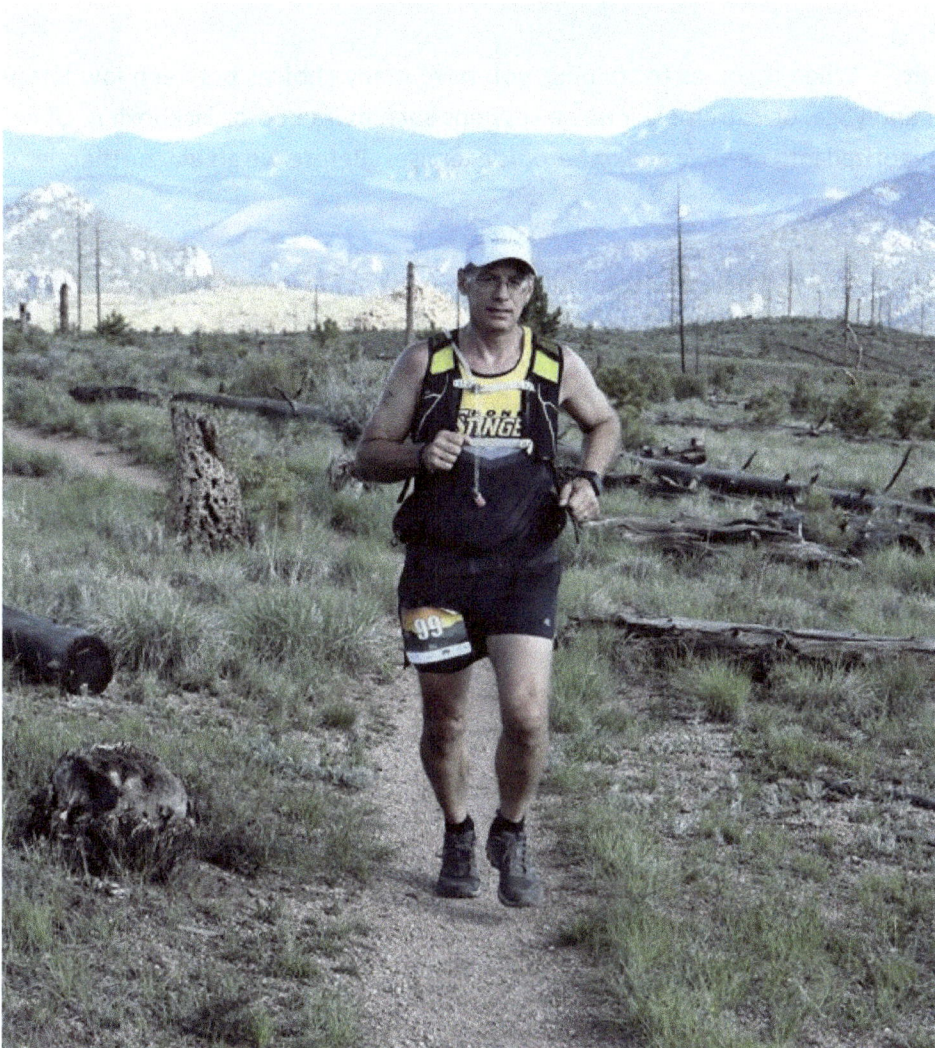

To avoid injury, train on a soft surface

Finally, if you just can't get outside to train, you can always go to your local gym and train on a treadmill. Most state-of-the-art machines will allow you to change grades, both uphill and downhill. This gives you the added advantage of running fartleks, base runs, tempo runs, recovery runs, and hill repeats. Modern treadmills can also monitor your heartrate and caloric burn during your training session.

Summary – Try all of the different training runs, but be sure to utilize proper warmup and cool-down techniques, as well as proper stretching and exercises as outlined in **Chapter 12 – Strength and Conditioning**.

Motivation

"The mind is the limit. As long as the mind can envision the fact that you can do something, you can do it, as long as you really believe 100 percent." – *Arnold Schwarzenegger*

Zone Training

Level of Intensity – When it comes to training, you have many choices between low intensity exercises such as t'ai chi and yoga, or extremely intense sessions such as Tae Bo or kickboxing. Of course, running can also be categorized into **aerobic** and **anaerobic** exercises. Before we go any further, let's define those terms:

- Aerobic exercise is defined as continuous activity performed for 15 minutes or longer, between approximately 60 percent and 80 percent of your maximum heart rate. The longer you exercise and the higher your heart rate, the more aerobic capacity and endurance you build. Aerobic activities burn more calories from fat than glycogen, compared to short, intense exercise.
- Anaerobic activity takes place in short bursts, and burns more glycogen than fat. Unlike aerobic activities which may last for hours, anaerobic activities may only last for minutes or seconds, as they eventually starve the body of much needed oxygen.

Perception or Reality – There are a number of scientific and non-scientific ways to gauge perceived and actual effort when you train. *Perceived effort* relates to how you *feel*. Granted, there will be days when repeated and identical workouts may seem much harder than the previous one, because you can judge your exercise intensity on how you *feel* during or after your workout.

Moderate Session – A workout with moderate intensity should make you sweat after about 10 minutes of activity, and increase your pulse and breathing rates. It should not, however, leave you completely out of breath or unable to carry on a conversation.

Intense Session – A vigorous or high intensity workout should cause you to sweat after just a couple of minutes of activity, leave you out of breath and make casual conversations difficult. You should never overexert yourself by pushing too hard. If you're too short of breath or in pain, your exercise intensity is higher than your current fitness level. If this happens, pull back from this level of intensity and gradually work up to the point at which you can handle the load. This may take days or even weeks to achieve.

Enter Science – While it is possible to monitor how you *feel*, there is a better way to scientifically train while improving your fitness level at the same time. This approach uses your **Maximum Heart Rate (MHR).** This is the maximum number of beats per minute that you should allow your heart to take, and is the best way to gauge your exercise intensity.

Enter Math – Before we begin, we need to answer two basic questions:
- What is maximum heart rate?
- What is YOUR maximum heart rate?

Maximum Heart Rate is defined as the upper limit of what the cardiovascular system can handle during an intense workout.

Your maximum heart rate is normally calculated using a formula based on your age. So, in all of its simplicity, here is the formula to calculate your maximum heart rate (MHR):

$$220 - Age = MHR$$

See? I told you it was a simple formula and it all starts with the "base number of 220." If you are 20 years old, your maximum heart rate should be a whopping 200 beats per minute, because the base number of *220 minus your age of 20 equals 200.* Therefore, a person at the age of 65 should have a maximum heart rate of 155. Simple math for now, but just wait, Math 2.0: Percentages, is coming up!

In The Zone – *Zone Training* has been around for years, but it's sometimes a hard concept to understand because of its complexity. Once again, however, it's really about the math. Zone Training is based on either a five-level zone range (most common) or a three-level zone range, and both are based on different levels of intensity. First, let's look at the five-level zones which we can use for our training program, and then we'll do a little math to figure out how your heart rate fits into these zones. For your convenience, I've also included the three-level heart rate zones. Let's break it down and look at some examples for each zone.

Five-level Heart Rate Zones –Most Common – Used by most watch manufacturers, such as Garmin and Polar. It consists of five zones beginning at 50% of your maximum heart rate, and goes up to 100% MHR.

Training Zone	Description
Zone 1	This zone is estimated at 50-60% of your maximum heart rate. This zone corresponds to an athlete's aerobic base and is typically reserved for a warmup and cool down.
Zone 2	This zone is estimated at 60-70% of your maximum heart rate. This is an aerobic zone where an athlete can run comfortably and utilize fat as a primary fuel source.
Zone 3	This zone is estimated at 70-80% of your maximum heart rate. This is the last aerobic zone before crossing the anaerobic threshold. Training in this zone is challenging but sustainable for most athletes with a healthy fitness level.
Zone 4	This zone is estimated at 80-90% of your maximum heart rate. This is an anaerobic zone which by definition implies the absence of oxygen resulting in a slight amount of fat metabolism. Therefore, our bodies are primarily using carbohydrates as a fuel source.
Zone 5	This zone is estimated at 90-100% of your maximum heart rate. This is the top heart rate level and will leave the athlete gasping for air after only 10 to 20 seconds of work.

Three-level Heart Rate Zones – Least Common – Used by some fitness and training companies such as NASM. These training zones begin at 65% of your MHR and go up to a maximum of 95%.

Training Zone	Description
Zone 1	This zone is estimated at 65-75% of your maximum heart rate. This zone corresponds to an athlete's aerobic base and is typically reserved for a warmup and cool down. Usually includes walking or jogging and recovery from the higher zones.
Zone 2	This zone is estimated at 76-85% of your maximum heart rate. This is an aerobic zone where an athlete can run comfortably and utilize fat as a primary fuel source. In this heart-rate model, this is known as the "lactate threshold" zone.
Zone 3	This zone is estimated at 86-95% of your maximum heart rate. This is an anaerobic zone which by definition implies the absence of oxygen resulting in a slight amount of fat metabolism. Therefore, our bodies are primarily using carbohydrates as a fuel source. Usually reserved for Peak and Interval training above lactate threshold levels.

I Hate Math! – For the following exercises, we'll calculate the Maximum Heart Rates using the five-level heart rate zones, as they are most commonly used.

George is a 45-year-old male and he wants to target Training Zone 3. George is an "average Joe" and thinks he can handle a sustained run in Zone 3 for 45 minutes. In the previous chart, George sees that Zone 3 is calculated on 70 to 80 percent of his MHR. Based on what we know, here is George's formula to get into Zone 3:

- George subtracts his age from 220 to get his maximum heart rate.
  220 – 45 = 175
- George multiplies his MHR (175) by 0.7 (70 percent) to determine the *lower* end of his target heart rate zone.
  175 x .70 = 123
- George multiplies his MHR (175) by .8 (80 percent) to determine the *upper* end of his target heart rate zone.
  175 x .80 = 140

George now knows that for his age, his heart rate for Zone 3 should be between 123 and 140 beats per minute! If you dislike calculating all of those numbers like I do, take a look at the next chart. It's based on five-year increments and shows the minimum and maximum beats per minute for each of the five zones.

Training Zones for You – In the table below, I've outlined the maximum heart rate that you should target for your age. For example, if you are 50 years old and are targeting Zone 2, your heart rate should be between 102 and 119 beats per minute. If you're below that range, congratulations! However, if you're over by more than 10%, you should slow your pace down until you're fit enough to be within that range. I've rounded these numbers into five-year intervals, but they should get you fairly close to your target. Remember, your "base number" is 220 minus your age.

Five-Stage Zone Chart (Three-Stage Zone Chart on next page for comparison)

Age	Base Number	Zone 1 50%-60%	Zone 2 60%-70%	Zone 3 70%-80%	Zone 4 80%-90%	Zone 5 90%-100%
20	200	100-120 bpm	120-140 bpm	140-160 bpm	160-180 bpm	180-200 bpm
25	195	98-117 bpm	117-137 bpm	137-156 bpm	156-176 bpm	176-195 bpm
30	190	95-114 bpm	114-133 bpm	133-152 bpm	152-171 bpm	171-190 bpm
35	185	93-111 bpm	111-130 bpm	130-148 bpm	148-167 bpm	167-185 bpm
40	180	90-108 bpm	108-126 bpm	126-144 bpm	144-162 bpm	162-180 bpm
45	175	88-105 bpm	105-123 bpm	123-140 bpm	140-158 bpm	158-175 bpm
50	170	85-102 bpm	102-119 bpm	119-136 bpm	136-153 bpm	153-170 bpm
55	165	83-99 bpm	99-116 bpm	116-132 bpm	132-149 bpm	149-165 bpm
60	160	80-96 bpm	96-112 bpm	112-128 bpm	128-144 bpm	144-160 bpm
65	155	78-93 bpm	93-109 bpm	109-124 bpm	124-140 bpm	140-155 bpm
70	150	75-90 bpm	90-105 bpm	105-120 bpm	120-135 bpm	135-150 bpm
75	145	73-87 bpm	87-102 bpm	102-116 bpm	116-131 bpm	131-145 bpm
80	140	70-84 bpm	84-98 bpm	98-112 bpm	112-126 bpm	126-140 bpm

Three-Stage Zone Chart – Use this chart if you do not use the Five-Stage Zone range

Age	Base Number	Zone 1 65%-75%	Zone 2 76%-85%	Zone 3 86%-95%
20	200	130-150 bpm	152-170 bpm	172-190 bpm
25	195	127-146 bpm	148-166 bpm	168-185 bpm
30	190	124-143 bpm	144-162 bpm	163-181 bpm
35	185	120-139 bpm	141-157 bpm	159-176 bpm
40	180	117-135 bpm	137-153 bpm	155-171 bpm
45	175	114-131 bpm	133-149 bpm	151-166 bpm
50	170	110-128 bpm	129-145 bpm	146-162 bpm
55	165	107-124 bpm	125-140 bpm	142-157 bpm
60	160	104-120 bpm	122-136 bpm	138-152 bpm
65	155	101-116 bpm	118-132 bpm	133-147 bpm
70	150	98-113 bpm	114-128 bpm	129-143 bpm
75	145	94-109 bpm	110-123 bpm	125-138 bpm
80	140	91-105 bpm	106-119 bpm	120-133 bpm

Automated Monitoring – You can check your beats per minute manually or by the use of a device such as a heart rate monitor. Most modern running watches can synchronize with a heart rate accessory such as a chest-strap monitor, but some even have a wrist heart rate monitor built in to them, such as these watches from Garmin.

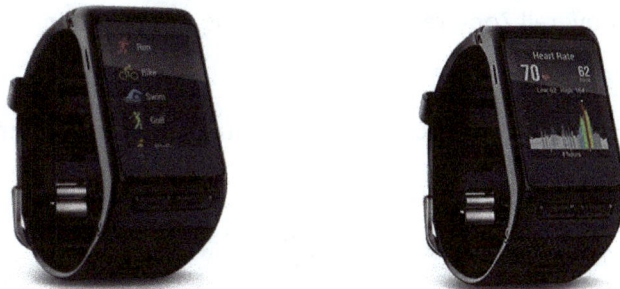

Use a battery powered heart rate monitor, either standalone or one that is synchronized to your watch or smart phone.

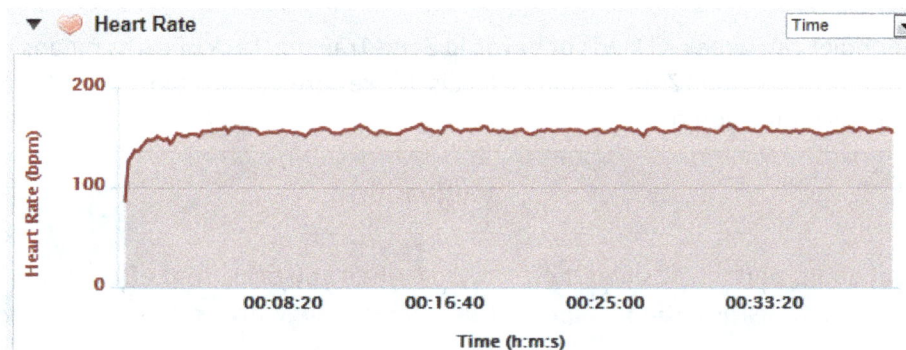

Manual Monitoring – Stop your run and immediately take your pulse for 15 seconds. Don't time it for a full minute because your heart will slow in that amount of time, giving you a false reading. Multiply your pulse by four to get your beats per minute.

George wants to calculate his heart rate to see which Zone he is running in. As soon as he's done with his run, he takes his pulse for 15 seconds. He counted 33 beats during those 15 seconds. He now multiplies the rate times four (4 x 15 = 60 seconds).

$$33 \times 4 = 132$$

From the chart on the previous page, he now knows that he was running in Zone 3, which for his age of 45, should be between 123 and 140.

Variables, Exceptions, and Excuses – We just took an in-depth look at Training Zones 1 through 5, but there are always other reasons that your heart rate might show an exception from one day to the next.

- **Medication** – Are you currently on any type of medication that can affect your heart rate, such as blood pressure medicines?

- **Temperature** – Extreme temperature, both hot and cold, can affect your heart rate. Take a sampling over several days or weeks to get an average.

- **Altitude** – Running at higher altitudes can put more stress on your cardiovascular system, because your oxygen levels are lower. Take this into account when you run at altitude.

- **Hill Running, Intervals, Tempo Runs, etc.** – Any training that forces an increase of heart rate is going to change your overall Zone rating. Consider this when training, and *average* the numbers for proper results.

- **Stress** – We all have stress in our daily lives, but try to minimize the stress before you take measurements.

- **Insomnia** – Lack of sleep can cause your body to work harder than it should have to. Try to get seven to 10 hours of sleep each night.

- **Illness** – If you're sick, your body is going to naturally work harder. If you don't feel good, don't push it or don't run at all until you do feel better.

- **Diet** – Poor diet can wreak all kinds of havoc in Zone Training. Lack of carbs means that you won't be able to reach or sustain Zone 4 training levels. Make sure you have lots of carbs, not just before a race, but each time you run!

Motivation

"It's not about perfect. It's about effort. And when you bring that effort every single day, that's where transformation happens. That's how change occurs." — *Jillian Michaels*

My Story

Face it, I'm a gadget guy. Coming from an IT background, I'm always interested in the latest, greatest technologies. I constantly look for an edge, to either make me better or make me think I am doing better. When I bought my first Timex Ironman watch, I thought it was the coolest thing ever. I could run a race and all I had to do was tap a button at each mile marker. Then I found out about watches that would measure the distance for me, and I wouldn't have to do anything but start it at the beginning of my race and stop it at the end! I ditched the Timex for a Garmin, and one thing led to another. Soon, I started purchasing all kinds of accessories for my watch. Solar chargers, so my watch could charge while I was out on ultramarathons, foot pods to measure my pace, and of course the chest-strap heart monitor. With newer technologies, most heart rate monitors are built in to the watch, eliminating the need for a chest strap.

Out of all the accessories I bought, the heart rate monitor feature was and still is, the best piece of running gear that I have. The heart rate monitor helped me analyze my fitness level, especially during the early stages of my training. I didn't have to use "perceived effort" at all because my heart rate monitor showed me exactly which Zone I was in and I could correlate that effort to how I felt.

As my fitness level increased, my average heart rate decreased. An accurate heart rate monitor can act as a coach, especially if it has a "virtual training partner" built in. The virtual training partner can "beep" an audible noise and tell you when you've entered or exited your targeted zone.

As I became more fit, I learned to depend on my monitor less and less, but I still use it in my early training sessions and once per month thereafter.

I urge all "average Joe" runners to invest in a good heart rate monitor, either standalone or integrated, and chart out your biological analytics to see where you really are in your Zone Training.

Finally, integrate your Cross-training with your Zone Training. You don't need to run to get into your target zones. You can achieve the same results by swimming, biking or many other aerobic (and anaerobic) activities.

Challenge!

Basic Instincts

When we opened this chapter, I told you about my breathing difficulties during my early training sessions. I took something as easy, natural and *basic*, and over-complicated it to the *nth* degree.

Your challenge: *As you read the last five chapters in this book, try to keep things as basic as possible. Running is hard enough as it is. Keep in touch with your senses, feelings and instincts, and don't make things more difficult than they need to be.*

Chapter 14 – Cross-training

My Story

Over the years, I've run thousands and thousands of miles. I've burned and consumed millions of calories, and climbed millions of feet of elevation. I'm proud of those accomplishments and feel that I've worked very hard for them. But, I also know that I'm lacking in one statistic that I've always *wanted* to achieve, but didn't make it a *priority* until later in my running career.

For years, I had a sleeping disorder. I tried to squeeze too many things into each day, and before I knew it, it would be 11:30 p.m., or 1:00 a.m. and I was planning to get up early to run or go to work. Sleep was not a priority! I was too busy doing this or that, so I'd be wound so tight that I couldn't sleep. Or, I'd wake up extra early to hit the pavement with my running shoes – day after day, week after week. I was one of those people who had a million reasons to keep training but didn't take the time to rest! Now I look back at my poor race results or my oft-injured body and have to wonder what my real potential would have been, had I received the rest that I needed. Once I learned the importance of a good night's rest, I gradually saw less frequent injuries and earned faster race times. I had changed very little in my workouts or diet – I only added rest – pure, simple sleep.

I finally had to *train* myself to go to bed at a specific time, just like getting up at a specific time to begin my day. One evening, I decided to buy a second alarm clock – designed to ring at 9:30 each night, marking the end of my day, and starting my journey to dreamland. When that alarm clock rang, I'd stop any stimulating activity I was doing, such as reading or watching TV. I'd simply sit in my recliner for a few minutes, close my eyes, take deep breaths – and *relax!* It only took a few minutes to feel relaxed enough to get up, brush my teeth, wash my face and go to bed.

After seven to 10 hours of sleep, my primary alarm clock would wake me each morning, and before I knew it, I was beginning to *feel good and rested!* Not only did my body feel better, but my stress levels went way down, and my thoughts had a greater level of clarity. I began to dream at night, something I'd rarely done in 10 or 12 years. This was due to the fact that I was finally reaching the REM cycle, the fifth and most important part of our normal sleep patterns.

Motivation

"Sleep is that golden chain that ties health and our bodies together." – *Thomas Dekker*

Cross-Training – Cross-training is defined as *"training in two or more sports in order to improve fitness and performance, especially in a main sport."*

Over the years, many athletes have excelled in single-sport training and activity. Swimmers did all or most of their training in the pool, while cyclists spent countless hours on their road or stationary bikes. And of course, runners spent time simply running endless mile after mile at the track, or hour after hour on the treadmill. Rarely did the athlete stray from their discipline. For instance, if the runner's goal or interest was a 5k or 10k race, they simply ran their specified goal distance. In any of these examples, if the athlete actually did any cross-training, it was more than likely a session or two per week of weight training. The mentality at the time was to focus on *specificity* rather than *overall health and balance* of the bodies' various systems.

In recent years, however, sports physiologists have determined the *entire* body reaps more benefits and creates a stronger, faster, more agile and more coordinated body through proper cross-training. The coaches and athletes soon recognized this fact and have developed strategies to enhance the athlete's core discipline. Well-planned cross-training allows the entire body to be trained as a *unified entity*, rather than individual parts. Let's take running, for example. Obviously, a runner needs strong legs to go the specified distance and pace. The arms are heavily involved as counter balance to keep the momentum going. The arms don't necessarily need a lot of lifting power, but they must be able to swing as long as the legs are in motion. This requires strong connective tissue in the shoulders and elbows. For shorter runs such as 400 meter or 1 mile races, leg strength and arm counter balance may be all you need. But when you get into medium and long distance running, you'll need to focus on your abdomen and back because they connect your upper and lower extremities. You'll need to work on muscle *groups* rather than *individual* muscles. This is where cross-training comes in – to train muscles that are neglected with the rigors of normal training. The key to successful training of any discipline is the ability to match it with one or more cross-training programs that *enhances* the main sport. This is one of the reasons that triathletes, particularly those participating at the Ironman levels, are usually considered the fittest of the fit. They train for running AND cycling AND swimming – a great program for success and whole-body fitness.

Under the Hood – When you consider the many components of an automobile, there are thousands of moving parts – the engine where the horsepower originates, the drivetrain and wheels that set the vehicle in motion, the cooling and heating systems that regulate the temperature, the weight and design of the car to keep it under control on the road, and the various on-board computer systems that keep all of these systems functioning in unison. All of these systems work *together,* to allow the car to run efficiently for a long time. One subsystem without the other will slow the car down or force it to break completely.

The same can be said of the human body – we need strong muscles to generate power; arms and legs that work together – fluidly and efficiently; a body that's conditioned to maintain a good working temperature without overheating; and a mind that's mentally sharp and can handle the entire workload of all the associated subsystems. Cross-training allows all of these systems to work together!

Back on page 181, I introduced a basic training plan for a startup running program. Twice per week, I recommended your choice of *rest* or *cross-training*. What exactly is cross-training? What's it used for? Why is it important? Which forms of cross-training are right for your program? Is cross-training important as you dial in on your upcoming race? These are all great questions, and like all of the other questions in this book, they demand to be answered. We're going to address these questions and more, but before we do, let's talk about one of the most important training concepts that you'll need to know.

Listen to Your Body – This book focuses on various training methodologies and concepts, myths and ideas, facts and opinions. One subject that I'd like to mention sooner, rather than later, is the subject of *rest*. As you know, your body constantly monitors all of your biological systems and communicates with your brain as to what your needs are. The brain tells you when you're hungry or thirsty, and lets you know when you have plenty of energy to burn. It also lets you know when you don't feel well and when you're tired. Most of us listen to our bodies when it comes to hunger and thirst. We go to the doctor and stay home from work when we're sick. But how many of us get the amount of sleep that we REALLY need? This world is a busy place and we seem to find a million reasons to keep going, despite the need for rest. How many of us really know *how* to relax? Rest is a crucial part of healthy living for all ages. Rest invigorates and rejuvenates your mind and body, regulates your mood, reduces your stress, stabilizes your immune system, and has a direct link to learning and memory functions.

Prioritize Your Sleeping Habits – Notice the word *habit*. Just like eating meals at regular intervals, take time to sleep. Do your best to keep it on a normal, repeatable schedule. Sleep, not your actual workouts, can be the focal point of your training regimen. Schedule your day around your night, not the other way around. Rest is even more important when you're tired or stressed, even if you just take an afternoon nap or simply a stroll around the neighborhood.

Sleep Suggestions from the Experts – Most doctors and physiologists recommend these important elements for a good night's rest:

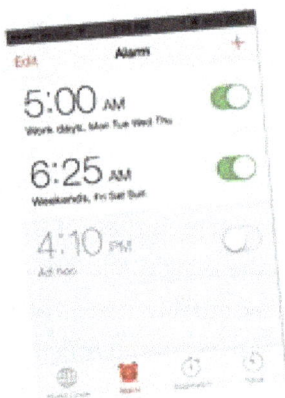

- Go to bed at the same time each night.
- Eliminate visual and audible stimulation just before bed time.
- Try to get seven to ten hours of sleep each night.
- Sleep in the most natural setting possible, with minimal or no artificial lighting.
- Turn down the thermostat – keep the air fresh and cool.
- Wake up with the sun if possible – experts agree that waking early yields better productivity, creativity, decreased stress and increased fitness.

Rest Days – In the last chapter, I presented the option of resting or cross-training on your off days. Once again, it's important to listen to your body. I normally schedule a cross-training day, one to two times per week, but if my body is fatigued, I'll simply take a break from physical activity, or might do just a light cross-training effort. Go ahead and schedule your cross-training days, but if you're feeling tired, your body is telling you that you need a break. Rest to prevent further fatigue and injuries from over-use. And don't feel bad about missing a workout – your body will thank you the next day! Remember - rest allows your body to recover.

Now that we know WHY we should cross-train, let's take a look at HOW we can cross-train. And believe me; you have an abundance of choices when it comes to cross-training. In this next segment, I'll categorize the different methods, give examples of each, and teach you different ways to help gain extra strength, flexibility and agility, all of which are needed to excel in your running program.

Benefits – Besides strength, balance, flexibility, and agility, cross-training offers two other huge benefits that are often disregarded – those being *injury prevention* and *active recovery.* Cross-training is especially important because it targets muscles and connective tissues that are often ignored during routine training. And these neglected tissues are often times the source of an injury, and can keep you out of training for months at a time, such as a back or hamstring injury. Remember, the larger the muscle, the longer it takes to heal. Cross-training helps to prevent injury by strengthening active and passive muscles alike.

Secondly, active recovery is the method of utilizing an alternative type of training to recover from your primary training objective. For instance, you may try aqua running (running in a swimming pool) to keep up your running fitness level and activity, but remove weight-bearing loads and joint impact from your training session. These methods allow expedient recovery because it increases the blood supply and necessary nutrients to your muscles without damaging the tissues further.

When we consider cross-training, the most popular method, by far, is weight training. And for good reason – it's readily available and can be done with or without weight in a modern gym, or in the convenience of your own home. It's so popular that I wrote an entire chapter on it – **Chapter 12 – Strength and Conditioning.** That chapter in and of itself, should give you all you need for weight training, other than the option to add more weight, sets or reps. I address strength training to increase muscle mass, reduce fat, and increase balance and stability. It also targets conditioning, the ability to increase cardio-aerobic capacity and quicken your body – all in one compact workout. With that in mind, I'll cover the remaining popular cross-training methods.

Cross-training choices – When it comes to cross-training, you have many choices and variables. As a runner, the core muscles you need to develop and maintain are of course, your legs. We'll start by looking at cross-training methods and exercises that will increase your lower body parts, and work our way up and out to the other muscle groups and extremities. Take a look at the next couple of pages where I outline the wide variety of cross-training techniques that you can do to enhance your running.

Use your imagination and train different muscles and muscle groups by mixing and matching some of the cross-training methods. Don't limit your own potential by running alone. Be sure to schedule two cross-training sessions per week, but if you're too tired for one of them, simply take a day off.

Motivation

"The best training program in the world is absolutely worthless without the will to execute it properly, consistently, and with intensity." *– John Romaniello*

Cross-training that focuses on your lower body:

- Running
- Dancing
- Walking your dog
- Walking
- Hiking
- Jazzercise

- Mountain biking
- Road biking
- Stationary bike
- Elliptigo ®
- Rollerblading
- Kettle bells

Cross-training that focuses on your upper body:

- Weight lifting
- Medicine balls
- Free weights
- Kettle bells
- Machine-assisted weights
- Rowing

- Planks
- Push-ups
- Pull-ups
- Curls
- Dips

Low Intensity Cross-training that focuses on your core muscles:

- Yoga
- t'ai chi
- Pilates
- Sit-ups
- Kettle bells

- Bridges
- Planks
- Side planks
- Medicine ball rotation

Cross-training that focuses on aerobics and cardio fitness:

- Tae Bo
- Boxing exercises / heavy bag, jump rope
- Kick boxing
- Martial arts
- Water sports
  - Swimming
  - Rowing or kayaking
  - Standup paddle-boarding
  - Water skiing
  - Aqua jogging
  - Water aerobics
- Winter sports
  - Downhill snow skiing
  - Cross country skiing
  - Ice skating

- Indoor sports
  - Stationary bike
  - Stair climber
  - Elliptical trainer
  - Basketball
  - Rowing
  - Treadmill

- Outdoor sports
  - Baseball
  - Football
  - Soccer
  - Racquetball
  - Volleyball
  - Tennis

> ## Motivation
>
> *"Desire is the key to motivation, but it's determination and commitment to an unrelenting pursuit of your goal - a commitment to excellence - that will enable you to attain the success you seek."*
> – Mario Andretti

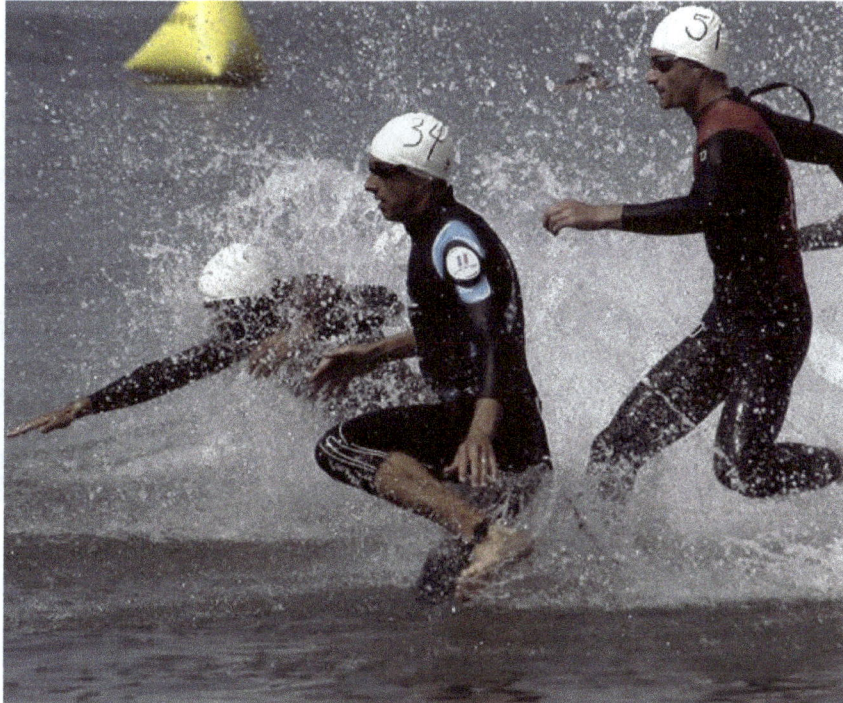

Consider water sports to enhance your running

Challenge!

Cross-Train

There are many different ways to cross-train to strengthen and enhance your body during your normal training routine, but cross-training can also be used for healing and active recovery between difficult training days. Use cross-training days wisely and always have a goal for each workout. How will this cross-training day affect your next running day? What benefits will it produce?

Your challenge: *Find ways to work different muscle groups, with other types of workouts. We'll soon be into **Chapter 16 – Training Plans**, and we'll find out how to mix daily running in with cross-training and rest days. Your challenge for this chapter is to find out what types of cross-training you would like to do and how it will fit into your running program. If you're a strong swimmer, for instance, you might consider water-based workouts to develop your core and upper body. Think of specific goals that you want to achieve – which brings us to the next chapter – **Setting Goals**.*

Chapter 15 – Setting Goals

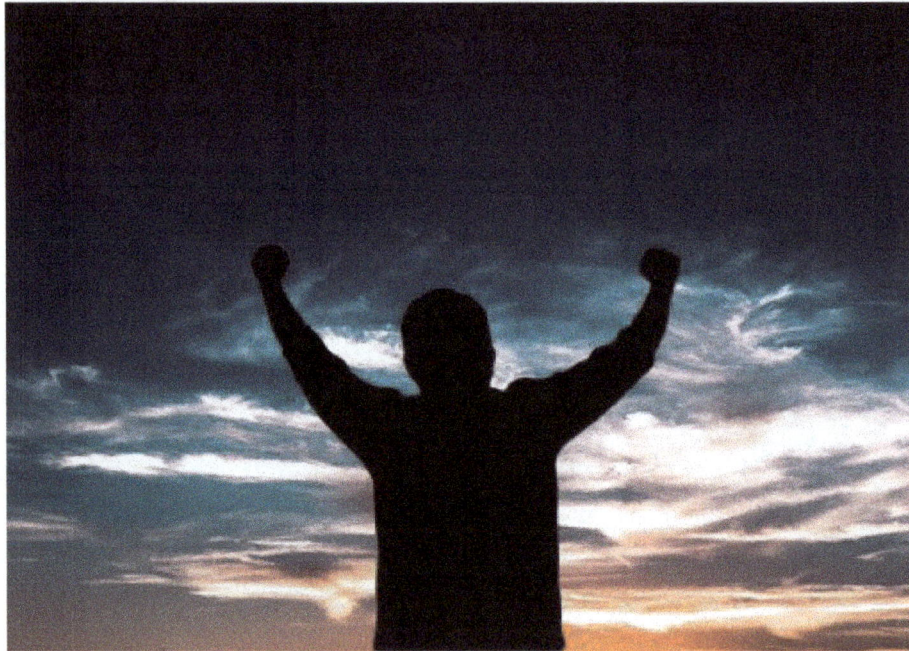

Back in **Chapter 5 – Sports Psychology**, we discussed how to set goals. What are your goals? Do you need goals? How do you turn your goals into reality?

When I started researching this chapter, I was astounded by the amount of information, philosophies, and concepts of goal setting. Some ideals were as simple as "Set a goal and achieve it," all the way to a 440 page, hardcover book that looked more like a Kennedy Assassination Inquiry.

As I pored over the various theories and hypotheses, I found that most experts agreed on these five elements:

Specific – You must know exactly what the end result should be. Do you want to run a 5k or a 50k? Without specificity, you cannot achieve your goal. When it comes to implementing a goal, you first have to define one. To reduce stress and frustration, keep the goal as simple and short as possible, but keep it exact and clear. Know the precise results that you seek. If you generalize or are unclear of your goals, you will most likely fail. Defining a goal is sometimes the most difficult part of this entire process. Lack of knowledge, lack of focus and lack of desire are the main reasons for failure. So, here is my advice when it comes to setting goals. Be clear and state exactly what you want from your goal. Since this a personal goal, you need to be self-motivating. Create a mantra for your goal such as: "I *will* run a 5k in 22 minutes and thirty seconds." Notice I didn't say "I *want* to run a 5k in 22 minutes and thirty seconds." Finally, stay focused on one goal at a time. Setting multiple goals will add complexity and increase the chance for failure.

> **Motivation**
>
> **"You can reach your goal only if you have one."** — *Bill Watts*

Measurable – You can measure your goal in a number of ways – How long does it take you to run your race? How much have you achieved since your previous goal? How much distance has been covered, etc.? Once you establish your exact, specific goal, you will be able to measure it. If your goal is still vague, continue to re-define it until it's clear. Can you measure it now? In the example above, we *specified* an exact distance, with an exact finish time. Now, you can set up baselines, benchmarks, and milestones as you go through your training. For example, early in your training, you can time yourself for a one-mile run. Next, add a second, and then a third mile. You can measure your time each week to see your setbacks or improvements. Ask questions that demand answers such as: "If I did have a setback, what was the cause and can I find a way to get around it, so I can get a new measurement?" or "If I improved, how much did I advance it?" or "Was I able to maintain the same pace throughout today's session?" Keep logs and personal statistics to measure your progress.

Attainable – All races can be difficult but most are attainable. Will power and motivation are a must. Believe in yourself! As humans, we have limits. While some of us have all the will power and confidence in the world, the hard facts may show us that we don't have the physical capabilities to attain our most aspired goals. When you set a goal, make sure that you consider how much time you can commit, what your physical attributes are, and base it on previous experiences if possible. Age, health, and many other elements can dictate whether or not your goal is achievable. Be careful not to set your goals too high, or have too many concurrent goals. If you shoot too high, you will demoralize your attitude and shatter your confidence. If this is your first time with goal-setting, use common sense and moderation. Use "baby steps" when necessary and use a series of smaller, less intimidating goals. However, you should also avoid the temptation for goals that are too easy. Keep small, but challenging goals in mind, and continue to raise the bar as you progress.

Time Based – What is your timeline for achieving your goal? Once again, specify your goal, and if you don't make it on the first pass, reschedule it. Whether your goal moves or not, make sure you keep it!

Your goal can only be achieved if it has an end in sight. Your goal should be time-based with a *reasonable* and *attainable* deadline. Pick a date and time and add enough buffers to allow for unexpected time away, illness, injuries or emergencies. Earlier in this chapter, we said, "I **WILL** run a 5k in 22 minutes and 30 seconds." A time-based plan will clearly state: "I **WILL** run a 5k in 22 minutes and 30 seconds at the Annual Turkey Trot, November 23rd." Having a clear-cut goal similar to this example, will increase your sense of urgency, and remove the temptations for an open-ended goal. Goals with no defined end, of course, would result in failure.

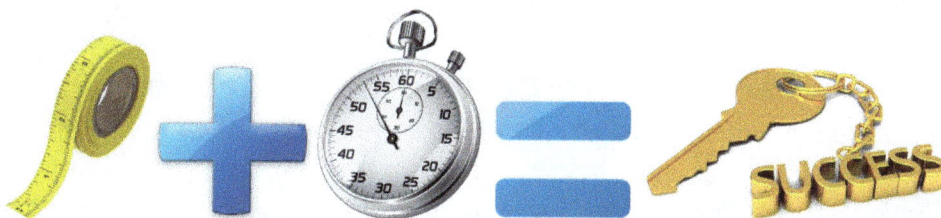

Motivation

"The key to winning is poise under stress." – *Paul Brown*

Documented – Keep logs of your training, races, and accomplishments. Write down your goals, successes and even your failures. Keep detailed logs on your activities, as well as your priorities. If you know how to use a spreadsheet, by all means keep your numbers in there for quick and accurate results.

If you specified your goal and found that it is measurable and attainable, create an ***action plan*** of your own on your computer or in a notebook. It doesn't matter how you keep your records, just make sure that you do. And hold yourself accountable! **Chapter 16 – Training Plans** will introduce you to new ways of documenting or journaling your runs. Unlike the creation of the goal, where you want to keep it short and simple, you'll want to document the details of your progress.

Finally, keep your documents handy and accessible. Place them in a visible area to remind yourself each day of your upcoming intents and events. Post a "Cliff Notes" version near your computer monitor, or on your bathroom mirror or refrigerator.

Tip

Always make your goals tangible and real by writing them down. This physical act alone will set the stage for the implementation and delivery of your goal. Make two copies – one to keep near you, and give another copy to a friend who can help you be accountable if you start to stray from your goal. If you're a "to-do list" type of person, jot down your list and don't be afraid to reprioritize when necessary. Always keep the end result within your vision!

Challenge!

Set a Goal

There's a saying: "Best-laid plans of mice and men oft go astray." In other words, if you don't have a solid plan, you are really setting yourself up for failure and certain misery. Running is difficult and if you don't plan your training properly, you probably won't succeed.

Your challenge: *Create a solid goal, one that's specific, measureable, and attainable. Document your goal and set a reasonable timeline. Once you have your goal, move on to the next chapter!*

Chapter 16 – Training Plans

My Story

The Marathon Owns You

During my years as a runner, I've learned a lot about pain, injury and suffering on the race course. I've experienced these discomforts at nearly every race distance. Early in my running, when I started with the 5k distance and gradually worked my way up to the five-mile distance, I touched base with all of them. As I morphed into the 10k and 10 mile distances, I became increasingly aware of how each extension of the distance required more and more effort from me. Eventually, I worked up to the half marathon distance and found that while it was achievable, it took so much more time and effort. I knew that running was no longer dependent on just putting one foot in front of the other. While the physical strength was still required, I soon found that I was now deep into the domain of the emotional and mental aspects of running.

Each time I "graduated" to a new running distance, I began to wonder what my limits really were. From the 5k to the 10k, I'd doubled my distance. From the five mile to the 10 mile, I'd done it again. Sure it was difficult, but each time I was able to summon the strength – mentally, emotionally and physically. Up until this point, things were pretty straightforward, and the learning curve was relatively static. Until then, I was able to dictate how far I ran and didn't really feel limited by time or distance.

But something changed when I attempted my first half marathon. I quickly found that I no longer controlled the distance – it controlled me. I was suddenly within its boundaries and power, not my own. And when I moved to the marathon distance, the difference in distance between 13.1 and 26.2 miles seemed like light years to me. It was no longer just a progression through longer training sessions – this was going to change the way I thought about running. In fact, it DID change my perceptions about running and the new requirements for the additional distance. Physicality alone was no longer the determining factor that I'd have to engage in. Instead of my body *allowing* me to run a certain distance, my mind had now taken control and was *telling* me how far I could go. It was telling me that pain was going to be the dominant feature. It was telling me that doubling the distance doesn't merely equal doubling the effort. I soon found out that the effort involved for each new distance was going to increase *exponentially*. It was no longer a flat rate or gentle learning curve. It was more like the Richter scale.

The Richter scale is built on a 1 to 10 scale with 1/10th fractions, such as 3.2, 3.3, etc. Logic would suggest that a 5.0 earthquake would be 10 times stronger than a 4.0 earthquake. Unfortunately, logic does not dictate and we find that the actual formula has the 5.0 earthquake being 31.6 times stronger than a 4.0 temblor.

...continued

My Story.... Continued

And so it is with adding more distance to your run. A change of distance from 5 miles to 10 miles is in reality twice as much, but the effort increases exponentially, much like the ratings of the 10 point Richter scale. This effort is known as **perceived exertion**. There are several well-known rating systems, but in essence, they all state that the longer you perform, the quicker you will encounter a meeting with "the wall." In reality, however, the rating can change when other variables come into play. These variables include the rate of decay – how fast your body is becoming inefficient in its processes, with decreasing oxygenation, and increasing internal temperature and lactate. When you start running the longer distances, you'll find that it's not just about doubling your time and distance. While the marathon is exactly twice as long as the half marathon, the perceived effort can and will be much more than that, and it requires tactical training. You can most likely do a 5k, 5-miler, 10k and even a 10-miler without a great deal of training. And you can probably even squeeze out a half marathon, although it will be slow and painful if you've never trained for one. You might have only run 11 miles in training for your half marathon and that will be enough to get you to the finish line.

The marathon is a completely different beast. If you're serious about running a marathon, you need to get serious with your training. At some point before your race, you will need to go the entire distance, not just for meeting the physical challenge, but to make sure that you're mentally prepared. We've all heard of "hitting the wall" in marathon running, when the physical barriers have been breached and you struggle not just to run, but to move forward in general.

The Wall

"The wall" – it is at this point, where **pain, fatigue, biological imbalances, fear, doubt** and **perception** all collide and tell you that you can go no further. You're done. Toast. *Fini*.

But is the wall imaginary, or does it really exist? In **Chapter 5 – Running Psychology and Chapter 6 – Running Physiology**, we looked at the mental and physical attributes of running. Indeed, we found that the wall really does exist and it's really no secret or unexpected reaction to distance running. When we run long distances, we break down, just like an old, high-mileage car, and the further we go, the more we risk other parts breaking down.

Most distance runners begin to feel the wall around 30 kilometers into the race, or about 18.6 miles. It's at this point where you've exhausted most of your glycogen stores and the chemical imbalances that are outside of your control have begun to erode. I've hit the wall many times in my running career and found ways to get through it, around it, or over each time. That takes physical strength as well as mental discipline. Over the years, I've learned to predict when it's going to hit and even learned to embrace it when it does.

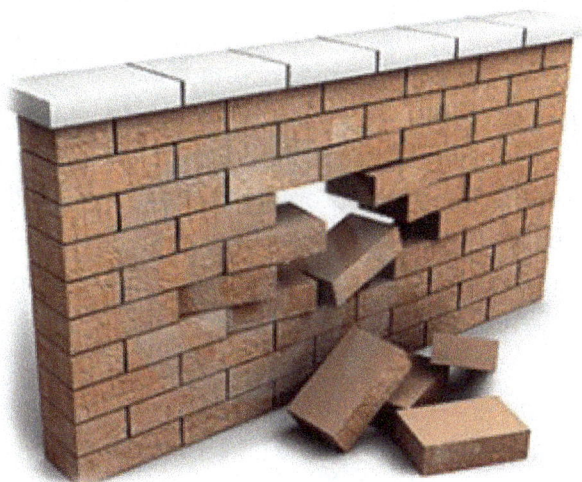

Analyzing the Wall

So let's break down the wall and find ways to get through the collision I just described.

- **Pain** – Pain at any distance is possible, depending on how far or how hard you run, what the course is like and how well you've prepared and convalesced when required. Expect pain, and embrace it – it's going to be with you at some point during the race. When you were training for this race, did you try to emulate the course, such as practicing on hills if it was a hilly race? Did you run on concrete to prepare for an inner city road course? Pain will not escape you come race day, but proper preparation can alleviate much of it and teach you how to deal with it.

- **Fatigue** – Of course you're going to get tired during the race. Much of this is because of the fuels that you're burning at the late stages of the race. Gone are the special glycogen stores that you accumulated during your taper (you did taper didn't you?). Fatigue goes hand-in-hand with pain, but can also be minimized through proper training, diet and sleep habits.

- **Biological Imbalances** – If you're like most "average Joes," you will thirst when you're already deficient in liquids. The key is to take on water or sports drinks BEFORE you feel thirsty. The onset of the wall is similar to thirst, in that it begins to happen before you start to feel it. And, even though you might not begin to feel the wall until around mile 18, your body has been at work for several miles, preparing for the inevitable collapse. If you didn't carbo-load over the week prior to your race, you can expect to start breaking down internally, and without even feeling it at mile eight. If you carbo-loaded properly, the invisible breakdown starts around mile 15, two or three miles in advance of the actual confrontation with the wall. Lower glycogen levels, increased lactate in the system and inefficient transport of oxygen are already pushing you towards it.
The wall is unavoidable for most "average Joes," but there are many things you can do to get past it. Start with a good diet throughout your training program. Don't carbo-load just the night before. If you're really doing it right, you will be consuming the proper amount of carbs, proteins and fats through your *entire* training program, you'll taper a week before, and you'll begin heavy loading of carbohydrates at least three days in advance of your run. Please don't worry about your weight!

You'll lose some of the additional weight during the race anyway. During the race, try to take on carbs, simple sugars for quick entry into your system, and gels that contain adequate amounts of ingestible and fast-absorbing carbs. The most important part of understanding the wall is to feel it first-hand. During your weeks and months of training up to your race, go looking for the wall. Your marathon training runs should include at least one encounter with it. There are a lot of varying opinions on this, but I personally recommend two or three runs of 22 to 24 miles and one run of the entire distance of 26.2 miles. Unless you are more than an "average Joe," you will hit the wall head-on. The experience is not pleasant, but it's important to know what it feels like and how you can push through it.

- **Fear, Doubt** and **Perception** – These are all "feeling" words and all manufactured in your mind. You can't do much to stop the pain, fatigue and biological imbalances, but there's plenty you can do to avoid fear, doubt and perception. You can avoid these feelings by actually pushing through the wall before race day. Practice doesn't make perfect, but with these three, it certainly helps to dispel them before race day. Get rid of them by going the distance in your training runs. Removing these three makes pain, fatigue and biological imbalances manageable once again. Do it not, and you will suffer.

Looking in From the Outside

In one of my running clubs, I saw a young man who had a great deal of potential. We'll call him Bob. Bob was just 24 years old and he ran like the wind when it came to 5ks and 10ks, harvesting age group awards nearly every time. One day he said he wanted to run a marathon, and I watched for several months as his running distances grew longer, and his race times decreased. He was getting stronger and faster, and he was averaging about 10 miles per day. On the weekend, he'd do a 15 or 16 miler, but never anything longer. He posted comments on his blog about how he was training for his first marathon on Labor Day. But something was amiss. Even though he was running nearly 300 miles per month, he was missing out on the most important aspect of the training program – running long and coming face-to-face with the wall. Labor Day came and went and I looked at the race results on the marathon website. His name wasn't listed – DNF. I later saw on the Garmin website that he did indeed start the race but stopped at 21.79 miles. Bob ran his first 10 or 12 miles VERY aggressively. This young bundle-of-hope-marathoner did just about everything wrong that he could have done for his first marathon.

- He never ran the complete distance during training (nothing over 16 miles)
  - He should have run at least one marathon distance training run to see how it feels, what to expect in pain tolerance and to establish a finish time estimate.

- He never ran the expected amount of time during his training (nothing beyond two hours and 35 minutes)
  - He should have run the full distance to establish his finish time estimate. For example, if his training run of 24 to 26 miles established the fact that he needed to be on his feet for four hours, he should experience at the very least, one training run of four hours or more. Instead, his longest run, in terms of time, was only two hours and 35 minutes, a far cry from what he should expect.

- He most likely didn't experience the wall during training.
  - Although I don't know this for a fact, I would assume that he didn't hit the wall because he just kept doing the same training week in and week out, each time stopping short of the wall. The marathon distance and the wall will humble you into changing your training tactics or convince you to quit altogether. I assume he didn't experience the wall, and figured that everything was "okay."

- Bob didn't do any cross-training during his buildup to the marathon. Cross-training is very important for all race distances. It helps development of non-running muscle groups and allows your entire body to work as one unit. This minimizes the risk of injury and allows the muscle groups used for running, to heal on "off" or "rest" days. Be sure to review – **Chapter 14 – Cross-Training** if you have questions or concerns.

- Although he probably didn't think about it at the time, he was putting in 300 miles per month, but most were "junk" miles because they didn't serve the purpose.
  - He would have been fine if his planned race had been a half marathon. He wouldn't have had to deal with the wall, he had several or many training runs covering or exceeding the distance and his pace was good. I mentioned earlier in this book that "junk miles are easily accumulated, but rarely meaningful." He would have been better off with a base of 200 miles per month that would have included a couple long runs of 22 to 24 miles.

- Bob went out way too aggressively on race day (he was running faster than his normal 5k pace)
  - In any marathon, especially your first one, you don't need to run like a bat out of Hell. Be patient and get up to speed gradually. Don't expect to run a 5k pace in the marathon as Bob did. Run the mile you are in and if you're running slower than you expect, don't try to "make up" time in the next mile. Instead, try to run a few seconds faster with each coming mile and focus on saving energy for the last five or six miles, when you'll need it the most.

Tip

To feel is to understand. Without experiencing the wall before race day, you are setting yourself up for a DNF (did not finish). While it's not a comfortable event to go through, I think that every marathon-hopeful should experience it at some point during their training. That requires running somewhere between 18 and 22 miles, the distance at which the wall usually rears its ugly head. During this encounter, basic math becomes difficult and you might even get confused on how many miles you have left to run!

Motivation

"Remember the feeling you get from a good run is far better than the feeling you get from sitting around wishing you were running." – *Sarah Condor*

In the previous chapter, we talked about goals, the importance of them, and how to create your own. But now, let's take it a step further, and create an *action plan* to help you achieve your goals.

To create a successful action plan, you must have a goal – a vision and a clear purpose, designed to take you from where you are today to where you want to be in the future. Only through proper planning can you achieve your goal.

To succeed in your plan, start by writing down everything, including your concepts, goals, successes and failures. Keep track of where you run, how far you run, and how you felt on that day. Was it raining? Were you sore from previous activities?

Log It – Start by creating a *runner's log*. The log can contain as much or as little information as you want to keep. More is better if you're a number cruncher, but it can also be a burden if you try to track too much.

I've seen (and used) many different types of running logs that vary from a single entry in a notebook to elaborate spreadsheets on computers. I'm going to furnish you with the basics – information you'll need to track in order to get to your personal goals. In this chapter, I'm going to introduce my training plan, which includes seven cycles in the program.

Motivation

"If you don't design your own life plan, chances are you'll fall into someone else's plan. And guess what they have planned for you? Not much." *– Jim Rohn*

To use my **7 Step Training Program**, you'll need to track these basic elements:

- **Calendar** – Create a calendar that shows which days you trained.
- **Distance** – Log how far you ran, walked, jogged, swam, or biked.
- **Time** – Write down how long you trained that day (or event).
- **Pace** – If this was biking, swimming or running, note the pace. If this was a cross-training day, note your reps and sets.
- **Type** – Categorize your effort. For instance, note if you ran hills, did a tempo run, or swam open water or pool laps.
- **Comments** – Use this space for personal comments. Something always comes up that doesn't fit in a predefined category.

Running Log

Month April   Year 2016

Week	Day	Distance	Time	Pace (Avg)	Pace (Best)	HR (Avg)	HR (Max)	Type	Route	Comments
1	SUN		: :							
	MON	X-train	: :							Cross-training (Swim)
	TUE	4 miles	: 35 : 24	8:51	8:18	125	141	Fartleks	Track	Felt sluggish, weather was nice
	WED	0	: :							
	THU	2 miles	: 22 : 40	11:20	9:03	140	156	Hills	Apex Park	Great run!
	FRI	11 miles	1 : 35 : 20	8:40	7:14	147	159	Progressions	River Run	Very cool weather but felt good!
	SAT		: :							
2	SUN		: :							
	MON		: :							
	TUE		: :							

To add detail, add the following elements to your log:

- Heart rate
- Resting heart rate
- Shoe type and mileage
- How you felt that day (emotionally)
- How you felt that day (physically)

- Route name
- Weather conditions
- Pre-activity calorie intake
- Calorie burn
- Current weight

You might have a separate "racing log" that can include:

- Division placement
- Overall placement

- Event name
- Personal records or milestones

Racing Log

Year **2015**

Date	Race Name	Distance	Time	Pace (Avg)	Pace (Best)	HR (Avg)	HR (Max)	Overall Place	Division Place	Comments
11/25	Turkey Day 5k	3.1 miles	: 25 :13	8:07	7:22	144	160	15/221	2/11	2nd in my age group! Sunny!
12/7	Santa Claus 10k	6.2 miles	: 53 :37	8:38	7:55	142	153	35/412	16/23	Didn't place but had fun anyway.
12/15	Snowman Stomper	10 mile	1 :27 :08	8:43	8:12	136	150	-	-	Fun run, no awards!
			: :							
			: :							

Turning Technical – If you're the type of person who struggles with manual daily logging of your activities, you can always turn to technology to gather most of the important attributes that you wish to track. As we saw in **Chapter 11 – Equipment and Safety,** there is a plethora of hardware, software and web-based technologies that can track the important features of your run. What's more, the technology-based solutions can keep historical statistics that are accessible at the click of a mouse or the touch on a tablet.

Tip

Managing Your Time

As with any long-term plan, you need to be able to manage the time that you have available. This means you need to be able to balance family, work, and personal time and it's not always an easy thing to do in this fast-paced world. Here are a few hints to help you manage your time:

- Plan your time a week in advance – block out sections of your day, and plan your activity well ahead of time.
- Be flexible with your time. Reschedule, but don't reduce your training time.
- Balance! Take time for family and work, but keep enough time to do the things you need to do to reach your goals. If this means running early in the morning, do it.
- Every lap, mile, step, or lift should have a purpose. Focus on moving forward and stay efficient. Train for your goal.
- Schedule for problems. Allow time for injuries, emergencies and unexpected events.
- Learn to disconnect. Put down the cell phone, disengage from social networking, and allow yourself to focus on the simpler things in life.

Thinking in Phases - Macrocycles and Mesocycles

There are seven phases in my running program that are known in their entirety as the *running macrocycle*, with each phase known as a *mesocycle*. In most training arenas, there are only 4 or 5 mesocycles, but I've also included the *Taper* and *Recovery* phases because I believe they are just as important in the overall macrocycle.

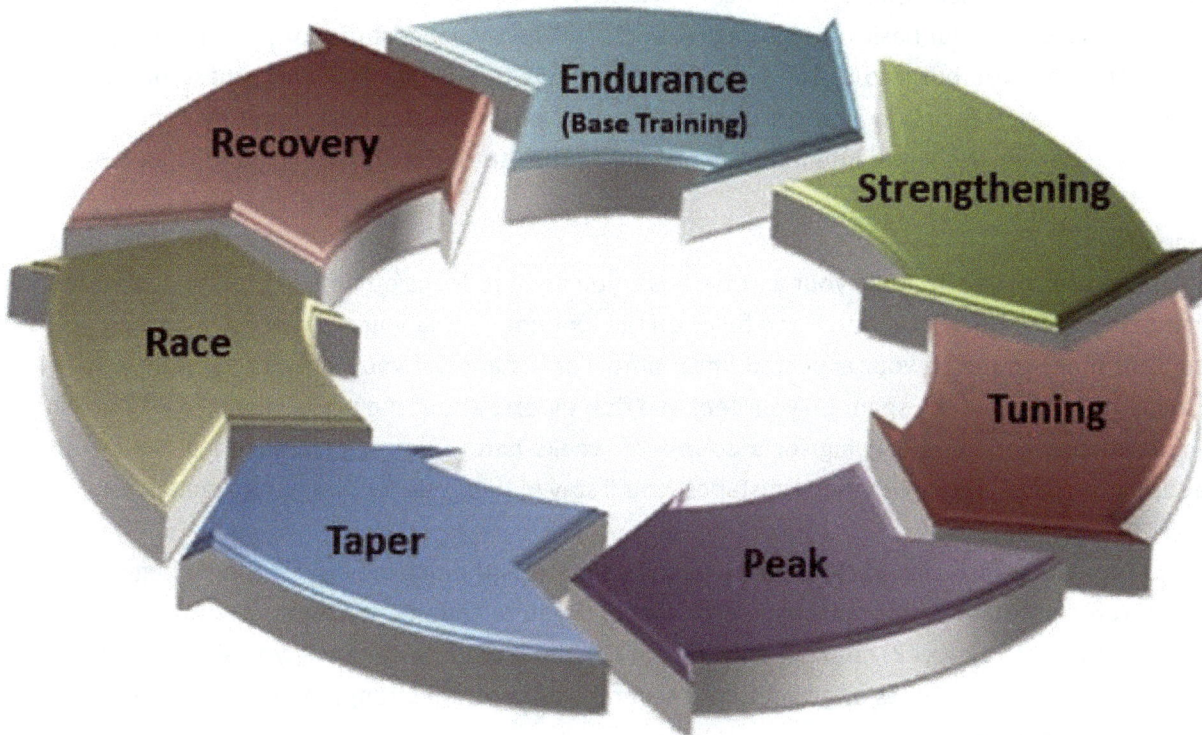

Each mesocycle is as important as its predecessor and its successor. For instance, you can't reach the Peak phase without first going through the Endurance (base training), Strengthening and Tuning cycles.

Similarly, you can't race effectively without a proper Taper cycle. Finally, before you start the buildup to your next macrocycle, you must restore your body and mind by going through the Recovery cycle.

Each time you build up for your next macrocycle, you need to spend the appropriate amount of time in each phase. Every macrocycle begins with the Endurance mesocycle and finishes with the Recovery mesocycle. Let's turn to the next page to look at the details of each mesocycle and learn the importance of them.

Motivation

"Once you make the decision that you will not fail, the heart and the body will follow." – *Kara Goucher*

The Master Plan

In this section, we'll cover the seven mesocycles that make up the macrocycle with a brief description, action plan, and Zone Training recommendation for each.

Endurance Mesocycle

This is the phase in which we build our base as described in **Chapter 13 – Training Basics**. Mix in some cross-training when you start to get comfortable with your running.

This is where your basic training begins, and it will be the longest part of your training program in terms of the time you put into it. The focus of this cycle is to build an endurance base of *stability* and *volume*. We will NOT focus on *intensity* during this initial phase. At this time, don't be concerned about how fast you can go. We'll dive into intensity training in the Strengthening, Tuning and Peak mesocycles.

Action Plan:
Build an aerobic base – To build your aerobic base, you need to focus on time in motion. Substitute your running GPS watch for a basic watch and focus on the amount of time you are putting in on long runs with consistent times to match your expected finish time. For instance, if you think you can run a 30 minute 5k, focus ONLY on the time spent on your feet and don't worry about the actual distance. Establish your 30-minute base and keep it going for a couple of weeks before you start measuring the distance or increasing the pace. If you're in the 5k distance, you'll stay in this cycle for one to two weeks, longer if you have NO aerobic base.

Your Endurance mesocycle should end and your Strengthening mesocycle should begin only when you can run comfortably for your planned distance. If you're training for a marathon, you'll be in this mesocycle for six to 12 weeks, and possibly longer. For the marathon distance, you should experience at least one long run of 22 miles or greater, and several weeks of the strengthening phase before starting the Tuning mesocycle.

Focus:
Form and Technique – Teach your body to run with the correct form as described in **Chapter 3 – What is Running?** Correct form and execution is important because it allows your body to work easier and more efficiently.

You may gradually increase your mileage until you can run your goal distance, but don't worry about increasing your pace yet – that will come in the next mesocycle.

Training Zone: You should be in Zone 1 for your warmups and cool-downs. During this phase, you should normally be in Zone 2, and occasionally reaching into Zone 3 for short periods of time while you push your cardiovascular system. (Refer to **Chapter 13 – Training Basics** for Training Zones.)

Motivation

"The man who thinks he can and the man who thinks he can't, are both right. Which one are you?" – *Henry Ford*

Strengthening Mesocycle

This phase is used for strengthening other parts of our body to match the strength in our legs. Friendly competition is fine, but you should not be racing at this point.

Action Plan:

Expand your strength – At this point, you continue with your aerobic training while you add tempo runs, hill runs, or longer intervals done at 5k race pace once or twice a week.

Focus:

Strength and Conditioning – Review the exercises and activities in **Chapter 12 – Strength and Conditioning**.

Cross-Train! – You should be cross-training at least two times per week, working with weights and activities that will strengthen your existing muscles and connective tissues. Add core and upper body activities to provide strength, coordination and balance. You will cross-train more during this phase than in any of the other mesocycles. Work on one-leg exercises that push your limits, with a focus on hips and core body improvements. Now is the chance for you to get strong!

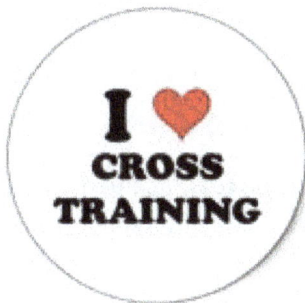

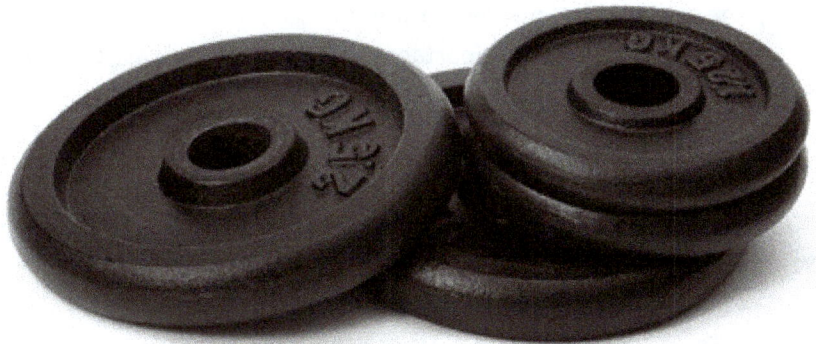

Pick Up the Pace – Your intensity should increase, but your overall mileage should remain at your intended goal distance. Pick one or two days per week to work on a faster pace. Concentrate on a turnover rate of 90 steps per foot, per minute. Fartleks and hill repeats are a good choice for this phase.

Training Zone: You should be in Zone 1 for your warmups and cool-downs. During this phase, you should normally be in Zone 3, and occasionally reaching into Zone 4 for short periods of time while you push your cardiovascular system. (Refer to **Chapter 13 – Training Basics** for Training Zones.)

> **Motivation**
>
> "I often hear someone say I'm not a real runner. We are all runners, some just run faster than others. I never met a fake runner." – *Bart Yasso*

Tuning Mesocycle

This mesocycle is probably the most important phase to determine your actual fitness level. It should be used for final preparation to test and fine tune your body before you hit your "peak." Test your limits – push the distance and the pace. Stay in Zone 4 as long as possible without injuring yourself.

With regards to injuries, this is probably the most risky mesocycle that you'll experience because you'll be increasing your pace to threshold levels, which can put major stressors on your body. The real danger may not be in the additional intensity, but could be more directly related to an absent, shortened, or ineffective recovery.

Action Plan:

During your hill repeats, intervals and fartleks, make sure you take additional time to cool down before the next repetition.

If you're going to race up to 10 miles, you should be able to cover the entire 10 miles at a pace that's about 15 to 30 seconds per mile slower than your intended goal pace. Run the entire distance two to four times during this cycle.

If you're going to race a half marathon or full marathon, you should be able to cover up to 90% of the distance at a pace that's 30 to 45 seconds per mile slower your intended goal pace. Half marathoners should run at least 12 miles, two to three times during this phase. Full marathoners should run at least 22 miles, one to two times during this phase.

Rest days are most important during this phase – as you increase your intensity, you can decrease your mileage.

Focus:

Intensity and Consistency – This is your last chance to fine tune your body using real race techniques. All systems are "go" at this point and you'll use the next two to four weeks to emulate live racing conditions.

Training Zone: You should be in Zone 1 for your warmups and cool-downs. During this phase, you should normally be in Zone 3, reaching into Zone 4 for extended periods of time. Attempt to stay in Zone 4 for at least 50% of your run. This will be difficult, but should be attainable. (Refer to **Chapter 13 – Training Basics** for Training Zones.)

> **Tip**
>
> Use the Tuning mesocycle to push your pace for extended lengths of time. Stay in Training Zone 4 for extended periods of time. Increase the intensity but lower your overall weekly mileage. The best training routines are tempo and progression runs for sustained threshold training. You will not benefit as much from fartleks and hill repeats at this point. (See page 233 for information on different running workouts.)

> **Motivation**
>
> **"Every time I step on the field, I'm going to give my whole heart regardless of the score."** – *Tim Tebow*

Peak Mesocycle

For weeks or months, you've been working hard with your base running program and cross-training. You have a goal and an action plan to accomplish it. You've finished your strengthening and tuning cycles and are now "race-ready" in the Peak mesocycle.

It's time to transform potential into reality and you can do that by entering a real race. This shouldn't be your goal race, but should be a race to test your finely honed skills, speed, and endurance.

Action Plan:

If your goal race is between 5 and 10 kilometer races, you should be able to enter a trial race, and run at full speed. If you fail to meet your goals, use the next couple of weeks before your "real" race to focus on intensity and consistency.

If your goal race is a half-marathon or full marathon, you should enter a race of that distance and run at least 90% of the race at race pace. Half marathoners should run at least 11 miles and full marathoners should run at least 22 miles at your goal pace. Again, if you miss your target pace, reduce your overall weekly mileage, but don't reduce the distance of your weekly long run; instead focus on intensity for that long run. If this is your first marathon, you should experience "hitting the wall" by running 18 to 22 miles. Be sure to review "My Story – the Marathon Owns You" at the beginning of this chapter.

Use the training schedules coming up later in this chapter to decide how and when to run your trial race. You need to make sure you have enough time to iron out the last few wrinkles and still give yourself enough time to rest through the Taper mesocycle.

Focus:

Real Race Experience – Use this mesocycle to gain practical experience at your target distance and pace. This is "dress rehearsal" for the actual run, using the actual equipment you'll be running with. Your diet should include plenty of carbs and you should be completely aware of dietary needs and how your body responds to the foods that you're eating. Everything you do at this point should mimic the big event.

Finally, don't be tempted to outrun your goal. In other words, if you've been training for a marathon, there is no point or purpose to go out and try to run a 30 miler. Likewise, if you've been training for a 10k race, don't try to run at 5k pace. These are the types of mistakes that can most certainly end in overuse injuries.

Training Zone: You should be in Zone 1 for your warmups and cool-downs. During this phase, you should run in trial races and spend most of your time in Zone 4, unless you are having physical issues staying in that zone. Attempt to stay in Zone 4 for at least 80% of your run. This will be very difficult, but if you've trained properly, it should be attainable. (Refer to **Chapter 13 – Training Basics** for Training Zones.)

> ### Motivation
>
> **"What you *get* by achieving your goals is not as important as what you *become* by achieving your goals."** — *Henry David Thoreau*

Taper Mesocycle

Sometimes, the simplest things turn out to be the most difficult. And so it can be true with this phase of the running program. After developing a plan and working hard for months on end, you find that your running became an integral part of your daily life – it became a habit. And now you're being asked to slow down and at some point, actually stop running before your big race. This mesocycle will test your patience more than any other phase in the program.

Instead of focusing on your upcoming race, focus on the taper itself. Know that you will benefit and run a better race if you taper properly. Your body will appreciate the much needed rest.

Action Plan:

So, this is how it works: Once you begin your taper cycle, you don't just stop running. You gradually decrease your mileage, but keep the intensity up until a few days or a week before your race. It's at that point, when you'll actually stop running altogether.

You can still use this time for light cross-training, but stay away from training that can interfere with your overall training. Long bike rides and heavy weight lifting should not be done at this time. Moderation is the key.

Half marathoners and full marathoners should cut their long runs by 50% at least one week before their race.

Also, if you're worried about weight gain during this time, shove those concerns aside. You'll be just fine on race day, and your body will adjust accordingly. Fuel up with carbs, but avoid foods with a lot of fat.

Long interval running is your best training method during this phase, as it continues to tax your cardiovascular system, but won't overload it.

Focus:

Maintenance and Pre-Race Recovery – Use this phase to maintain your intensity, but not your distance. Distance should be reduced gradually during the taper cycle, but don't reduce the intensity until a week or so before your race. Once you've hit the Peak mesocycle it will take about three weeks before your fitness level starts to diminish, so you don't need to worry about showing up at the start line "out of shape."

Training Zone: You should be in Zone 1 for your warmups and cool-downs. Early on in the taper, you should reduce your distance, but stay in Zone 4 as much as possible, unless you are having physical issues staying in that zone. Attempt to stay in Zone 4 for at least 80% of your run. Halfway through your taper cycle, reduce your mileage AND your intensity up until race day. (Refer to **Chapter 13 – Training Basics** for Training Zones.)

> **Motivation**
>
> ***"Every accomplishment starts with the decision to try."*** – *Unknown*

Race Mesocycle

Congratulations! After months of blood, sweat and tears, your big day has arrived, and now it's time to put all you've rehearsed to the test. **Chapter 17 – Running Your Race** will give you much more insight on what you can expect on the days leading up to the day of the race, and the days following the race, so I won't elaborate in this section. Instead, I'll give you your *Action Plan* and *Focus* for this mesocycle.

Action Plan:

First of all, make sure you show up at the start line relaxed and ready to go. If you're running late, you will most likely be out of focus and you don't need that additional stress. Be early and give yourself the time you need to stretch and warm up properly, just like you did in your training.

Race day can conjure up all kinds of emotions which will trigger adrenaline in your body. The release of this hormone activates the body's "fight or flight" response, causing air passages to dilate. It also causes the blood vessels to contract in an effort to redirect blood towards major muscle groups, in preparation of "the fight." Finally, adrenaline decreases the body's ability to feel pain, which is why you can keep running. This can be a good thing if you're aware of the effects of this powerful hormone; however, it can also cause you to run at a faster pace than you trained for. In other words, don't "go out too fast." Be patient and stay within your training pace. We'll talk about this more in the next chapter.

Focus:

Turnover – The word of the day is "turnover." Focus on a turnover rate of 90 to 94 steps per minute, per foot, and more if you can handle it. Keep your form intact from start to finish. The Endurance mesocycle taught you to rely on good form throughout your training program but you'll have to constantly monitor it on race day.

Training Zone: You should be in Zone 1 for your warmups and cool-downs. If you're running in distances longer than 13.1 miles, you might not want to do a warmup, instead using the first mile as your warmup. It's counterproductive to waste precious, limited energy on a warmup when you're running a long race. During the race you should spend most of your time in Zone 4. Attempt to stay in Zone 4 for at least 90% of your run. (Refer to **Chapter 13 – Training Basics** for Training Zones.)

Motivation

"You have to wonder at times what you're doing out there. Over the years, I've given myself a thousand reasons to keep running, but it always comes back to where it started. It comes down to self-satisfaction and a sense of achievement." – *Steve Prefontaine*

Recovery Mesocycle

Race day has come and gone. Now what? You may find that habits really are hard to break. You set a big goal and finally accomplished it, but it shouldn't end there. Even if you didn't meet your goals and swore you'd never do it again, you should try to keep an open mind. Most first-time "average Joe" runners go through this, sometimes multiple times. But for now, take the time to heal physically and mentally. Your body has gone through a very brutal experience, but it may be the mind that suffers longer. You may encounter "the blues," a state of psychological depression that could last much longer than your physical pain. Expect this – it's a normal response when you quit doing something that you've grown accustomed to after a long period of time. If you're like most of us, you need to "reboot" your systems and get a fresh start.

The recovery mesocycle marks the end of your macrocycle. Rest, relax, and recover – recover physically and mentally. Don't start your next cycle until you are free from pain and burnout. When you're ready to start up again, schedule your next race and plan out your entire macrocycle.

Recovery Explained – I'm hoping that after your race you'll want to start your running program all over again, once you've healed from your wounds. With that in mind, you shouldn't just *stop* training. Treat your recovery as an "active rest cycle," – meaning no races, no heavy lifting, no hard training, and no fretting over which training zone you think you should be in. Instead, light exercise and jogging will be good for your mind and soul, once you are pain-free again. This is a perfect time to engage in cross-training such as swimming or biking.

First-time runners may take longer to reestablish their will to run again, but experienced runners are quite the opposite. They'll be scoping out the race website for the next available race they can sign up for!

Actual recovery times will vary according to your age, the distance you ran, the effort you put into your race, and your body's ability to fully recover. For some, it may take a couple of days before they can walk normally again, and some might take a couple of weeks. Either way, I recommend that you take one to two weeks off from hard running or workouts if you ran distances between a 5k and 10 mile race. If you ran a half marathon or longer, take three to four weeks off before starting your next macrocycle. Remember, light jogging and workouts are fine and I urge you to do them, but please don't race until your body and mind are fully functional again.

Freaks! – There are some people out there who have the innate ability to run marathons week after week. My friend Keith, whom I've referred to several times in this book, ran over 30 marathons in one year. Most of his times were good enough to qualify for the Boston Marathon. Personally, I've run a couple of back-to-back marathons (or longer) in a single weekend. When conditioned properly, the body can tolerate long stretches of endurance activities, but there is a point at which you will need to recover. Since we're all different and have different endurance and pain thresholds, only you can determine how soon and how often you can run. If you're a "freak," consider yourself blessed!

Every goal must have a plan to succeed. Let's turn to the next page and start the planning process.

Motivation

"Breakdowns can create breakthroughs. Things fall apart so they can fall together." – *Unknown*

Planning Your Macrocycle

Back in **Chapter 15 – Setting Goals,** we talked about what we wanted to achieve. Before you can plan your running macrocycle, you must first set your goals. Earlier in this chapter, we defined our action plan to accomplish our goals. Let's now focus on the actual training program that will drive the action plan.

Are you going to run two marathons this year? Are you going to start with a 5k, go up to the 10k or 10 mile distance, and finish out your season with a competitive half marathon? How will you know when to "peak" for your upcoming race? When should you start your fine-tuning?

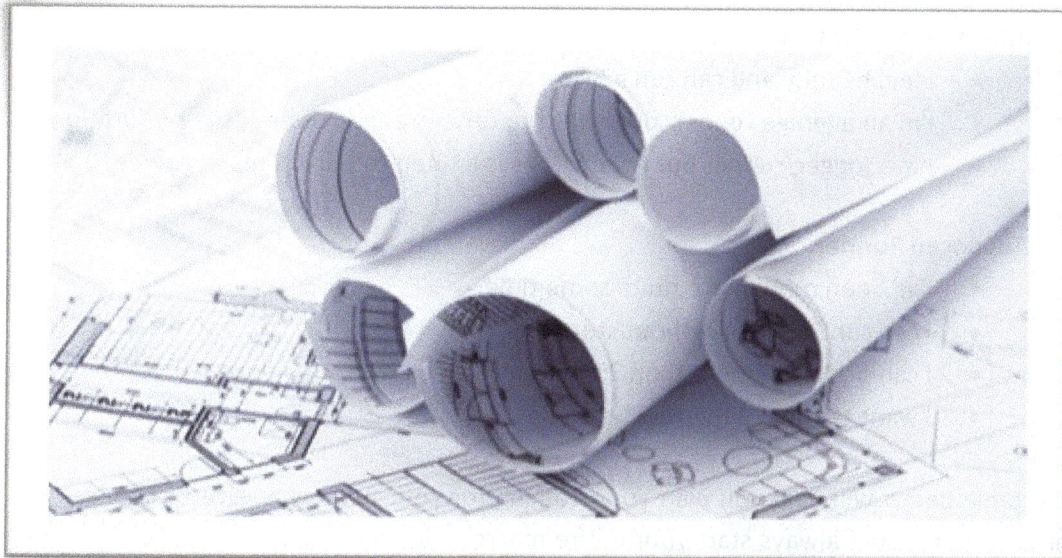

Tip
Bringing a plan to life

I started training 6 months before the 2009 St. George Marathon, with a gradual buildup to my intended pace and distance. That summer, I ran quite a few 5k and 10k races to "feel the burn" of competitive running. I also focused on the "Yasso 800s" mentioned earlier in this book and set a goal to run a sub-3-hour marathon. That year, I took the time to create an actual training plan and followed every detail of it, including cross-training and recovery days. Even though I didn't consider myself to be a gifted runner, I was still able to meet my goal because I trained with VERY SPECIFIC plans to guide me. Because I had a plan, I was able to meet my goal and finish in less than three hours. I could not have accomplished this by simply running every day – I had to *create* and *follow* my plan.

Motivation

"Give me six hours to chop down a tree and I will spend the first four sharpening the axe." – *Abraham Lincoln*

In **Chapter 12 – Strength and Conditioning**, we talked about different levels of fitness as we enter our running program. Since we all might be at different points in our training, let's review them and give some examples to help you assess your current fitness level.

- **Beginning Runner:**
    - I feel overweight or unhealthy and need a place to start
    - I consider myself healthy but have never run regularly
    - I haven't run in a long time
    - I'm a jogger/runner but my mileage is limited to 1 to 5 miles per week

- **Intermediate Runner:**
    - I feel healthy and can run a 5k or 10k
    - I'm an average runner, but I want to raise my level of intensity or duration
    - I'm a jogger/runner but my mileage is limited to 5 to 25 miles per week

- **Advanced Runner:**
    - I've been running for quite some time
    - I can run 15 miles without stopping
    - I can or do run more than 25 miles per week without injury
    - I want to run competitively

The table below will help you plan your training for your upcoming race or race season. Please remember that you should always start your entire macrocycle completely rested. Your body and mind need time to recover from possible physical *and* mental fatigue (injury or burnout). The table lists each of the seven mesocycles in the first column, and the weekly TOTAL shows the duration of the entire macrocycle. All schedules include Recovery time to complete the macrocycle. To calculate the actual training time, subtract the Recovery phase from the TOTAL.

Macrocycle / Mesocycle Duration

Mesocycle	5k	10k	10 mile	Half Marathon	Marathon
Endurance	4 Weeks	5 Weeks	6 Weeks	10 Weeks	14 Weeks
Strengthening	4 Weeks	4 Weeks	6 Weeks	10 Weeks	14 Weeks
Tuning	2 Weeks	2 Weeks	3 Weeks	3 Weeks	4 Weeks
Peak	1 Week	1 Week	10 Days	2 Weeks	3 Weeks
Taper	2 Days	4 Days	5 Days	10 Days	2 Week
Race	Race	Race	Race	Race	Race
Recovery	1 Week	10 Days	2 Weeks	3 Weeks	4 Weeks
TOTAL	**12 Weeks**	**14 Weeks**	**19 Weeks**	**30 Weeks**	**41 Weeks**

In this example, the marathon training cycle is 37 weeks plus 4 weeks recovery to make up the entire 41-week macrocycle.

Once you've identified your starting point – *Beginner, Intermediate* or *Advanced* – you'll need to assemble your plan by developing your own macrocycle. On the next page, we'll start by following one of the plans that meets your current level of fitness.

You'll notice right away that the duration of the *Beginner, Intermediate* and *Advanced* plans are the same for any given distance, but the frequency and total mileage increases with each subsequent plan.

For instance, the *Beginner* and the *Advanced* marathon training plans are both 41 weeks in duration, but the *Beginner* plan only has four days of running per week, whereas the *Advanced* plan features six days of running with nearly three times the mileage per week. The *Advanced* plans may also feature multiple Cross-training days as well as "two-a-days" in which you are challenged with two runs per day. The *Intermediate* plan falls somewhere in between the *Beginner* and *Advanced* plans.

Tuning and Peak macrocycles will be fairly static across all levels because you can only peak for so long. The longest of your training phases will be early on, during the first two mesocycles. The Recovery mesocycle is similar on all three groups.

Key differences in the training plans are:

- Beginner
    - Run four days per week
    - Cross-train one day per week
    - Rest two days per week

- Intermediate
    - Run five days per week
    - Cross-train one day per week
    - Rest one day per week

- Advanced
    - Run six days per week
    - AND cross-train two days per week
    - Rest one day per week
    - Increased mileage compared to Beginner and Intermediate

Motivation

"It's important to know that at the end of the day it's not the medals you remember. What you remember is the process – what you learn about yourself by challenging yourself, the experiences you share with other people, the honesty the training demands – those are things nobody can take away from you whether you finish twelfth or you're an Olympic Champion."
– Silken Laumann

Custom Training Plans

I just described *how long* your training plans might take. Now, let's focus on *what* your training should be made of, including recovery days, easy and hard running days, long run days and cross-training days. I'll try to make it as easy as possible by creating a training plan for each of the categories above. We'll start with Beginner 5k and work all the way up to Advanced Marathon.

> **Tip**
>
> **Beginning Level Runners – Please Read!!!** If you're just starting out with your running, please review page 187 and make sure you can run for 20 minutes BEFORE you start any of these training plans.

Mesocycle
Endurance
Strengthening
Tuning
Peak
Taper (light running)   Taper (no running)
Race
Recovery

I've color-coded the training plans by their associated mesocycle. Suggested distances for the day are also included. For example, "Easy 1M" means an easy run of one mile for that day. "Tempo 3.5 mi." would describe a 3.5 mile Tempo run.

Week	Sunday	Monday	Tuesday	Wednesday	Thursday	Friday	Saturday
1					Easy 1mi.	Rest	Easy .5 mi
2	Rest	Easy 1.5 mi.	Cross-train	Hills 1 mi.	Easy 2 mi.	Rest	Easy 1.5 mi.
3	Rest	Easy 1.5 mi.	Cross-train	Hills 1.5 mi.	Easy 2 mi.	Rest	Medium 1.5 mi.
4	Rest	Easy 2 mi.	Cross-train	Hills 2 mi.	Easy 2 mi.	Rest	Medium 2.5 mi.
5	Rest	Medium 2 mi.	Cross-train	Hills 2.5 mi.	Easy 2 mi.	Rest	Medium 2.5 mi.
6	Rest	Medium 2 mi.	Cross-train	Fartleks 2.5 mi.	Easy 2 mi.	Rest	Tempo 2.5 mi.
7	Rest	Medium 3 mi.	Cross-train	Intervals 2 mi.	Easy 2.5 mi.	Rest	Tempo 3 mi.
8	Rest	Medium 3.5 mi.	Cross-train	Tempo 2 mi.	Easy 1 mi.	Rest	Hills 2.5 mi.
9	Rest	Easy 3 mi.	Cross-train	Hill Repeats 1 mi.	Easy 3 mi.	Rest	Tempo 3.5 mi.
10	Rest	Easy 1.5 mi.	Cross-train	Tempo 3.1 mi.	Easy 3 mi.	Rest	Practice 5k Race
11	Rest	Easy 2 mi.	Cross-train	Tempo 3.1 mi.	Easy 2 mi.	Rest	Tempo 3 mi.
12	Rest	Progression 2.5 mi.	Cross-train	Easy 2 mi.	Easy 1 mi.	Rest	5k Race
13	Recovery	Recovery	Recovery	Recovery	Recovery	Recovery	Recovery

Each day of your training calendar has a purpose. Cross-training days should be used for weight lifting, swimming, or biking. Use cross-training days to strengthen muscles, joints and ligaments that are NOT primarily used for running. If you are injured or severely fatigued, use your cross-training days for recovery.

The Endurance cycle usually consists of easy and medium effort runs. Use this cycle to gradually build up your body and condition it properly.

The Strengthening cycle will begin to fill with varying degrees of difficulty, including hills, hill repeats, fartleks, and tempo runs. Weight lifting is highly recommended for your cross-training during this mesocycle.

The Tuning and Peak mesocycles will include difficult runs with a focus on hill repeats, tempo runs, and progression runs.

For clarification purposes, here is a brief description of each of the workout types you'll see in the upcoming training calendars.

Easy – This is part of your **base** running to establish your endurance. A base run is a fairly short to moderate length run at a runner's natural gait and pace. This run does not need to be particularly challenging, but it should be done frequently, and should be the foundation of your aerobic capacity, endurance, and running economy. See page 191 for more details on the base run.

Medium – This is part of the **base** run and can be treated the same as an easy run, but you should try to get into Zone 3 for about 75% of your run. Push your cardio system a bit more on these days to where conversations are difficult.

Long – This is also a base run, meaning you implement your natural gait and pace. Nothing fancy, you just run a long distance. I don't include long runs on 5k or 10k plans. See page 196 for details.

Tempo – This is defined as the fastest pace that can be sustained for one hour by a very fit individual. More or less, it's the fastest pace that can be sustained for 20 minutes in less fit runners. See page 193 for details.

Hills – Hill running is comprised of a combination of up- and downhill running of various grades and distances. This is the "free-form" of hill running, with no set structure. Refer to page 194 for details.

Hill Repeats – The idea of hill repeats is to choose a moderately steep hill (four to six percent grade) with 30- to 45-second speed bursts, from bottom to top. See page 195 for more information.

Intervals – They consist of repeated segments of moderate- to fast-paced running separated by slow running or walking for a brief recovery. Read page 191 for more information.

Fartleks – If you're feeling good, you simply speed up for as long as you can, and if you start to fatigue you simply slow down. Read more about this run on page 192.

Progression – The concept is to start out at your slower than your natural pace, and gradually build to a strong finish. See page 194 for details.

Beginner Training Plans – 5K to Marathon

In this section, we'll take a look at training plans for beginners from a 5k to the marathon distance. Each of the plans includes at least one cross-training day, two rest days, and one easy day, although you will be challenged by the remainder of the days. Each plan will also feature a practice run or a real race. Use this day to sign up for a race similar to the one you'll do on race day. If you don't sign up for a race that day, try to emulate race conditions with a strong tempo or progression workout.

The training plans also feature a race that you should consider entering towards the end of your Strengthening mesocycle. These special races offer a great chance to enter a trial race and benchmark your efforts. They can really put you into a racing frame of mind. They're highlighted in orange and begin in the 10k training plan. **NOTE:** If you're already running a specific distance, feel free to jump into the training plan at the distance you've already done. For instance, if you're already running half marathons, your entry point to the marathon training plan would be at a distance of 13 miles.

Level: Beginner   **Distance:** 5k
Macrocycle Time: 12 weeks + 1 week Recovery   **Peak Maximum Mileage:** 9.5 miles in 7 days
About This Plan: This training plan starts with short distances and finishes with three consecutive weekends of fast-paced tempo runs to train you for your first 5k.

Week	Sunday	Monday	Tuesday	Wednesday	Thursday	Friday	Saturday
1					Easy 1 mi.	Rest	Easy .5 mi
2	Rest	Easy 1.5 mi.	Cross-train	Hills 1 mi.	Easy 2 mi.	Rest	Easy 1.5 mi.
3	Rest	Easy 1.5 mi.	Cross-train	Hills 1.5 mi.	Easy 2 mi.	Rest	Medium 1.5 mi.
4	Rest	Easy 2 mi.	Cross-train	Hills 2 mi.	Easy 2 mi.	Rest	Medium 2.5 mi.
5	Rest	Medium 2 mi.	Cross-train	Hills 2.5 mi.	Easy 2 mi.	Rest	Medium 2.5 mi.
6	Rest	Medium 2 mi.	Cross-train	Fartleks 2.5 mi.	Easy 2 mi.	Rest	Tempo 2.5 mi.
7	Rest	Medium 3 mi.	Cross-train	Intervals 2 mi.	Easy 2.5 mi.	Rest	Tempo 3 mi.
8	Rest	Medium 3.5 mi.	Cross-train	Tempo 2 mi.	Easy 1 mi.	Rest	Hills 2.5 mi.
9	Rest	Easy 3 mi.	Cross-train	Hill Repeats 1 mi.	Easy 3 mi.	Rest	Tempo 3.5 mi.
10	Rest	Easy 1.5 mi.	Cross-train	Tempo 3.1 mi.	Easy 3 mi.	Rest	Practice 5k Race
11	Rest	Easy 2 mi.	Cross-train	Tempo 3.1 mi.	Easy 2 mi.	Rest	Tempo 3 mi.
12	Rest	Progression 2.5 mi.	Cross-train	Easy 2 mi.	Easy 1 mi.	Rest	**5k Race**
13	Recovery	Recovery	Recovery	Recovery	Recovery	Recovery	Recovery

Level: Beginner
Distance: 10k
Macrocycle Time: 14 weeks + 10 days Recovery
Peak Maximum Mileage: 19.2 miles in 7 days
About This Plan: Similar to the 5k training plan, this one is loaded with hills and tempo runs to build strength in each of the last six weekends. This plan is the ultimate challenge for any first-time 10k runner! It builds with intensity and distance, but has many recovery points. Be sure to honor the rest days to avoid overuse injuries. If you're already running 5k's you can enter this training plan at week 10.

Week	Sunday	Monday	Tuesday	Wednesday	Thursday	Friday	Saturday
1			Cross-train	Easy .5 mi.	Easy 1 mi.	Rest	Easy .5 mi.
2	Rest	Easy 1.5 mi.	Cross-train	Hills 1 mi.	Easy 2 mi.	Rest	Easy 1.5 mi.
3	Rest	Easy 2 mi.	Cross-train	Hills 1.5 mi.	Easy 2 mi.	Rest	Medium 2 mi.
4	Rest	Easy 3 mi.	Cross-train	Hills 2.5 mi.	Easy 3 mi.	Rest	Medium 3 mi.
5	Rest	Medium 3 mi.	Cross-train	Hills 3 mi.	Easy 4 mi.	Rest	Medium 3.5 mi.
6	Rest	Medium 3.5 mi.	Cross-train	Hills 3.5 mi.	Easy 2 mi.	Rest	Medium 4 mi.
7	Rest	Medium 3.5 mi.	Cross-train	Hills 4 mi.	Easy 3 mi.	Rest	Medium 4.5 mi.
8	Rest	Medium 4 mi.	Cross-train	Fartleks 3.5 mi.	Easy 3 mi.	Rest	Tempo 4.5 mi.
9	Rest	Medium 4 mi.	Cross-train	Intervals 4 mi.	Easy 4 mi.	Rest	Tempo 5 mi.
10	Rest	Medium 5 mi.	Cross-train	Hills 5 mi.	Easy 5 mi.	Rest	5k Race
11	Rest	Easy 6 mi.	Cross-train	Hill Repeats 1.5 mi.	Easy 6 mi.	Rest	Tempo 5 mi.
12	Rest	Easy 3 mi.	Cross-train	Progression 5 mi.	Easy 3 mi.	Rest	Practice 10k Race
13	Rest	Progression 6 mi.	Cross-train	Tempo 6.2 mi.	Easy 4 mi.	Rest	Tempo 6 mi.
14	Rest	Easy 3 mi.	Easy 4 mi.	Easy 2 mi.	No running	No Running	**10k Race**
15	Recovery	Recovery	Recovery	Recovery	Recovery	Recovery	Recovery
16	Recovery	Recovery	Recovery				

Motivation

"Efforts and courage are not enough without purpose and direction." *– John F. Kennedy*

Level: Beginner   **Distance:** 10 miles

Macrocycle Time: 19 weeks + 2 weeks Recovery   **Peak Maximum Mileage:** 35 miles in 10 days

About This Plan: This plan is for the serious beginner and is a perfect plan to help you "upgrade" to half marathons and full marathons at a later date. The focus of this plan is to expand your endurance with plenty of hills and long runs. If you don't want to run a "practice" race at the end of week 16, do another "long 10-miler" instead. You don't need to race, but you should cover the distance in several consecutive weekends. If you're already running 10k's you can enter this training plan at week 12.

Week	Sunday	Monday	Tuesday	Wednesday	Thursday	Friday	Saturday
1						Easy .5 mi.	Rest
2	Rest	Easy 1.5 mi.	Cross-train	Hills 1 mi.	Easy 2 mi.	Rest	Easy 1.5 mi.
3	Rest	Easy 1.5 mi.	Cross-train	Hills 1.5 mi.	Easy 2 mi.	Rest	Medium 1.5 mi.
4	Rest	Easy 2 mi.	Cross-train	Hills 2 mi.	Easy 2M	Rest	Medium 2.5 mi.
5	Rest	Easy 3 mi.	Cross-train	Hills 2.5 mi.	Easy 3 mi.	Rest	Medium 3 mi.
6	Rest	Medium 3 mi.	Cross-train	Hills 3 mi.	Easy 4 mi.	Rest	Medium 3.5 mi.
7	Rest	Medium 3.5 mi.	Cross-train	Hills 3.5 mi.	Easy 2 mi.	Rest	Medium 4 mi.
8	Rest	Medium 4 mi.	Cross-train	Fartleks 3.5 mi.	Easy 2 mi.	Rest	Medium 5 mi.
9	Rest	Medium 5 mi.	Cross-train	Intervals 4 mi.	Easy 2.5 mi.	Rest	Medium 6 mi.
10	Rest	Medium 6 mi.	Cross-train	Progression 5 mi.	Easy 3 mi.	Rest	Long 7 mi.
11	Rest	Medium 7 mi.	Cross-train	Hills 4 mi.	Easy 5 mi.	Rest	Tempo 7 mi.
12	Rest	Medium 6 mi.	Cross-train	Hill Repeats 1 mi.	Easy 6 mi.	Rest	10k Race
13	Rest	Medium 8 mi.	Cross-train	Hills 4 mi.	Easy 7 mi.	Rest	Long 9 mi.
14	Rest	Medium 7 mi.	Cross-train	Progression 5 mi.	Easy 8 mi.	Rest	Tempo 9 mi.
15	Rest	Hills 3 mi.	Cross-train	Hill Repeats 2 mi.	Easy 9 mi.	Rest	Long 10 mi.
16	Rest	Easy 8 mi.	Cross-train	Progression 6 mi.	Easy 8 mi.	Rest	Practice 10 mi. Race
17	Rest	Easy 5 mi. or Rest	Cross-train	Progression 6 mi.	Easy 4 mi.	Rest	Tempo 10 mi.
18	Rest	Easy 7 mi.	Easy 5 mi.	No Running	No running	No Running	**10 mi. Race**
19	Recovery	Recovery	Recovery	Recovery	Recovery	Recovery	Recovery
20	Recovery	Recovery	Recovery	Recovery	Recovery	Recovery	Recovery

Level: Beginner **Distance:** Half marathon – 13.1 miles
Macrocycle Time: 27 weeks + 3 weeks Recovery **Peak Maximum Mileage:** 57 miles in 2 weeks
About This Plan: This plan is specifically designed to build strength and endurance. It's loaded with hill running, repeats, fartleks, intervals and progression runs. This will be a very challenging plan for any beginner because of the increasing difficulty week after week. The Tuning mesocycle is especially difficult because of the long and tempo runs every weekend. I've tried to soften the plan by adding shorter distances during the week, but it will still challenge you! Prepare for week 22 – it will be a tough one with 33 very hard miles. If you're already running 10 miles, enter the training plan on week 20.

Week	Sunday	Monday	Tuesday	Wednesday	Thursday	Friday	Saturday
1				Easy .5 mi.	Easy 1 mi.	Rest	Easy 1.5 mi.
2	Rest	Easy 1.5 mi.	Cross-train	Hills 1.5 mi.	Easy 1.5 mi.	Rest	Easy 2 mi.
3	Rest	Easy 2 mi.	Cross-train	Hills 2.5 mi.	Easy 1 mi.	Rest	Easy 3 mi.
4	Rest	Easy 2.5 mi.	Cross-train	Hills 3.5 mi.	Easy 1.5 mi.	Rest	Easy 4 mi.
5	Rest	Easy 3 mi.	Cross-train	Hills 4.5 mi.	Easy 1.5 mi.	Rest	Medium 4 mi.
6	Rest	Easy 3.5 mi.	Cross-train	Hills 5 mi.	Easy 2 mi.	Rest	Medium 5 mi.
7	Rest	Easy 4 mi.	Cross-train	Hills 5.5 mi.	Easy 2 mi.	Rest	Medium 6 mi.
8	Rest	Easy 4.5 mi.	Cross-train	Hills 6 mi.	Easy 2 mi.	Rest	Medium 7 mi.
9	Rest	Easy 5 mi.	Cross-train	Hills 7 mi.	Easy 3 mi.	Rest	Medium 8 mi.
10	Rest	Medium 5.5 mi.	Cross-train	Hills 8 mi.	Easy 4 mi.	Rest	5k Race
11	Rest	Medium 6 mi.	Cross-train	Hill Repeats 1 mi.	Easy 2 mi.	Rest	Medium 9 mi.
12	Rest	Medium 6.5 mi.	Cross-train	Fartleks 7 mi.	Easy 2 mi.	Rest	Long 10 mi.
13	Rest	Medium 7 mi.	Cross-train	Intervals 5 mi.	Easy 2.5 mi.	Rest	Long 10 mi.
14	Rest	Medium 7.5 mi.	Cross-train	Progression 8 mi.	Easy 3 mi.	Rest	10k Race
15	Rest	Medium 8 mi.	Cross-train	Hill Repeats 1.5 mi.	Easy 4 mi.	Rest	Long 11 mi.
16	Rest	Medium 8.5 mi.	Cross-train	Fartleks 8 mi.	Easy 4.5 mi.	Rest	Long 12 mi.
17	Rest	Medium 9 mi.	Cross-train	Intervals 6 mi.	Easy 5 mi.	Rest	Tempo 7 mi.
18	Rest	Medium 9 mi.	Cross-train	Progression 10 mi.	Easy 4 mi.	Rest	Tempo 8 mi.
19	Rest	Medium 9 mi.	Cross-train	Hills 7 mi.	Easy 5 mi.	Rest	Tempo 9 mi.

Beginner – Half marathon 13.1 miles (continued)

Week	Sunday	Monday	Tuesday	Wednesday	Thursday	Friday	Saturday
20	Rest	Easy 8 mi.	Cross-train	Hill Repeats 2 mi.	Easy 6 mi.	Rest	10 mi. Race
21	Rest	Easy 4 mi.	Cross-train	Hills 4 mi.	Easy 5 mi.	Rest	Long 13 mi.
22	Rest	Easy 7 mi.	Cross-train	Progression 9 mi.	Easy 8 mi.	Rest	Tempo 9 mi.
23	Rest	Easy 5 mi.	Cross-train	Progression 11 mi.	Easy 9 mi.	Rest	Tempo 11 mi.
24	Rest	Easy 9 mi.	Cross-train	Progression 6 mi.	Easy 3 mi.	Rest	Practice Half Marathon
25	Rest	Easy 5 mi. or Rest	Cross-train	Progression 6 mi.	Easy 4 mi.	Rest	Tempo 10 mi.
26	Rest	Easy 10 mi.	Cross-train	Easy 7 mi.	Easy 4 mi.	Rest	Tempo 10 mi.
27	Rest	No Running	No Running	No Running	No running	No Running	**Half Marathon Race**
28	Recovery	Recovery	Recovery	Recovery	Recovery	Recovery	Recovery
29	Recovery	Recovery	Recovery	Recovery	Recovery	Recovery	Recovery
30	Recovery	Recovery	Recovery	Recovery	Recovery	Recovery	Recovery

Tip
Turkey Day "Warm Up"

Despite having successful and reasonably fast long-distance runs, I really sucked at the 5k distance. During the marathon, you can warm up during the first few miles. There really isn't a need for the "average Joe" runner to do strides before a marathon. For us, running before the marathon is a waste of precious energy. During most of my races, my first mile was actually one of my slower miles.

Over the course of a few years, I ran a number of 5ks but was always disappointed in my time. The problem was that I was treating the 5k as I did my longer distances. I had been accustomed to using the first mile as a warm up. While others were blowing past me, I was struggling to get up to the pace that I expected myself to go.

I finally decided to enter a Thanksgiving Day "Turkey Trot" in 2012 with a different strategy. I decided to run an "easy" seven miles to the start line and try to time it so I would get there just minutes before the race began. I arrived at the race about five minutes before the National Anthem was sung, grabbed my bib and arrived at the start line. As it turned out, it was, and to this day, is still my fastest 5k. I was normally running 21 to 24 minute 5k races up to that point. On that day however, I ran a 20:54 on what I thought was a tough course. I won my age group and smiled all the way home on my seven-mile return jog after the race.

Level: Beginner **Distance:** Marathon – 26.2 miles
Macrocycle Time: 37 weeks + 4 Recovery weeks **Peak Maximum Mileage:** 102 miles in 3 weeks
About This Plan: This is the ultimate training plan for a runner at any fitness level. It consists of a 14-week Endurance mesocycle, followed immediately by a 14-week Strengthening mesocycle. During these two mesocycles, you'll really need to hit the gym to build the core muscles you'll need late in a long-distance race. Focus on form throughout the entire length of your long runs.

Week	Sunday	Monday	Tuesday	Wednesday	Thursday	Friday	Saturday
1	Rest	Easy .5 mi.	Cross-train	Easy 1 mi.	Easy 1 mi.	Rest	Easy 1.5 mi.
2	Rest	Easy 1.5 mi.	Cross-train	Hills 1.5 mi.	Easy 1 mi.	Rest	Easy 2 mi.
3	Rest	Easy 2 mi.	Cross-train	Hills 2.5 mi.	Easy 2 mi.	Rest	Easy 3 mi.
4	Rest	Easy 2.5 mi.	Cross-train	Hills 3.5 mi.	Easy 2.5 mi.	Rest	Easy 4 mi.
5	Rest	Easy 3 mi.	Cross-train	Hills 4.5 mi.	Easy 2.5 mi.	Rest	Medium 4 mi.
6	Rest	Easy 3.5 mi.	Cross-train	Hills 5 mi.	Easy 3 mi.	Rest	Medium 5 mi.
7	Rest	Easy 4 mi.	Cross-train	Hills 5.5 mi.	Easy 3 mi.	Rest	Medium 6 mi.
8	Rest	Easy 4.5 mi.	Cross-train	Hills 6 mi.	Easy 4 mi.	Rest	Medium 7 mi.
9	Rest	Easy 5 mi.	Cross-train	Hills 7 mi.	Easy 3 mi.	Rest	Medium 8 mi.
10	Rest	Easy 5.5 mi.	Cross-train	Hills 8 mi.	Easy 4 mi.	Rest	Medium 9 mi.
11	Rest	Easy 6 mi.	Cross-train	Hill Repeats 1 mi.	Easy 4.5M	Rest	Medium 9 mi.
12	Rest	Easy 6.5 mi.	Cross-train	Fartleks 7 mi.	Easy 5 mi.	Rest	Long 10 mi.
13	Rest	Easy 7 mi.	Cross-train	Intervals 5 mi.	Easy 4 mi.	Rest	Long 10 mi.
14	Rest	Easy 7.5 mi.	Cross-train	Progression 4 mi.	Easy 3 mi.	Rest	5k Race
15	Rest	Easy 5 mi.	Cross-train	Hill Repeats 2 mi.	Easy 4 mi.	Rest	Long 11 mi.
16	Rest	Easy 5.5 mi.	Cross-train	Fartleks 8 mi.	Easy 4.5 mi.	Rest	Long 12 mi.
17	Rest	Easy 6 mi.	Cross-train	Intervals 6 mi.	Easy 5 mi.	Rest	Tempo 7 mi.
18	Rest	Easy 6.5 mi.	Cross-train	Progression 5 mi.	Easy 4 mi.	Rest	Tempo 8 mi.
19	Rest	Easy 7 mi.	Cross-train	Hills 7 mi.	Easy 5 mi.	Rest	Tempo 9 mi.
20	Rest	Easy 7.5 mi.	Cross-train	Hills 5 mi.	Easy 4 mi.	Rest	Long 13 mi.

Beginner – Marathon 26.2 miles (continued)

At this point, you're more than halfway through your Marathon training plan. If you're feeling overwhelmed, move your rest days around to accommodate your schedule, but try to keep the weekly mileage that has been prescribed. If you're suffering from an overuse injury, back off or stop the training. If it's serious, reschedule your goal, but don't cancel it. If you're already running half marathons you can enter this training plan at week 25.

Week	Sunday	Monday	Tuesday	Wednesday	Thursday	Friday	Saturday
21	Rest	Easy 8 mi.	Cross-train	Progression 6 mi.	Easy 5 mi.	Rest	Long 14 mi.
22	Rest	Easy 8 mi.	Cross-train	Hill Repeats 1.5 mi.	Easy 4 mi.	Rest	Long 15 mi.
23	Rest	Easy 8.5 mi.	Cross-train	Fartleks 5 mi.	Easy 6 mi.	Rest	Long 12 mi.
24	Rest	Easy 9 mi.	Cross-train	Progression 7 mi.	Easy 4 mi.	Rest	Long 13 mi.
25	Rest	Easy 9.5 mi.	Cross-train	Intervals 4 mi.	Easy 5 mi.	Rest	Long 14 mi.
26	Rest	Easy 7 mi.	Cross-train	Hill Repeats 2 mi.	Easy 6 mi.	Rest	Long 15 mi.
27	Rest	Easy 7.5 mi.	Cross-train	Progression 6 mi.	Easy 5 mi.	Rest	Long 16 mi.
28	Rest	Easy 8 mi.	Cross-train	Hills 4 mi.	Easy 5 mi.	Rest	10k Race
29	Rest	Easy 7 mi.	Cross-train	Progression 7 mi.	Easy 5 mi.	Rest	Long 18 mi.
30	Rest	Easy 7.5 mi.	Cross-train	Progression 8 mi.	Easy 4 mi.	Rest	Long 20 mi.
31	Rest	Easy 7 mi.	Cross-train	Hill Repeats 3 mi.	Easy 5 mi.	Rest	Long 15 mi.
32	Rest	Easy 8 mi.	Cross-train	Hills 4 mi.	Easy 6 mi.	Rest	Half Marathon Race
33	Rest	Easy 9 mi.	Cross-train	Hills 5 mi.	Medium 5 mi.	Rest	Long 20 mi.
34	Rest	Medium 6 mi.	Cross-train	Progression 6 mi.	Medium 3 mi.	Rest	Long 25 mi.
35	Rest	Easy 5 mi. or Rest	Cross-train	Progression 6 mi.	Easy 4 mi.	Rest	Tempo 20 mi.
36	Rest	Easy 10 mi.	Cross-train	Easy 7 mi.	Easy 4 mi.	Rest	Easy 15 mi.
37	No Running	No Running	No Running	No Running	No running	No Running	Marathon Race
38	Recovery	Recovery	Recovery	Recovery	Recovery	Recovery	Recovery
39	Recovery	Recovery	Recovery	Recovery	Recovery	Recovery	Recovery
40	Recovery	Recovery	Recovery	Recovery	Recovery	Recovery	Recovery
41	Recovery	Recovery	Recovery	Recovery	Recovery	Recovery	Recovery

Intermediate Training Plans – 5k to Marathon

In this section, we'll look at training plans for intermediate runners from a 5k to the marathon distance. Each of the plans includes one "cross-training" day, one rest day, and at least one easy day. Each plan will also feature a practice run. Use this day to sign up for a race similar to the one you'll do on race day. If you don't sign up for a race that day, try to emulate race conditions with a strong tempo or progression workout.

Level: Intermediate **Distance:** 5k
Macrocycle Time: 12 weeks + 1 week Recovery **Peak Maximum Mileage:** 10.5 miles in 7 days
About This Plan: This training plan starts with short distances and finishes with three consecutive weekends of fast-paced tempo runs to train you for your first 5k.

Week	Sunday	Monday	Tuesday	Wednesday	Thursday	Friday	Saturday
1					Easy 1 mi.	Easy 1 mi.	Easy .5 mi.
2	Rest	Easy 1.5 mi.	Cross-train	Hills 1 mi.	Easy 2 mi.	Easy 2 mi.	Easy 1.5 mi.
3	Rest	Easy 1.5 mi.	Cross-train	Hills 1.5 mi.	Easy 2 mi.	Easy 2 mi.	Medium 1.5 mi.
4	Rest	Easy 2 mi.	Cross-train	Hills 2 mi.	Easy 2 mi.	Easy 2 mi.	Medium 2.5 mi.
5	Rest	Medium 2 mi.	Cross-train	Hills 2.5 mi.	Easy 2 mi.	Easy 2 mi.	Medium 2.5 mi.
6	Rest	Medium 2 mi.	Cross-train	Fartleks 2.5 mi.	Easy 2 mi.	Easy 2.5 mi.	Tempo 2.5 mi.
7	Rest	Medium 3 mi.	Cross-train	Intervals 2 mi.	Easy 2.5 mi.	Easy 2.5 mi.	Tempo 3 mi.
8	Rest	Medium 3.5 mi.	Cross-train	Tempo 2 mi.	Easy 1 mi.	Easy 2 mi.	Hills 2.5 mi.
9	Rest	Easy 3 mi.	Cross-train	Hill Repeats 1 mi.	Easy 3 mi.	Easy 2 mi.	Tempo 3.5 mi.
10	Rest	Easy 1.5 mi.	Cross-train	Tempo 3.1 mi.	Easy 3 mi.	Easy 1 mi.	Practice 5k Race
11	Rest	Easy 2 mi.	Cross-train	Tempo 3.1 mi.	Easy 2 mi.	Easy 1 mi.	Tempo 3 mi.
12	Rest	Progression 2.5 mi.	Cross-train	Easy 2 mi.	Easy 1 mi.	Rest	**5k Race**
13	Recovery	Recovery	Recovery	Recovery	Recovery	Recovery	Recovery

---

Motivation

"Doing the best at this moment puts you in the best place for the next moment." – *Oprah Winfrey*

Level: Intermediate **Distance:** 10k
Macrocycle Time: 14 weeks + 10 days Recovery **Peak Maximum Mileage:** 23.2 miles in 7 days
About This Plan: Similar to the 5k training plan, this one is loaded with hills and tempo runs to build strength in each of the last six weekends. This is similar to the Beginner 10k plan, but you're now running five days per week instead of four days. As with all plans, be sure to honor the rest days to avoid overuse injuries. If you're already running 5k's you can enter this training plan at week 10.

Week	Sunday	Monday	Tuesday	Wednesday	Thursday	Friday	Saturday
1			Cross-train	Easy .5 mi.	Easy 1 mi.	Easy 1 mi.	Easy .5 mi.
2	Rest	Easy 1.5 mi.	Cross-train	Hills 1 mi.	Easy 2 mi.	Easy 2 mi.	Easy 1.5 mi.
3	Rest	Easy 2 mi.	Cross-train	Hills 1.5 mi.	Easy 2 mi.	Easy 2 mi.	Medium 2 mi.
4	Rest	Easy 3 mi.	Cross-train	Hills 2.5 mi.	Easy 3 mi.	Easy 3 mi.	Medium 3 mi.
5	Rest	Medium 3 mi.	Cross-train	Hills 3 mi.	Easy 4 mi.	Easy 4 mi.	Medium 3.5 mi.
6	Rest	Medium 3.5 mi.	Cross-train	Hills 3.5 mi.	Easy 2 mi.	Easy 2 mi.	Medium 4 mi.
7	Rest	Medium 3.5 mi.	Cross-train	Hills 4 mi.	Easy 3 mi.	Easy 3 mi.	Medium 4.5 mi.
8	Rest	Medium 4 mi.	Cross-train	Fartleks 3.5 mi.	Easy 3 mi.	Easy 2.5 mi.	Tempo 4.5 mi.
9	Rest	Medium 4 mi.	Cross-train	Intervals 4 mi.	Easy 4 mi.	Easy 3 mi.	Tempo 5 mi.
10	Rest	Medium 5 mi.	Cross-train	Hills 5 mi.	Easy 5 mi.	Rest	5k Race
11	Rest	Easy 6 mi.	Cross-train	Hill Repeats 1.5 mi.	Easy 6 mi.	Easy 4 mi.	Tempo 5 mi.
12	Rest	Easy 3 mi.	Cross-train	Progression 5 mi.	Easy 3 mi.	Rest	Practice 10k Race
13	Rest	Progression 6 mi.	Cross-train	Tempo 6.2 mi.	Easy 4 mi.	Easy 4 mi.	Tempo 6 mi.
14	Rest	Easy 3 mi.	Easy 4 mi.	Easy 2 mi.	No running	No Running	**10k Race**
15	Recovery	Recovery	Recovery	Recovery	Recovery	Recovery	Recovery
16	Recovery	Recovery	Recovery				

Motivation

"Never put an age limit on your dreams." – Dara Torres

Level: Intermediate **Distance:** 10 miles
Macrocycle Time: 19 weeks + 2 weeks Recovery **Peak Maximum Mileage:** 40 miles in 10 days
About This Plan: This plan is very challenging with many variations of workouts, including hills, progression runs, fartleks and tempo runs. Eat healthy and hydrate often, as this plan will surely stress your body. If you're already running 10k's you can enter this training plan at week 12.

Week	Sunday	Monday	Tuesday	Wednesday	Thursday	Friday	Saturday
1						Easy .5 mi.	Rest
2	Rest	Easy 1.5 mi.	Cross-train	Hills 1 mi.	Easy 2 mi.	Easy 2 mi.	Easy 1.5 mi.
3	Rest	Easy 1.5 mi.	Cross-train	Hills 1.5 mi.	Easy 2 mi.	Easy 2 mi.	Medium 1.5 mi.
4	Rest	Easy 2 mi.	Cross-train	Hills 2 mi.	Easy 2 mi.	Easy 2 mi.	Medium 2.5 mi.
5	Rest	Easy 3 mi.	Cross-train	Hills 2.5 mi.	Easy 3 mi.	Easy 3 mi.	Medium 3 mi.
6	Rest	Medium 3 mi.	Cross-train	Hills 3 mi.	Easy 4 mi.	Easy 4 mi.	Medium 3.5 mi.
7	Rest	Medium 3.5 mi.	Cross-train	Hills 3.5 mi.	Easy 2 mi.	Easy 2 mi.	Medium 4 mi.
8	Rest	Medium 4 mi.	Cross-train	Fartleks 3.5 mi.	Easy 2 mi.	Easy 2 mi.	Medium 5 mi.
9	Rest	Medium 5 mi.	Cross-train	Intervals 4 mi.	Easy 2.5 mi.	Easy 2.5 mi.	Medium 6 mi.
10	Rest	Medium 6 mi.	Cross-train	Progression 5 mi.	Easy 3 mi.	Easy 3 mi.	Long 7 mi.
11	Rest	Medium 7 mi.	Cross-train	Hills 4 mi.	Easy 5 mi.	Easy 4 mi.	Tempo 7 mi.
12	Rest	Medium 6 mi.	Cross-train	Hill Repeats 1 mi.	Easy 6 mi.	Rest	10k Race
13	Rest	Medium 8 mi.	Cross-train	Hills 4 mi.	Easy 7 mi.	Easy 4 mi.	Long 9 mi.
14	Rest	Medium 7 mi.	Cross-train	Progression 5 mi.	Easy 8 mi.	Easy 5 mi.	Tempo 9 mi.
15	Rest	Hills 3 mi.	Cross-train	Hill Repeats 2 mi.	Easy 9 mi.	Easy 6 mi.	Long 10 mi.
16	Rest	Easy 8 mi.	Cross-train	Progression 6 mi.	Easy 8 mi.	Rest	Practice 10 mi. Race
17	Rest	Easy 5 mi. or Rest	Cross-train	Progression 6 mi.	Easy 5 mi.	Easy 4 mi.	Tempo 10 mi.
18	Rest	Easy 7 mi.	Easy 5 mi.	No Running	No running	No Running	**10 mi. Race**
19	Recovery	Recovery	Recovery	Recovery	Recovery	Recovery	Recovery
20	Recovery	Recovery	Recovery	Recovery	Recovery	Recovery	Recovery

Level: Intermediate
Macrocycle Time: 27 weeks + 3 weeks Recovery

Distance: Half marathon – 13.1 miles
Peak Maximum Mileage: 61 miles in 2 weeks

About This Plan: This plan is specifically designed to build strength and endurance for the Intermediate runner and features three challenging races leading up to the half marathon, including 5k, 10k and 10 mile preparatory races. Give special attention to week 23 as it features 42 miles of difficult running. If you're already running 10 miles, enter the training plan on week 20.

Week	Sunday	Monday	Tuesday	Wednesday	Thursday	Friday	Saturday
1				Easy .5mi.	Easy 1 mi.	Easy 1 mi.	Easy 1.5 mi.
2	Rest	Easy 1.5 mi.	Cross-train	Hills 1.5 mi.	Easy 1.5 mi.	Easy 1 mi.	Easy 2 mi.
3	Rest	Easy 2 mi.	Cross-train	Hills 2.5 mi.	Easy 1 mi.	Easy 1 mi.	Easy 3 mi.
4	Rest	Easy 2.5 mi.	Cross-train	Hills 3.5 mi.	Easy 1.5 mi.	Easy 1.5 mi.	Easy 4 mi.
5	Rest	Easy 3 mi.	Cross-train	Hills 4.5 mi.	Easy 1.5 mi.	Easy 1.5 mi.	Medium 4 mi.
6	Rest	Easy 3.5 mi.	Cross-train	Hills 5 mi.	Easy 2 mi.	Easy 2 mi.	Medium 5 mi.
7	Rest	Easy 4 mi.	Cross-train	Hills 5.5 mi.	Easy 2 mi.	Easy 2 mi.	Medium 6 mi.
8	Rest	Easy 4.5 mi.	Cross-train	Hills 6 mi.	Easy 2 mi.	Easy 2 mi.	Medium 7 mi.
9	Rest	Easy 5 mi.	Cross-train	Hills 7 mi.	Easy 3 mi.	Easy 3 mi.	Medium 8 mi.
10	Rest	Medium 5.5 mi.	Cross-train	Hills 8 mi.	Easy 4 mi.	Rest	5k Race
11	Rest	Medium 6 mi.	Cross-train	Hill Repeats 1 mi.	Easy 2 mi.	Easy 2 mi.	Medium 9 mi.
12	Rest	Medium 6.5 mi.	Cross-train	Fartleks 7 mi.	Easy 2 mi.	Easy 2 mi.	Long 10 mi.
13	Rest	Medium 7 mi.	Cross-train	Intervals 5 mi.	Easy 2.5 mi.	Easy 2 mi.	Long 10 mi.
14	Rest	Medium 7.5 mi.	Cross-train	Progression 8 mi.	Easy 3 mi.	Rest	10k Race
15	Rest	Medium 8 mi.	Cross-train	Hill Repeats 1.5 mi.	Easy 4 mi.	Easy 4 mi.	Long 11 mi.
16	Rest	Medium 8.5 mi.	Cross-train	Fartleks 8 mi.	Easy 4.5 mi.	Easy 4.5 mi.	Long 12 mi.
17	Rest	Medium 9 mi.	Cross-train	Intervals 6 mi.	Easy 5 mi.	Easy 5 mi.	Tempo 7 mi.
18	Rest	Medium 9 mi.	Cross-train	Progression 10 mi.	Easy 4 mi.	Easy 4 mi.	Tempo 8 mi.
19	Rest	Medium 9 mi.	Cross-train	Hills 7 mi.	Easy 5 mi.	Easy 5 mi.	Tempo 9 mi.

Intermediate – Half Marathon 13.1 Miles (Continued)

Week	Sunday	Monday	Tuesday	Wednesday	Thursday	Friday	Saturday
20	Rest	Easy 8 mi.	Cross-train	Hill Repeats 2 mi.	Easy 6 mi.	Rest	10 Mile Race
21	Rest	Easy 4 mi.	Cross-train	Hills 4 mi.	Easy 5 mi.	Easy 5 mi.	Long 13 mi.
22	Rest	Easy 7 mi.	Cross-train	Progression 9 mi.	Easy 8 mi.	Easy 5 mi.	Tempo 9 mi.
23	Rest	Easy 5 mi.	Cross-train	Progression 11 mi.	Easy 9 mi.	Easy 6 mi.	Tempo 11 mi.
24	Rest	Easy 9 mi.	Cross-train	Progression 6 mi.	Easy 2 mi.	Rest	Practice Half Marathon
25	Rest	Easy 5M or Rest	Cross-train	Progression 6 mi.	Easy 4 mi.	Easy 5 mi.	Tempo 10 mi.
26	Rest	Easy 10 mi.	Cross-train	Easy 7 mi.	Easy 4 mi.	Rest	Tempo 10 mi.
27	Rest	No Running	No Running	No Running	No running	No Running	Half Marathon Race
28	Recovery	Recovery	Recovery	Recovery	Recovery	Recovery	Recovery
29	Recovery	Recovery	Recovery	Recovery	Recovery	Recovery	Recovery
30	Recovery	Recovery	Recovery	Recovery	Recovery	Recovery	Recovery

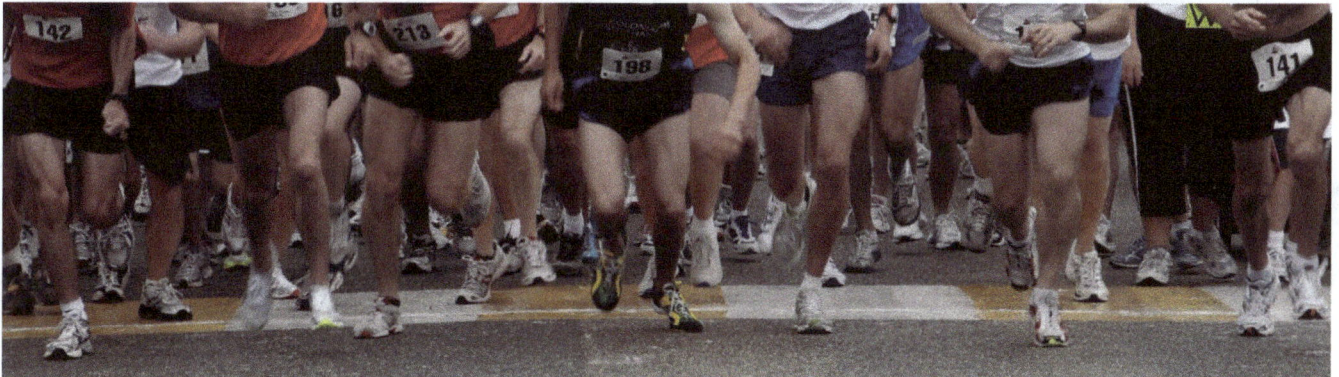

Motivation

"Never let the fear of striking out get in your way." – *Babe Ruth*

Level: Intermediate   **Distance:** Marathon – 26.2 miles
Macrocycle Time: 37 weeks + 4 Recovery weeks   **Peak Maximum Mileage:** 117 miles in 3 weeks
About This Plan: This is the ultimate training plan for a runner at any fitness level. It consists of a 14 week Endurance mesocycle, followed immediately by a 14 week Strengthening mesocycle. Work on core muscle groups throughout your training utilizing key cross-training days. This plan also features three races of various lengths leading up to your marathon.

Week	Sunday	Monday	Tuesday	Wednesday	Thursday	Friday	Saturday
1	Rest	Easy .5 mi.	Cross-train	Easy 1 mi.	Easy 1 mi.	Easy 1 mi.	Easy 1.5 mi.
2	Rest	Easy 1.5 mi.	Cross-train	Hills 1.5 mi.	Easy 1 mi.	Easy 1 mi.	Easy 2 mi.
3	Rest	Easy 2 mi.	Cross-train	Hills 2.5 mi.	Easy 2 mi.	Easy 2 mi.	Easy 3 mi.
4	Rest	Easy 2.5 mi.	Cross-train	Hills 3.5 mi.	Easy 2.5 mi.	Easy 2 mi.	Easy 4 mi.
5	Rest	Easy 3 mi.	Cross-train	Hills 4.5 mi.	Easy 2.5 mi.	Easy 2.5 mi.	Medium 4 mi.
6	Rest	Easy 3.5 mi.	Cross-train	Hills 5 mi.	Easy 3 mi.	Easy 3 mi.	Medium 5 mi.
7	Rest	Easy 4 mi.	Cross-train	Hills 5.5 mi.	Easy 3 mi.	Easy 3 mi.	Medium 6 mi.
8	Rest	Easy 4.5 mi.	Cross-train	Hills 6 mi.	Easy 4 mi.	Easy 4 mi.	Medium 7 mi.
9	Rest	Easy 5 mi.	Cross-train	Hills 7 mi.	Easy 3 mi.	Easy 3 mi.	Medium 8 mi.
10	Rest	Easy 5.5 mi.	Cross-train	Hills 8 mi.	Easy 4 mi.	Easy 4 mi.	Medium 9 mi.
11	Rest	Easy 6 mi.	Cross-train	Hill Repeats 1 mi.	Easy 4.5 mi.	Easy 4.5 mi.	Medium 9 mi.
12	Rest	Easy 6.5 mi.	Cross-train	Fartleks 7 mi.	Easy 5 mi.	Easy 5 mi.	Long 10 mi.
13	Rest	Easy 7 mi.	Cross-train	Intervals 5 mi.	Easy 4 mi.	Easy 4 mi.	Long 10 mi.
14	Rest	Easy 7.5 mi.	Cross-train	Progression 4 mi.	Easy 2 mi.	Rest	5k Race
15	Rest	Easy 5 mi.	Cross-train	Hill Repeats 2 mi.	Easy 4 mi.	Easy 4 mi.	Long 11 mi.
16	Rest	Easy 5.5 mi.	Cross-train	Fartleks 8 mi.	Easy 4.5 mi.	Easy 4.5 mi.	Long 12 mi.
17	Rest	Easy 6 mi.	Cross-train	Intervals 6 mi.	Easy 5 mi.	Easy 5 mi.	Tempo 7 mi.
18	Rest	Easy 6.5 mi.	Cross-train	Progression 5 mi.	Easy 4 mi.	Easy 4 mi.	Tempo 8 mi.
19	Rest	Easy 7 mi.	Cross-train	Hills 7 mi.	Easy 5 mi.	Easy 5 mi.	Tempo 9 mi.
20	Rest	Easy 7.5 mi.	Cross-train	Hills 5 mi.	Easy 4 mi.	Easy 4 mi.	Long 13 mi.

Intermediate – Marathon 26.2 Miles (Continued)

At this point, you're more than half way through your marathon training plan. If you're feeling overwhelmed, move your rest days around to accommodate your schedule, but try to keep the weekly mileage that has been prescribed. If you're suffering from an overuse injury, back off or stop the training. If it's serious, reschedule your goal, but don't cancel it. If you're already running half marathons you can enter this training plan at week 25.

Week	Sunday	Monday	Tuesday	Wednesday	Thursday	Friday	Saturday
21	Rest	Easy 8 mi.	Cross-train	Progression 6 mi.	Easy 5 mi.	Easy 5 mi.	Long 14 mi.
22	Rest	Easy 8 mi.	Cross-train	Hill Repeats 1.5 mi.	Easy 4 mi.	Easy 4 mi.	Long 15 mi.
23	Rest	Easy 8.5 mi.	Cross-train	Fartleks 5 mi.	Easy 6 mi.	Easy 5 mi.	Long 12 mi.
24	Rest	Easy 9 mi.	Cross-train	Progression 7 mi.	Easy 4 mi.	Easy 4 mi.	Long 13 mi.
25	Rest	Easy 9.5 mi.	Cross-train	Intervals 4 mi.	Easy 5 mi.	Easy 5 mi.	Long 14 mi.
26	Rest	Easy 7 mi.	Cross-train	Hill Repeats 2 mi.	Easy 6 mi.	Easy 4 mi.	Long 15 mi.
27	Rest	Easy 7.5 mi.	Cross-train	Progression 6 mi.	Easy 5 mi.	Easy 5 mi.	Long 16 mi.
28	Rest	Easy 8 mi.	Cross-train	Hills 4 mi.	Easy 5 mi.	Rest	10k Race
29	Rest	Easy 7 mi.	Cross-train	Progression 7 mi.	Easy 5 mi.	Easy 4 mi.	Long 18 mi.
30	Rest	Easy 7.5 mi.	Cross-train	Progression 8 mi.	Easy 4 mi.	Easy 4 mi.	Long 20 mi.
31	Rest	Easy 7 mi.	Cross-train	Hill Repeats 3 mi.	Easy 5 mi.	Easy 5 mi.	Long 22 mi.
32	Rest	Easy 8 mi.	Cross-train	Hills 4 mi.	Easy 6 mi.	Easy 5 mi.	Long 16 mi.
33	Rest	Easy 9 mi.	Cross-train	Hills 5 mi.	Easy 5 mi.	Rest	Half Marathon Race
34	Rest	Medium 6 mi.	Cross-train	Progression 6 mi.	Medium 6 mi.	Rest	Long 25 mi.
35	Rest	Easy 5 mi. or Rest	Cross-train	Progression 6 mi.	Easy 6 mi.	Rest	Tempo 20 mi.
36	Rest	Easy 10 mi.	Cross-train	Easy 7 mi.	Easy 4 mi.	Rest	Easy 15 mi.
37	No Running	No Running	No Running	No Running	No running	No Running	Marathon Race
38	Recovery	Recovery	Recovery	Recovery	Recovery	Recovery	Recovery
39	Recovery	Recovery	Recovery	Recovery	Recovery	Recovery	Recovery
40	Recovery	Recovery	Recovery	Recovery	Recovery	Recovery	Recovery
41	Recovery	Recovery	Recovery	Recovery	Recovery	Recovery	Recovery

Advanced Training Plans – 5k to Marathon

The training plans in this section are for Advanced runners that can run 25 miles per week. The level of intensity increases by adding a sixth day of running and cross-training two times, every two weeks. If you begin to struggle in these plans, go back to the Intermediate plans and gradually work back up to the Advanced levels.

Level: Advanced   **Distance:** 5k
Macrocycle Time: 12 weeks + 1 week Recovery   **Peak Maximum Mileage:** 14.5 miles in 7 days
About This Plan: This training plan starts with short distances and finishes with three consecutive weekends of fast-paced tempo runs to train you for your first 5k.

Week	Sunday	Monday	Tuesday	Wednesday	Thursday	Friday	Saturday
1					Easy 1 mi.	Easy 1 mi.	Easy .5 mi.
2	Rest	Easy 1.5 mi.	Easy 1.5 mi. Cross-train	Hills 1 mi.	Easy 2M Cross-train	Easy 1 mi.	Easy 1.5 mi.
3	Rest	Easy 1.5 mi.	Easy 1.5M Cross-train	Hills 1.5 mi.	Easy 2 mi.	Easy 2 mi.	Medium 1.5 mi.
4	Rest	Easy 2 mi.	Easy 2M Cross-train	Hills 2 mi.	Easy 2M Cross-train	Easy 2 mi.	Medium 2.5 mi.
5	Rest	Medium 2 mi.	Easy 2M Cross-train	Hills 2.5 mi.	Easy 2 mi.	Easy 2 mi.	Medium 2.5 mi.
6	Rest	Medium 2 mi.	Easy 2M Cross-train	Fartleks 2.5 mi.	Easy 2M Cross-train	Easy 2 mi.	Tempo 2.5 mi.
7	Rest	Medium 3 mi.	Easy 3M Cross-train	Intervals 2 mi.	Easy 2.5 mi.	Easy 2.5 mi.	Tempo 3 mi.
9	Rest	Medium 3.5 mi.	Easy 3.5M Cross-train	Tempo 2 mi.	Easy 1M Cross-train	Easy 2 mi.	Hills 2.5 mi.
9	Rest	Easy 3 mi.	Easy 3M Cross-train	Hill Repeats 1 mi.	Easy 3 mi.	Easy 3 mi.	Tempo 3.5 mi.
10	Rest	Easy 1.5 mi.	Easy 1.5M Cross-train	Tempo 3.1 mi.	Easy 3M Cross-train	Easy 2 mi.	Practice 5k Race
11	Rest	Easy 2 mi.	Easy 2M Cross-train	Tempo 3.1 mi.	Easy 2 mi.	Easy 2.5 mi.	Tempo 3 mi.
12	Rest	Progression 2.5 mi.	Easy 2.5M Cross-train	Easy 2 mi.	Easy 1 mi.	Rest	**5k Race**
13	Recovery	Recovery	Recovery	Recovery	Recovery	Recovery	Recovery

---

Motivation

"I'm racing against me. As long as I come across the finish line, I'll be okay." – *Ruben Studdard*

Level: Advanced   **Distance:** 10k
Macrocycle Time: 14 weeks + 10 days Recovery   **Peak Maximum Mileage:** 27.2 miles in 7 days
About This Plan: Similar to the 5k training plan, this one is loaded with hills and tempo runs to build strength in each of the last six weekends. This is a fast paced training plan and will quickly build up your cardio system. Focus on strength and conditioning exercises on all of your cross-training days. Be sure to honor the rest days to avoid overuse injuries. If you're already running 5k's you can enter this training plan at week 10.

Week	Sunday	Monday	Tuesday	Wednesday	Thursday	Friday	Saturday
1			Easy 1.5 mi. Cross-train	Easy .5 mi.	Easy 1M Cross-train	Easy 2 mi.	Easy .5 mi.
2	Rest	Easy 1.5 mi.	Easy 1.5 mi. Cross-train	Hills 1 mi.	Easy 2 mi.	Easy 2 mi.	Easy 1.5 mi.
3	Rest	Easy 2 mi.	Easy 2M Cross-train	Hills 1.5 mi.	Easy 2M Cross-train	Easy 2 mi.	Medium 2 mi.
4	Rest	Easy 3 mi.	Easy 3M Cross-train	Hills 2.5 mi.	Easy 3 mi.	Easy 3 mi.	Medium 3 mi.
5	Rest	Medium 3 mi.	Easy 3M Cross-train	Hills 3 mi.	Easy 4M Cross-train	Easy 4 mi.	Medium 3.5 mi.
6	Rest	Medium 3.5 mi.	Easy 3.5M Cross-train	Hills 3.5 mi.	Easy 2 mi.	Easy 2 mi.	Medium 4 mi.
7	Rest	Medium 3.5 mi.	Easy 3.5M Cross-train	Hills 4 mi.	Easy 3M Cross-train	Easy 3 mi.	Medium 4.5 mi.
8	Rest	Medium 4 mi.	Easy 4M Cross-train	Fartleks 3.5 mi.	Easy 3 mi.	Easy 3 mi.	Tempo 4.5 mi.
9	Rest	Medium 4 mi.	Easy 4M Cross-train	Intervals 4 mi.	Easy 4M Cross-train	Easy 4 mi.	Tempo 5 mi.
10	Rest	Medium 5 mi.	Easy 5M Cross-train	Hills 5 mi.	Easy 5 mi.	Rest	5k Race
11	Rest	Easy 6 mi.	Easy 6M Cross-train	Hill Repeats 1.5 mi.	Easy 6M Cross-train	Easy 5 mi.	Tempo 5 mi.
12	Rest	Easy 3 mi.	Easy 6M Cross-train	Progression 5 mi.	Easy 3 mi.	Rest	Practice 10k Race
13	Rest	Progression 6 mi.	Easy 5M Cross-train	Tempo 6.2 mi.	Easy 4M Cross-train	Easy 3 mi.	Tempo 6 mi.
14	Rest	Easy 3 mi.	Easy 3 mi.	Easy 2 mi.	No running	No Running	10k Race
15	Recovery	Recovery	Recovery	Recovery	Recovery	Recovery	Recovery
16	Recovery	Recovery	Recovery				

Motivation

"One man practicing sportsmanship is far better than 50 preaching it." – *Knute Rockne*

Level: Advanced   **Distance:** 10 miles
Macrocycle Time: 19 weeks + 2 weeks Recovery   **Peak Maximum Mileage:** 45 miles in 10 days
About This Plan: This plan is for the Advanced runner and will put you well on your way to the world of distance running. Progression runs and hill repeats will give you strength in a short amount of time. If you don't want to run a "practice" race at the end of week 16, do another "Long 10-miler" instead. If you do sign up for a 10-mile race at the end of week 16, make sure you rest during the next few days. If you're already running 10k's you can enter this training plan at week 12.

Week	Sunday	Monday	Tuesday	Wednesday	Thursday	Friday	Saturday
1						Easy .5 mi.	Rest
2	Rest	Easy 1.5 mi.	Easy 1.5M Cross-train	Hills 1 mi.	Easy 2 mi.	Easy 2M Cross-train	Easy 1.5 mi.
3	Rest	Easy 1.5 mi.	Easy 1.5M Cross-train	Hills 1.5 mi.	Easy 2 mi.	Easy 2 mi.	Medium 1.5 mi.
4	Rest	Easy 2 mi.	Easy 2M Cross-train	Hills 2 mi.	Easy 2 mi.	Easy 2M Cross-train	Medium 2.5 mi.
5	Rest	Easy 3 mi.	Easy 3M Cross-train	Hills 2.5 mi.	Easy 3 mi.	Easy 3 mi.	Medium 3 mi.
6	Rest	Medium 3 mi.	Easy 3M Cross-train	Hills 3 mi.	Easy 4 mi.	Easy 4M Cross-train	Medium 3.5 mi.
7	Rest	Medium 3.5 mi.	Easy 3.5M Cross-train	Hills 3.5 mi.	Easy 2 mi.	Easy 2 mi.	5k Race
8	Rest	Medium 4 mi.	Easy 4M Cross-train	Fartleks 3.5 mi.	Easy 2 mi.	Easy 2 mi. Cross-train	Medium 5 mi.
9	Rest	Medium 5 mi.	Easy 4 mi. Cross-train	Intervals 4 mi.	Easy 2.5 mi.	Easy 2.5 mi.	Medium 6 mi.
10	Rest	Medium 6 mi.	Easy 6 mi. Cross-train	Progression 5 mi.	Easy 3 mi.	Easy 3 mi. Cross-train	Long 7 mi.
11	Rest	Medium 7 mi.	Easy 7 mi. Cross-train	Hills 4 mi.	Easy 5 mi.	Easy 5 mi.	Tempo 7 mi.
12	Rest	Medium 6 mi.	Easy 6 mi. Cross-train	Hill Repeats 1 mi.	Easy 2 mi.	Rest	10k Race
13	Rest	Medium 8 mi.	Easy 8 mi. Cross-train	Hills 4 mi.	Easy 7 mi.	Easy 5 mi. Cross-train	Long 9 mi.
14	Rest	Medium 7 mi.	Easy 7 mi. Cross-train	Progression 5 mi.	Easy 8 mi.	Easy 6 mi.	Tempo 9 mi.
15	Rest	Hills 3 mi.	Easy 3 mi. Cross-train	Hill Repeats 2 mi.	Easy 9 mi.	Easy 5 mi. Cross-train	Long 10 mi.
16	Rest	Easy 8 mi.	Easy 8 mi. Cross-train	Progression 6 mi.	Easy 8 mi.	Rest	Practice 10 mi. Race
17	Rest	Easy 5 mi. or Rest	Easy 5 mi. Cross-train	Progression 6 mi.	Easy 5 mi.	Easy 4 mi.	Tempo 10 mi.
18	Rest	Easy 7 mi.	Easy 5 mi.	No Running	No running	No Running	10 mi. Race
19	Recovery	Recovery	Recovery	Recovery	Recovery	Recovery	Recovery
20	Recovery	Recovery	Recovery	Recovery	Recovery	Recovery	Recovery

Level: Advanced **Distance:** Half marathon – 13.1 Miles
Macrocycle Time: 27 weeks + 3 weeks Recovery **Peak Maximum Mileage:** 77.1 miles in 2 weeks
About This Plan: This long training plan prepares you for the half marathon distance, and can be a base for full marathon and ultramarathon races. With only one rest day per week, you will be challenged every day. Be sure to adjust workouts if you start to feel fatigued or are facing an injury. Prescribed hill running for the first ten weeks guarantees that you'll show up at the start line feeling strong! If you're already running 10 miles, enter the training plan on week 20.

Week	Sunday	Monday	Tuesday	Wednesday	Thursday	Friday	Saturday
1				Easy .5 mi.	Easy 1 mi.	Easy 1 mi. Cross-train	Easy 1.5 mi.
2	Rest	Easy 1.5 mi.	Easy 1.5 mi. Cross-train	Hills 1.5 mi.	Easy 1.5 mi.	Easy 1.5 mi.	Easy 2 mi.
3	Rest	Easy 2 mi.	Easy 2 mi. Cross-train	Hills 2.5 mi.	Easy 1 mi.	Easy 1 mi. Cross-train	Easy 3 mi.
4	Rest	Easy 2.5 mi.	Easy 2.5 mi. Cross-train	Hills 3.5 mi.	Easy 1.5 mi.	Easy 1.5 mi.	Easy 4 mi.
5	Rest	Easy 3 mi.	Easy 3 mi. Cross-train	Hills 4.5 mi.	Easy 1.5 mi.	Easy 1.5 mi. Cross-train	Medium 4 mi.
6	Rest	Easy 3.5 mi.	Easy 3.5 mi. Cross-train	Hills 5 mi.	Easy 2 mi.	Easy 2 mi.	Medium 5 mi.
7	Rest	Easy 4 mi.	Easy 4 mi. Cross-train	Hills 5.5 mi.	Easy 2 mi.	Easy 2 mi. Cross-train	Medium 6 mi.
8	Rest	Easy 4.5 mi.	Easy 4.5 mi. Cross-train	Hills 6 mi.	Easy 2 mi.	Easy 2 mi.	Medium 7 mi.
9	Rest	Easy 5 mi.	Easy 5 mi. Cross-train	Hills 7 mi.	Easy 3 mi.	Easy 3 mi. Cross-train	Medium 8 mi.
10	Rest	Medium 5.5 mi.	Easy 5.5 mi. Cross-train	Hills 8 mi.	Easy 4 mi.	Rest	5k Race
11	Rest	Medium 6 mi.	Easy 6 mi. Cross-train	Hill Repeats 1 mi.	Easy 2 mi.	Easy 2 mi. Cross-train	Medium 9 mi.
12	Rest	Medium 6.5 mi.	Easy 6.5 mi. Cross-train	Fartleks 7 mi.	Easy 2 mi.	Easy 2 mi.	Long 10 mi.
13	Rest	Medium 7 mi.	Easy 7 mi. Cross-train	Intervals 5 mi.	Easy 2.5 mi.	Easy 2.5 mi. Cross-train	Long 10 mi.
14	Rest	Medium 7.5 mi.	Easy 6 mi. Cross-train	Progression 8 mi.	Easy 3 mi.	Rest	10k Race
15	Rest	Medium 8 mi.	Easy 6 mi. Cross-train	Hill Repeats 1.5 mi.	Easy 4 mi.	Easy 4 mi. Cross-train	Long 11 mi.
16	Rest	Medium 8.5 mi.	Easy 8.5 mi. Cross-train	Fartleks 8 mi.	Easy 4.5 mi.	Easy 4.5 mi.	Long 12 mi.
17	Rest	Medium 9 mi.	Easy 9 mi. Cross-train	Intervals 6 mi.	Easy 5 mi.	Easy 5 mi. Cross-train	Tempo 7 mi.
18	Rest	Medium 9 mi.	Easy 6 mi. Cross-train	Progression 10 mi.	Easy 4 mi.	Easy 4 mi.	Tempo 8 mi.
19	Rest	Medium 9 mi.	Easy 9 mi. Cross-train	Hills 7 mi.	Easy 5 mi.	Easy 5 mi. Cross-train	Tempo 9 mi.

Advanced – Half Marathon 13.1 Miles (Continued)

Week	Sunday	Monday	Tuesday	Wednesday	Thursday	Friday	Saturday
20	Rest	Easy 8 mi.	Easy 8M Cross-train	Hill Repeats 2 mi.	Easy 6 mi.	Rest	10 mi. Race
21	Rest	Easy 8 mi.	Easy 8M Cross-train	Hills 4 mi.	Easy 5 mi.	Easy 5 mi. Cross-train	Long 13 mi.
22	Rest	Easy 7 mi.	Easy 6 mi. Cross-train	Progression 9 mi.	Easy 8 mi.	Easy 5 mi.	Tempo 9 mi.
23	Rest	Easy 5 mi.	Easy7 mi. Cross-train	Progression 11 mi.	Easy 9 mi.	Easy 2 mi. Cross-train	Tempo 11 mi.
24	Rest	Easy 9 mi.	Easy 7 mi. Cross-train	Progression 6 mi.	Easy 3 mi.	Rest	Practice Half Marathon
25	Rest	Easy 5 mi. or Rest	East 8 mi. Cross-train	Progression 6 mi.	Easy 4 mi.	Easy 4 mi. Cross-train	Tempo 10 mi.
26	Rest	Easy 10 mi.	Easy 8 mi. Cross-train	Easy 7 mi.	Easy 4 mi.	Rest	Tempo 10 mi.
27	Rest	No Running	No Running	No Running	No running	No Running	**Half Marathon Race**
28	Recovery	Recovery	Recovery	Recovery	Recovery	Recovery	Recovery
29	Recovery	Recovery	Recovery	Recovery	Recovery	Recovery	Recovery
30	Recovery	Recovery	Recovery	Recovery	Recovery	Recovery	Recovery

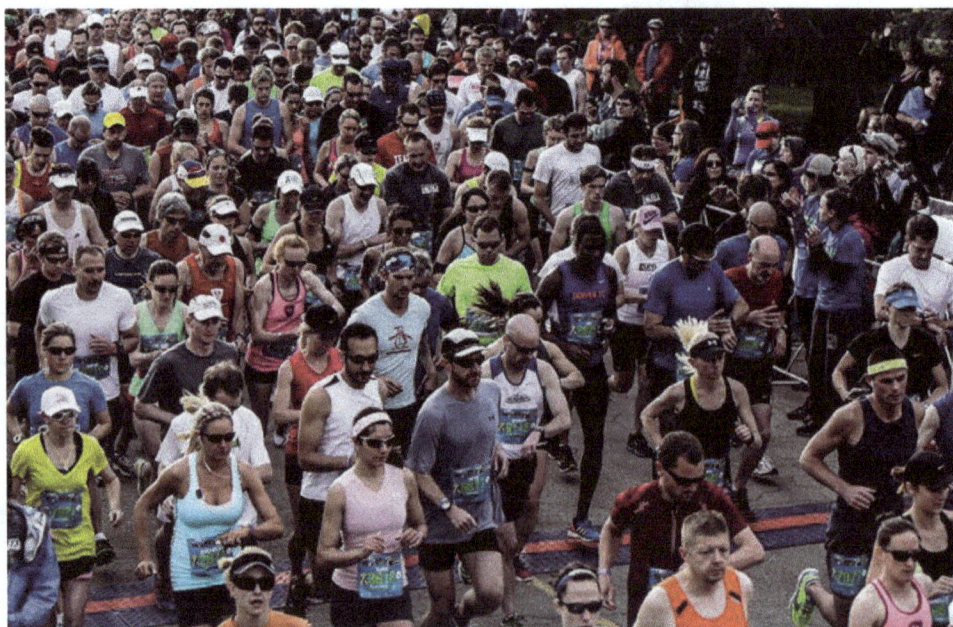

Motivation

"Yes, there may be suffering—in fact, it's certain there will be—but it serves to heighten our joy. It makes us grateful to be alive"– *Marshall Ulrich*

Level: Advanced **Distance:** Marathon – 26.2 miles
Macrocycle Time: 37 weeks + 4 Recovery weeks **Peak Maximum Mileage:** 133.1 miles in 3 weeks
About This Plan: This is the ultimate training plan for the Advanced marathon runner. It consists of a 14 week Endurance mesocycle, followed immediately by a 14 week Strengthening mesocycle. In this plan, you'll benefit from real races including a 5k, 10k and half marathon before running your full marathon. Focus on form throughout the plan and don't give up when you experience "the wall" during your long runs of 18 miles or more. Enter this plan at week 25 if you're already running half marathons.

Week	Sunday	Monday	Tuesday	Wednesday	Thursday	Friday	Saturday
1	Rest	Easy .5 mi.	Easy .5 mi. Cross-train	Easy 1 mi.	Easy 1 mi.	Easy 1 mi. Cross-train	Easy 1.5 mi.
2	Rest	Easy 1.5 mi.	Easy 1.5 mi. Cross-train	Hills 1.5 mi.	Easy 1 mi.	Easy 1 mi.	Easy 2 mi.
3	Rest	Easy 2 mi.	Easy 2 mi. Cross-train	Hills 2.5 mi.	Easy 2 mi.	Easy 2 mi. Cross-train	Easy 3 mi.
4	Rest	Easy 2.5 mi.	Easy 2.5 mi. Cross-train	Hills 3.5 mi.	Easy 2.5 mi.	Easy 2.5 mi. Cross-train	Easy 4 mi.
5	Rest	Easy 3 mi.	Easy 3 mi. Cross-train	Hills 4.5 mi.	Easy 2.5 mi.	Easy 2.5 mi.	Medium 4 mi.
6	Rest	Easy 3.5 mi.	Easy 3.5M Cross-train	Hills 5 mi.	Easy 3 mi.	Easy 3 mi. Cross-train	Medium 5 mi.
7	Rest	Easy 4 mi.	Easy 4 mi. Cross-train	Hills 5.5 mi.	Easy 3 mi.	Easy 3 mi.	Medium 6 mi.
8	Rest	Easy 4.5 mi.	Easy 4.5 mi. Cross-train	Hills 6 mi.	Easy 4 mi.	Easy 4 mi. Cross-train	Medium 7 mi.
9	Rest	Easy 5 mi.	Easy 5 mi. Cross-train	Hills 7 mi.	Easy 3 mi.	Easy 3 mi.	Medium 8 mi.
10	Rest	Easy 5.5 mi.	Easy 5.5 mi. Cross-train	Hills 8 mi.	Easy 4 mi.	Easy 4 mi. Cross-train	Medium 9 mi.
11	Rest	Easy 6 mi.	Easy 6 mi. Cross-train	Hill Repeats 1 mi.	Easy 4.5 mi.	Easy 4.5 mi.	Medium 9 mi.
12	Rest	Easy 6.5 mi.	Easy 6.5 mi. Cross-train	Fartleks 7 mi.	Easy 5 mi.	Easy 5 mi. Cross-train	Long 10 mi.
13	Rest	Easy 7 mi.	Easy 7 mi. Cross-train	Intervals 5 mi.	Easy 4 mi.	Easy 4 mi.	Long 10 mi.
14	Rest	Easy 7.5 mi.	Easy 7.5 mi. Cross-train	Progression 4 mi.	Easy 3 mi.	Rest	5k Race
15	Rest	Easy 5 mi.	Easy 5 mi. Cross-train	Hill Repeats 2 mi.	Easy 4 mi.	Easy 4 mi. Cross-train	Long 11 mi.
16	Rest	Easy 5.5 mi.	Easy 5.5 mi. Cross-train	Fartleks 8 mi.	Easy 4.5 mi.	Easy 4.5 mi.	Long 12 mi.
17	Rest	Easy 6 mi.	Easy 6 mi. Cross-train	Intervals 6 mi.	Easy 5 mi.	Easy 5 mi. Cross-train	Tempo 7 mi.
18	Rest	Easy 6.5 mi.	Easy 6.5 mi. Cross-train	Progression 5 mi.	Easy 4 mi.	Easy 4 mi.	Tempo 8 mi.
19	Rest	Easy 7 mi.	Easy 7 mi. Cross-train	Hills 7 mi.	Easy 5 mi.	Easy 5 mi. Cross-train	Tempo 9 mi.
20	Rest	Easy 7.5 mi.	Easy 7.5 mi. Cross-train	Hills 5 mi.	Easy 4 mi.	Easy 4 mi.	Long 13 mi.

Advanced – Marathon 26.2 Miles (Continued)

Week	Sunday	Monday	Tuesday	Wednesday	Thursday	Friday	Saturday
21	Rest	Easy 8 mi.	Easy 8 mi. Cross-train	Progression 6 mi.	Easy 5 mi.	Easy 3 mi. Cross-train	Long 14 mi.
22	Rest	Easy 8 mi.	Easy 8 mi. Cross-train	Hill Repeats 1.5 mi.	Easy 4 mi.	Easy 4 mi.	Long 15 mi.
23	Rest	Easy 8.5 mi.	Easy 8.5 mi. Cross-train	Fartleks 5 mi.	Easy 6 mi.	Easy 6 mi. Cross-train	Long 12 mi.
24	Rest	Easy 9 mi.	Easy 9 mi. Cross-train	Progression 7 mi.	Easy 4 mi.	Easy 4 mi.	Long 13 mi.
25	Rest	Easy 9.5 mi.	Easy 9.5 mi. Cross-train	Intervals 4 mi.	Easy 5 mi.	Easy 5 mi. Cross-train	Long 14 mi.
26	Rest	Easy 7 mi.	Easy 7 mi. Cross-train	Hill Repeats 2 mi.	Easy 6 mi.	Easy 6 mi.	Long 15 mi.
27	Rest	Easy 7.5 mi.	Easy 7.5 mi. Cross-train	Progression 6 mi.	Easy 5 mi.	Easy 4 mi. Cross-train	Long 16 mi.
28	Rest	Easy 8 mi.	Easy 8 mi. Cross-train	Hills 4 mi.	Easy 5 mi.	Rest	10k Race
29	Rest	Easy 7 mi.	Easy 7 mi. Cross-train	Progression 7 mi.	Easy 5 mi.	Easy 5 mi. Cross-train	Long 18 mi.
30	Rest	Easy 7.5 mi.	Easy 7.5 mi. Cross-train	Progression 8 mi.	Easy 5 mi.	Easy 4 mi.	Long 20 mi.
31	Rest	Easy 7 mi.	Easy 7 mi. Cross-train	Hill Repeats 3 mi.	Easy 5 mi.	Rest	Long 22 mi.
32	Rest	Easy 8 mi.	Easy 8 mi. Cross-train	Hills 4 mi.	Easy 6 mi.	Easy 6 mi. Cross-train	Long 16 mi.
33	Rest	Easy 9 mi.	Easy 9 mi. Cross-train	Hills 5 mi.	Medium 5 mi.	Rest	Half Marathon Race
34	Rest	Medium 6 mi.	Easy 6 mi. Cross-train	Progression 6 mi.	Medium 3 mi.	Easy 3 mi. Cross-train	Long 25 mi.
35	Rest	Easy 5 mi. or Rest	Easy 5 mi. Cross-train	Progression 6 mi.	Easy 4 mi.	Easy 4 mi.	Tempo 20 mi.
36	Rest	Easy 10 mi.	Easy 10 mi. Cross-train	Easy 7 mi.	Easy 4 mi.	Rest	Easy 15 mi.
37	No Running	No Running	No Running	No Running	No running	No Running	Marathon Race
38	Recovery	Recovery	Recovery	Recovery	Recovery	Recovery	Recovery
39	Recovery	Recovery	Recovery	Recovery	Recovery	Recovery	Recovery
40	Recovery	Recovery	Recovery	Recovery	Recovery	Recovery	Recovery
41	Recovery	Recovery	Recovery	Recovery	Recovery	Recovery	Recovery

Motivation

"Under any circumstance, simply do your best, and you will avoid self-judgment, self-abuse and regret." *– Miguel Angel Ruiz*

Challenge!

Review

This chapter was like a marathon – the longest chapter in the book. Similar to a marathon, it took a lot of work and knowledge to create your very own traing plan. I've given you starter plans for you to use and adjust as needed, however if you adjust the daily schedule, try to avoid changing the weekly mileage. The gradual buildup to your eventual goal is centered on the weekly mileage and time on your feet.

Throughout this book, I've stressed the importance of setting goals and executing a specific plan to achieve your running goals. Remember, EVERY workout has a purpose, and EVERY mile must be run according to your training plan – don't run unnecessary junk miles! If you run hard, you should do it because it's in your plan for that day. If you rest or cross-train, you should do it because it's in the plan for that particular day.

MARATHONERS: If you plan on running a full marathon, review **Chapter 5 – Running Psychology** to establish the mental strength you'll need to push through the "wall." Continue on to **Chapter 6 – Running Physiology** and re-read the entire chapters so you know what your body is doing and WHY it's doing it. The knowledge of these two chapters will help you push through the "wall." Of course, neither chapter will help you unless you train properly

Your Challenge:
1) *Create a goal.*
2) *Create a plan (or use a plan that I've provided).*
3) *Document everything.*
4) *Follow the 7 Step Running Macrocycle – it's a proven method.*
5) *Feel free to adjust your daily plan, but avoid changing your weekly mileage.*
6) *If you're hurt or burned out, adjust your timeline, but don't change your goal. If you can't run your September half marathon, simply reschedule another a few months down the road.*
7) *Stay focused – Stick to the plan and honor your rest or cross-training days. Avoid "running streaks" to accumulate mileage.*
8) *ENJOY your running and remember why you started running in the first place.*

Your day is near! Turn to the next chapter and RUN YOUR RACE!

Chapter 17 – Running Your Race

You've covered a lot of ground in this book – from history, nutrition and health, all the way through the endless options in the training plans. You defined your goals and developed your project plan. You've done all the legwork, so to speak, except for the big race itself.

You've worked hard in your training, and hopefully, you'll show up to the start line fresh and optimistic for an outstanding performance.

This section will focus on the days leading up to the race, the race itself with post-race activities and expectations.

One of the most important things you can take away from your journey is this: Your race might not turn out the way you expected on race day. A lot of things can come up and keep you from reaching your goal, but don't let it get you down. Be proud of your accomplishments! Don't be discouraged if things don't go exactly as planned on your first attempt. They rarely do! The point is to learn and grow from your experiences and let running and other exercises forge your future to keep you healthy for the rest of your life. This book is not just about running – it's to help you manage a healthy and happy lifestyle. Running is just the bonus you get from your lifestyle changes!

I'd like to touch on a few things before we get to "race day." Those things, being the importance of the taper, nutrition, and hydration leading up to the big day. Let's break them down into three separate topics, so we can focus on each one independently.

The Taper

Obviously, you want to show up at the start line fit from your months of training, and well-rested. I've already stated it multiple times in this book, but please "honor the taper." Take advantage of the rest that you'll need to finish the race. You've gained an incredible amount of knowledge and built a fitness program that has left you strong and lean. Don't throw it all away now by adding more miles and fatigue. Your running program has tuned and refined your running abilities, and I promise that you will NOT lose your fitness by taking a few days off during the taper mesocycle. So once again, if your taper mesocycle calls for 3 days of "no running," simply do not run for 3 days. Instead, focus on the taper itself and prepare your body for the laborious event just a few days away!

Sleep is a wonderful thing, but some of us just can't seem to get enough of it, especially the night before a big race. My advice to you: Don't worry about sleep the night before the race. If you don't sleep because you're so excited, you really can't do much about it. Alcohol and sleep aids won't do you much good, and in fact they may make for a miserable day out on the course, so avoid them. Focus more on the nights of two, three and four days before the race. So, if you're wide awake in the wee hours of the night before your race, don't try to sleep. Just try to relax – this is normal for many runners, so just accept it. If you had plenty of rest the nights before, you should be just fine.

Nutrition

During your training, you should have been eating the proper amounts of carbs, fat and proteins, as we saw in **Chapter 10 – Nutrition.** You should have also "rehearsed" meals before your other races and long runs. By now, you should know what fuels your body and know what didn't work. During this most important week, the week of the taper, you should take great care in fueling your body, with an abundance of carbs and proteins and an avoidance of fats. You'll need fuels from complex sugar sources such as pastas and grains. And don't worry about gaining weight – you'll work off much of what you gained during your race.

Finally, you should know what your bowel habits are like during your training. If it took twelve hours for your pasta to "process," you should make sure that you eat twelve hours in advance of the start on race day. Eat foods that you're familiar with and foods that gave you plenty of energy during your training. The eve of the race is not the time to go out with friends and try new foods. Stick to foods that fuel you effectively.

Hydration

Of course, you should always be hydrated, but it's ever so important in the 24 to 48 hours leading up to the start of your race. Drink adequate amounts of water and sports drinks at the tune of six to eight ounces per hour, the day before the race. You'll know if you're hydrated properly if there is no sloshing of liquids in your stomach, and your urine is clear. Dark yellow urine before the big race is a recipe for disaster.

The Day Before

Typically, most races will have an expo before the race. This is a great time to relax, but try to get to the Expo early. For one thing, you may need to purchase gels or other supplies and you don't want to find out that your favorite vendor ran out. Better yet, purchase important gels and recovery drinks well ahead of the expo.

If your race does offer an expo, try to listen to the guest speaker if they have one. They can offer a wealth of information that can help you on the course.

Pick up your race packet, bib, safety pins and race information. READ the race information as there may be changes in the course or other last-minute deviations. Some vendors offer "pace bands" that go on your wrist and show predicted mile splits. Grab a couple of the bands that are close to your expected finish time, and put it with your supplies the night before.

If you can, try to drive the course to get familiar with it. Build a strategy in your mind and imagine how you'll attack that next big hill, or avoid going down a steep hill too fast.

Check the weather forecast and be prepared for inclement conditions. Be sure to use the "20-degree" rule mentioned earlier in this book. It can make or break your running experience.

The Night Before

During the evening hours, try to relax as much as possible. Avoid loud or stressful situations and keep the TV or radio down low. Quiet conditions can help you relax on a night when it may seem that sleep is impossible.

Eat early and take your normal medications. Avoid alcohol, caffeine and food that might disrupt your bowel functions. Prepare your body to race!

Be prepared by laying out your clothes, attaching your bib to your shirt or shorts. And remember, this ain't a rodeo – the bib goes on the FRONT, not the back of your clothing. The race directors want you to wear it on the front so they can verify your finish if their timing system goes down. Some smaller races don't use timing systems, so it becomes even more important to put it on the front side.

In an effort to help you prepare, I've made up this handy little checklist that can be used for any length of race. Feel free to make a copy of it and use it the night before. Your watch and MP3 player are charged, right?

Runner's Checklist					
FOOTWARE		**CLOTHING**		**ACCESSORIES**	
	Training shoes		Training shirt		BodyGlide, Aquaphor, etc.
	Race day shoes		Training shorts		Nipple guards
	Socks		Warm-up jacket and pants		Watch, HR monitor
	Band-Aids		Racing shorts		Hat, visor, sweat band
			Racing shirt		Arm warmers, sleeves
HYDRATION			Wind breaker, trash bag		Waist pouch and belt
	Water belt		Sports bra		MP3 player if allowed
	Water bottles		Underwear		Sunglasses
	Electrolyte drinks		20 degree rule clothing		Bib, safety pins
NUTRITION		**RECOVERY**		**EXTRAS**	
	Gel packs, gummy bears		Foam roller		GPS watch
	Electrolyte snacks		The "stick" roller		Reflective gear
	Electrolyte drinks		Compression socks		Sunscreen, lip balm
	Recovery drink		Blister kit		Small amount of cash

Finally, go to bed early. Even if you can't fall asleep for a while, the best thing you can do is simply relax.

Race Day is Here!

The big day that you've been preparing for is finally here and you're about to begin your race. If this is your first time, be prepared for a bit of uneasiness and chaos. This is a day when you can expect the unexpected.

As I pointed out in the prologue of this book, I found my very first race experience to be very rushed and chaotic. I didn't know about putting out my running clothes the night before. I didn't know that the lines at the porta-pots would be a mile long. I didn't know anything about race day. Simply put, I didn't know what I didn't know, so that's why I'd like to share my experiences with you now.

Early Morning

Eat a light meal, high in carbohydrates, at least two hours before your race is scheduled to begin. Caffeine is okay and may even help with your race. Try to empty your bowels before you race, and begin drinking 6 to 8 ounces of water or sports drink as soon as you get up. If you feel like showering, although it might seem to be counter-productive, by all means do it if it makes you feel more comfortable. It's a great way to wake up and prepare for the battle ahead.

Make sure you read your race instructions one more time before boarding the bus (if they have them) for final instructions. Get to the bus on time – there's no greater stressor than thinking you're going to miss your ride to the start line.

Make sure your bib is secured to your clothing with all four safety pins. Take a trash bag if it's cold or windy, and build a makeshift windbreaker out of it while you're standing at the start line.

Have a plan with an estimated time and location to meet your loved ones! Do this before the race. If you aren't sure, put your cell phone in your fuel belt pouch, and call your friends or family about 30 minutes before you get to the finish line.

Prepare Mentally

Your body is fully prepared for the race, but is your mind ready? Now's a good time to focus on deep breathing exercises. Quietly stating your mantra and visualizing the race course can calm your nerves. Try to clear your mind and de-stress before the start.

At the Starting Line

Try to stay warm and dry as long as possible. Many races have warm staging areas or even campfires to stay warm. Don't let your muscles get cold – wear sweatshirts and pants and place them in the gear bag to return to the finish area. Alternatively, you can wear "throw-away" sweats that you can discard on the side of the road, once the race begins. Please be courteous to others when you throw them to the side so that you don't trip somebody. Also, know that most of these clothes are given to charities by the race organizer, so don't expect to get them back. Stretch properly, like you did in your training program. Warm up if this is a short enough race that you won't burn extra energy.

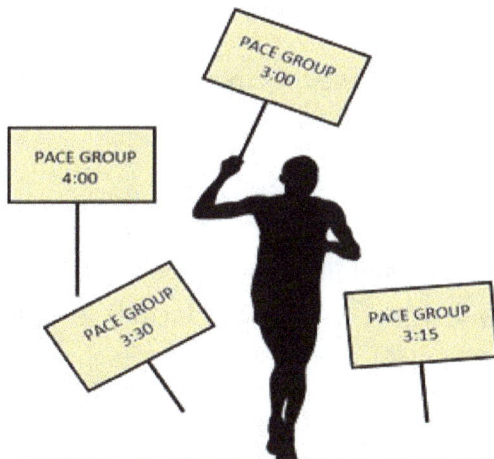

If you want to run a certain pace, most big races have "pace groups." Watch for runners with balloons or banners that have expected finisher times.

Pace groups are great for maintaining your goal pace and building camaraderie during the race. Be sure to join your pace group early, so you don't have to catch up during the race. If your pace group loses you, try to tag along with the next one that's moving at your pace.

Tip

How you get through a race:

- Run with your head; be smart about your pace early on.
- Run with your legs; keep in touch with your turnover.
- Run with your heart; keep going when your head and legs are telling you that you can go no further.

Motivation

"The miracle isn't that I finished. The miracle is that I had the courage to start." – John Bingham

Runners Beware

Many of the smaller races, especially the benefit races, offer entries for dogs and strollers. While they are welcomed in these races, they normally go to the back of the pack at the start line. Also, please note that not all races allow MP3 players with earbuds. Your race director will put this information in the race guidelines, and you may get sanctioned or completely disqualified if you're caught wearing them.

Many of the races don't have enough porta-pots at the start line or on the course. Please use discretion when the need arrives.

Finally, a final bit of etiquette – be courteous to other runners. Just like you, they worked very hard to get to the start line. Help others if they need assistance, and cheer them on for the greater good! Please show respect by being quiet and taking your hat off during the National Anthem.

The Race

Remember to go out slow and run the pace that you trained for, and visualize the course as you go. Focus on 90 to 94 steps per minute, just like you did in your training, and keep your running form consistent throughout the race. Make sure your watch is running at the start and stopped at the finish. Hit all the water stops along the way and consume gels or other nutrients every five miles of your race. Break the race up into manageable parts instead of the entire distance. For instance, focus on the sign about a half mile ahead and just get to that point before you focus on another object in the distance. Stay focused on each mile split to stay consistent with each segment. If the road has a great deal of camber on the side of the road, try to run on the opposite side for a while so your feet, ankles, knees and hips don't get sore.

If you see other runners in trouble, try to help or encourage them. Sometimes a kind word is all it takes to get going again.

The Finish

When you get to the finish line, collect your medal and stay on your feet if possible. Begin your recovery with appropriate food and beverages within 30 minutes of finishing. This will help re-energize your body and lead to a faster recovery. Finish knowing that you trained hard for this very moment. Embrace it, celebrate it. And then go cheer for the other runners!

After Your Race

Immediately after the race, stay on your feet until your blood pressure stabilizes. Hydrate as soon as possible by drinking water or sports drinks. High protein recovery drinks such as chocolate milk are also recommended. Be sure to eat plenty of carbs too, as they need to be replenished soon after your race.

Motivation

"A great accomplishment shouldn't be the end of the road, just the beginning point for the next leap forward." – *Harvey Mackay*

If you have access to ice or a massage, seek it out and get treatment to keep the inflammation down and return the blood flow to your lower extremities.

You'll most likely be sore that night and the following day; however, the worst pain may occur two or three days after your race. This is to be expected and can be minimized by taking ice or cold water baths and anti-inflammatory drugs like Ibuprofen to reduce the swelling in your muscles. Try to stay active by taking short therapeutic walks to keep the blood flowing to your legs.

If you're like most "average Joes," you'll most likely start searching for more races. Be sure to wait until you're fully recovered – physically and emotionally – so you don't face overuse injuries or mental burnout. Take the time to enjoy your accomplishment!

Challenge!

Evaluate

You've come a long way – from learning the definition of running to how running affects the mind, body and soul. You got an inside glimpse of great runners from the past and the present and looked at the benefits of running from mental, physical, emotional and social perspectives. You've studied the importance of proper health and nutrition, and found out what happens when you suffer from mental or physical fatigue. In the middle chapters of the book, we looked at the importance of having the right equipment to keep you safe and efficient.

Finally, you were able to set your goals and create your very own training plan, based on the proven method of the 7 Step Macrocyle program that I introduced to you. This set the wheels into motion, so you could train properly to achieve your goals.

Why did you start running? Were you trying to lose weight or did you just want to get in shape? Did you achieve your goals? At this point, I would hope that you achieved most of your goals and that you take the time to look in the mirror and evaluate yourself.

Your challenge: *When you look in the mirror, acknowledge your accomplishments and setbacks. Evaluate your experience and make adjustments to be even more successful next time. Turn the page and learn how to extend your running successes into other phases of your life!*

Motivation

"Your mind will answer most questions if you learn to relax and wait for the answer."
– *William S. Burroughs*

Chapter 18 – Extending Your Goals

We're on the final section of the book, but it doesn't have to be the end. Now is the time to ink the chapters of your running life. When you finish your first race, you may be hesitant to enter another one. Maybe you didn't meet your time goal and maybe you didn't even finish. That's okay because this isn't just about running, remember? This is about creating or enhancing a happy, healthy lifestyle. It's a personal commitment to YOU. Even if you never enter another race, at the very least, try to continue your fitness program, whether it's running, biking, swimming or any other type of physical activity. Do it for yourself and your family. And urge them to adopt a fitness program of their own!

Many of us will face injuries or burnout at some point and while you don't want to give up your fitness, you might want to take a hiatus from running or build up to something bigger. Or if you're bored with your running program and need to expand your horizons, you'll be thrilled to know that there are tons of options.

Some of these options might include changing the distance of your running program to greater (or lesser) distances. You can also change gears and look at variations of the sport including **Mud Runs, Warrior Dashes,** and **Spartan Races.** These are extreme racing programs that feature running with challenging obstacles. They can revive a stagnant running program and put the fun back into your training. Moreover, the entire family can get involved and everyone can compete together.

You can also switch to **duathlons, triathlons** and **biking,** with a choice of mountain or road biking. When you're facing an injury or burnout, or simply want to add more to your life, take a good look at these options.

Volunteers Needed

If you find yourself unable to compete, you can always volunteer at the races! Race directors are always looking for motivated, energetic people to help at the aid stations and cheer for the runners. Finally, ALWAYS thank the volunteers, police and paramedics. Without them, we wouldn't be able to run races in towns or the big cities. Many of them would rather be out there running with us, but for many different reasons, aren't able to. And of course, some are happy just helping out and watching the runners. Either way, you should make them feel appreciated and give them a great big "Thank you!" when you pass by them.

Parting Thoughts

When I first started running, I did it because I didn't feel good. I was overweight and unhealthy and needed something in my life to give it a boost. I didn't realize it at the time, but I forged my first goal when Keith convinced me to run. I had no idea that I would someday run an ultramarathon. I had no idea that it would lead me to goal after goal after goal. And that includes the penning of this book. I urge you as Keith urged me, to keep your dreams alive, extend your goals, and enhance your life with a fitness program that keeps you healthy and happy for years to come.

> **Motivation**
>
> **"Methinks that the moment my legs began to move, my thoughts began to flow."**
> — *Henry David Thoreau*

Values vs. Obsession

Don't let your obsession for running take over your life. Keep it balanced with your job, your spare time and your family. Consider travel destinations and family vacations when making your travel plans.

Pride vs. Humility

When you first start running, you'll find that you're proud of your accomplishments, but as you migrate to longer runs, such as half-marathons, full-marathons and ultramarathons, you'll see that your pride is displaced by humility. The longer distances can humble even the most prepared athlete. Be humble – stay humble.

Camaraderie

When you're done with your race, high five and cheer for the others who are still coming in. If someone wants to high five you during the race, accept their congratulations! Thank the volunteers for their efforts! Smile and be happy, enjoy the experience!

Pick up trash or move dangerous obstacles such as branches, barbed wire, etc., from the race course. It's not going to slow you down that much and could be a game changer for someone else.

Running Clubs

Again, this is a great way to stay motivated by running with others. Running in a group can help keep you safe too! Running clubs provide a great social network in a setting that supports your fitness levels and goals. These clubs usually offer different activities such as beginning running programs, regular group or training runs, distance training programs, organized racing teams, local calendar events, and much more. It's a great way to start or extend your running lifestyle by learning from experienced runners.

Charity Races

Get involved in non-profit events and charity races. These events can bring much-needed funding for research and awareness for groups that are trying to raise money for the greater good. This includes foundations for cancer research and other fundraising organizations. It's a great way to get motivated for a cause while increasing your fitness. Be aware, however, of organizations that are focusing more on the "branding" of their research instead of the actual benefits that the charity creates. Do your own research and make sure your donation will be used for the intended purpose.

Additional Inspiration

Many people inspired and motivated me during the writing of this book. My father, Gordon "Fuzz" Watts, my friend Keith Panzer and many others whom I personally know or simply know about; they all contributed in some way. But no one contributed more than the other runners out there, the "average Joes." These are the middle of the pack or even the back of the pack runners. No one suffers more than they do; I know because I've been there. I have more respect for these runners than I do for the elite runners because they're NOT gifted or talented. They inspire because they know that *winning* isn't nearly as important as *finishing*.

I know a few elite runners who never seem to be satisfied, despite winning it all. I also know a lot of "average Joes" who are perfectly content because they were able to finish today and let tomorrow take care of itself.

At a Turkey Trot 5k, I met a young, talented 11-year-old boy and he beat me by about 30 seconds. I saw him at the finish line, cheering the other runners on. I was at a "flat spot" in my book, and while he was motivating the other runners, he also motivated me to get back to writing. It just goes to show you that anyone at any age can motivate you, and the motivation doesn't just stop at running. It can spread to other facets of your life. So go out and motivate, go out and inspire. You never know whose life you're going to touch.

Live to run, run to live...

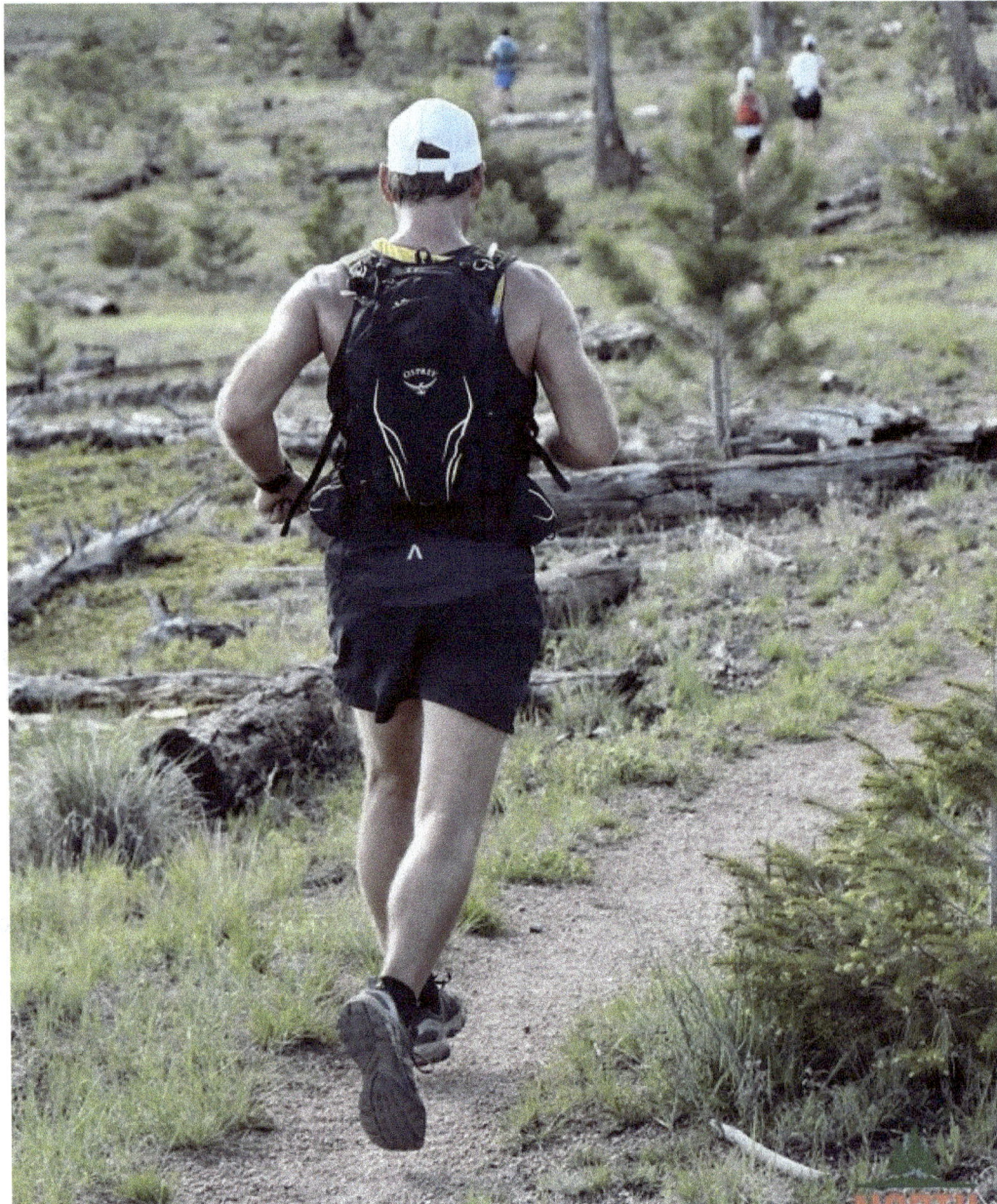

Running the 2021 North Fork 50-Miler in Colorado – Happy Trails!

Glossary

ATP – Adenosine triphosphate is considered by biologists to be the most important component of energy production. It is the high-energy molecule that stores the energy that the human body uses to function.

DNF – Acronym for "did not finish."

Femur – The large bone in your upper leg, also known as the *thighbone*.

Fibula – The smaller of the two bones in your lower leg.

Glycogen – Glycogen is the main form of glucose storage in the human body. Glucose that isn't immediately used by the body is stored as glycogen. Most of the glycogen is stored in the liver, and a small amount is stored in muscle tissue. During intense or lengthy exercise, available glucose is expended and the body is then able to use the glycogen stores to provide energy for the body.

Ketone bodies – Acetone, acetoacetate, and beta-hydroxybutyrate are chemicals that the body manufactures when there is not enough insulin in the blood. The function of ketone bodies is to convert fatty acids into water-soluble substrates that are easier to transport and metabolize in the body.

Lactate – Lactate is produced when your body burns glucose. Often confused with lactic acid, this lactate is then reprocessed by the body back into glucose and used as fuel. Excess lactate is sent to other parts of the body. When there is an excess of lactate, it raises your blood lactate levels.

Lactate Threshold – The lactate threshold is the exercise intensity at which lactate starts to accumulate in the blood stream

Macrocycle – By common definition, a macrocycle is normally made up of smaller *mesocycles* within its entirety. A macrocycle is usually thought of as long cycle such as 6 months, 1 year or 2 years in length.

Metabolism – Metabolism is the total of all the chemical reactions an organism needs to survive. It can also refer to the processing and transport of chemicals, enzymes and substances between different cells in the body.

Mesocycle – A mesocycle is analogous to a *phase* of an entire production cycle, known as a macrocycle. A mesocycle is usually thought to have a life cycle of 1 week to 2 months. A third cycle or phase, known as a *microcycle* normally has a duration of 7 days or less. (Microcycles are not referenced in this book.)

Mitochondria – Known as the energy creators of the cell, they act as a processing system that admits nutrients into the cells, breaks them down and creates energy-rich molecules to be used by the cells. This process is known as *cellular respiration*. (See page 58)

Mitochondrial Biogenesis – This is the process by which new mitochondria are formed in the cell, usually during environmental stimuli or stress in the cells.

Negative Split – A negative split is defined as the second portion completed in a faster time than the first portion. For example, Joe had a negative split when he ran the first half of his marathon in 2 hours, and the second half in 1 hour and 50 minutes.

PR – Personal record or personal best time for a given distance.

PTSD – Post Traumatic Stress Disorder is categorized as mental illness that develops after a person is exposed to one or more traumatic events.

RICE – RICE is a form of therapy used to alleviate pain and swelling. It is simply an acronym for: **R**est, **I**ce, **C**ompression and **E**levation.

Tibia – The larger of the two bones in your lower leg, also known as the *shinbone*.

VO2 max – VO2 max is simply a measure of the maximum volume of oxygen that an athlete can use. It is measured in milliliters per kilogram of body weight per minute (ml/kg/min). See the bottom of page 49 for an easy-to-understand description of VO2 max.

ACKNOWLEDGEMENT

Admittedly, I'm not a writer. I work in the Information Technology business to pay the bills, and I run to relieve the stress of everyday life. So, when I decided to write this book, I assembled a collage of notes and thoughts strewn about in a notebook. I finally starting transcribing these into my word processing program, but it still lacked clarity in many ways.

To the rescue came my niece, **Kristen Bashaw**, professional editor extraordinaire! She somehow made sense of my efforts and helped me reorganize many pages of this book. Thanks Kristen, for the fantastic advice and dedicated hard work to help me finish this project. It's been an awesome experience, and I am grateful for you, and deeply indebted to you.

Many thanks to **Doug Davis** of Vandavauk Photography, friend and photographer, for taking many of the photos in the book and attempting to teach me how to use Photoshop. Thanks to my son **Billy Watts** who redesigned the front and back covers for the book.

I'd like to give a very special "thank you" to **Keith Panzer** – as a long-time friend and fellow runner, Keith is the one who first introduced me to running as a way of life. He also posed for many of the pictures in the "Strength and Conditioning" chapter of this book.

Finally, thanks to my wife **Jeanne**, and the friends and family members who have supported and encouraged me in this journey! I believe that having faith in a higher power has given me the grace and guidance to help me through some very difficult times and bring this book to fruition.

Credits – Text **Also includes charts and tables if applicable**

Definition of "run" on page 11: American Psychological Association (APA): run. (n.d.). *Dictionary.com Unabridged*. Retrieved February 02, 2016 from Dictionary.com website http://dictionary.reference.com/browse/run
Chicago Manual Style (CMS): run. Dictionary.com. *Dictionary.com Unabridged*. Random House, Inc. http://dictionary.reference.com/browse/run (accessed: February 02, 2016).
Modern Language Association (MLA): "run". *Dictionary.com Unabridged*. Random House, Inc. 02 Feb. 2016. <Dictionary.com http://dictionary.reference.com/browse/run>.

"Tip" on page 13 was adapted from *The International Journal of Sports Physiology and Performance – May 2013*. Reprinted with permission.

"Short Distance Runners" on pages 23 and 24 was adapted from "Roger Bannister." *Wikipedia, The Free Encyclopedia*. Author: Wikipedia contributors. Date of last revision: 25 January 2016, Date retrieved: 4 February 2016

Permanent link: https://en.wikipedia.org/w/index.php?title=Roger_Bannister&oldid=701638966
Page Version ID: 701638966. Reprinted with permission.

"Who Runs Ultramarathons?" on page 28, 29 - Ultramarathon runner Marshall Ulrich adapted from private E-mail correspondence with Marshall and Heather Ulrich. Printed with permission.

"Dick Hoyt and his son Rick" on page 37 adapted from private E-mail correspondence with "Team Hoyt." Printed with permission.

"Physiology" on page 45, 46 was adapted from "Human brain." *Wikipedia, The Free Encyclopedia*. Author: Wikipedia contributors. Date of last revision: 4 February 2016, Date retrieved: 4 February 2016 Permanent link: https://en.wikipedia.org/w/index.php?title=Human_brain&oldid=703205244
Page Version ID: 703205244 Reprinted with permission.

"Cardiac Arrest" on page 63, 64 was adapted from "Cardiac Arrest during Long Distance Running Races," printed by the *New England Journal of Medicine* in 2012. Reprinted with permission.

"What Does Fitness Mean?" on page 162 was adapted from information gathered from the *United States Department of Health and Human Services*.

© "My Story" throughout this book developed by William Watts

© "Tips" throughout this book developed by William Watts

© Tables on pages: 110-112, 124, 126, 188, 189, 199, 200, 230, 258 developed by William Watts

© "Training Plans" on pages 234 to 254 developed by William Watts

Credits – Photography   Also includes graphics and icons if applicable.

© William Watts: pages 3, 6, 7, 13, 16, 17, 18, 20, 24, 32, 35, 38, 43, 44, 46, 48, 49, 54, 58, 61, 63, 67, 68, 70, 71, 72, 73, 74, 76, 79, 86, 87, 88, 89, 98, 99, 101, 102, 105, 106, 107, 108, 109, 110, 111, 112, 113, 115, 122, 124, 125, 126, 127, 128, 130, 132, 134, 136, 137, 138, 140, 141, 142, 144, 145, 146, 147, 148, 149, 150, 151, 152, 153, 154, 155, 156, 157, 179, 188, 189, 190, 192, 195, 197, 199, 200, 201, 202, 206, 210, 211, 212, 215, 218, 219, 220, 221, 223, 229, 232, 245,252, 260, front cover, back cover

Foreword: Photo of Bill Watts and Marshall Ulrich by Jeanne Watts

Page 8: "Discobolus." *Wikipedia*. Wikimedia Foundation, n.d. Web. 14 Feb. 2016.

Page 10: Wikipedia contributors. "Eliud Kipchoge." *Wikipedia, The Free Encyclopedia*. Wikipedia, The Free Encyclopedia, 2 Jan. 2022. Web. 9 Jan. 2022.

Page 18: "Usain Bolt." *Wikipedia*. Wikimedia Foundation, n.d. Web. 19 Feb. 2017.

Page 25: "Steve Prefontaine." *Wikipedia*. Wikimedia Foundation, n.d. Web. 16 Feb. 2016.

Page 28: Photo of Marshall Ulrich – *Marshall Ulrich* 27 Feb 2016 - Special thanks to Marshall and Heather Ulrich for contributing such detailed facts for this book. Be sure to visit them at www.marshallulrich.com

Page 29: "Marshall Ulrich's 220 pound elephant" - *Ben Jones* 25 Feb 2016 – Special thanks to Heather Ulrich for contributing this photograph, and Ben Jones for reprint permission.

Page 33: "Trail Running." *Wikipedia*. Wikimedia Foundation, n.d. Web. 16 Feb. 2016.

Page 34: "Titus Canyon." *Wikipedia*. Wikimedia Foundation, n.d. Web. 16 Feb. 2016.

Pages 37, 264: ."Dick Hoyt and his son Rick" – Special thanks to Dick, Rick, Kathy and all of Team Hoyt for providing great pictures and additional inspiration! Be sure to visit them at www.teamhoyt.com.

Page 53: By Adrian Grycuk - Own work, CC BY-SA 3.0 pl, https://commons.wikimedia.org/w/index.php?curid=32152574.

Page 54: "When Things Go Terribly Wrong" – Photo by Jeanne Watts

Page 56: "Dehydration" – Baines, Christofer P. "USMC-100612-M-3240B-303.jpg." *Wikimedia*. N.p., n.d. Web. 22 Feb. 2016. (Marine Corps Public Domain photo)

Page 64: Cardiac Arrest - "Heart." *Wikipedia*. Wikimedia Foundation, n.d. Web. 23 Feb. 2016.

Page 85: "Circulatory System." *Wikipedia*. Wikimedia Foundation, n.d. Web. 25 Feb. 2016.

Page 95: By Flickr user Alan Cordova - Paula & Isla Radcliffe on FlickrOriginally uploaded to the English Wikipedia at Image: Paula & Isla Radcliffe 2007 NYC.jpg, CC BY 2.0, https://commons.wikimedia.org/w/index.php?curid=4831627

Page 119: By AJ Guel - originally posted to Flickr as Arian Foster, CC BY 2.0, https://commons.wikimedia.org/w/index.php?curid=12191360

Page 120: "Scott Jurek" By Windriverwild - Own work, CC BY-SA 3.0, https://commons.wikimedia.org/w/index.php?curid=33988096

Page 155 – "Foam Roller" pictures of Jeanne Watts by Bill Watts

Pages 166-178: "Exercise photos" – All photos of Keith Panzer by Doug Davis, Vandavauk Photography.

Page 182: "By http://www.marines.mil/unit/mcbjapan/PublishingImages/2010/Sep10/IMG_1967.jpg, Public Domain, https://commons.wikimedia.org/w/index.php?curid=22963546.

Page 183: "Yoga." *Wikipedia*. Wikimedia Foundation, n.d. Web. 07 Mar. 2016.

Page 209: By J Krabbe at English Wikipedia - Transferred from en.wikipedia to Commons., Public Domain, https://commons.wikimedia.org/w/index.php?curid=2198416

Page 264: Photo purchased by Bill Watts from the Bear Chase 50 Mile Race of 2021

Page 278: Photo of Bill Watts near Jones Pass, Clear Creek County, Colorado by Jeanne Watts, 31 July, 2020.

Index

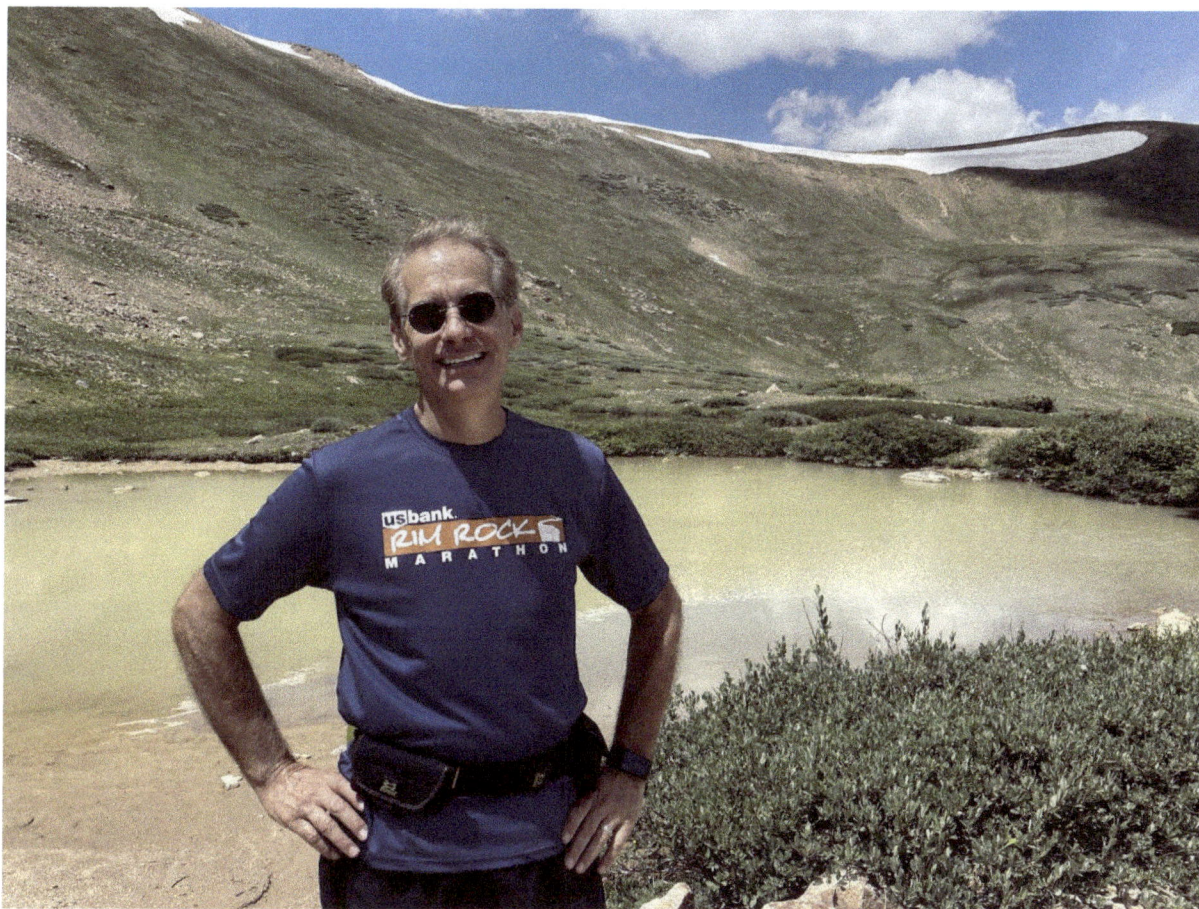

About the Author

Bill Watts is an avid outdoor enthusiast and experienced, but self-proclaimed "average" runner.

Born in a small town in northwest Nebraska, he was involved in high school sports. He played football, baseball, and was on the wrestling and track teams but admits he absolutely hated running at that time. 25 years later, he entered his first 10k race and has since entered over 350 races, from 5k street races all the way up to 50-mile trail races. He's raced in over 100 marathons in the past 20 years and estimates that he's logged about 80,000 miles in that time.

Watts won the highly coveted RRCA Grand Masters Marathon championship in both Colorado and Wyoming in 2017, and the RRCA Senior Grand Masters 50k championship in Colorado during his 2019 running campaign. He also has several sub-three-hour marathons on his resume, all after the age of 51.

During the summer of 2017, Watts ran the entire Colorado Trail, covering 516 miles and more than 92,000' of elevation gain in just 13 days from Durango to Denver, CO. He completed the Colorado Trail again in the summer of 2022, this time in the opposite direction, from Denver to Durango.

Watts works in the Information Technology business as a Systems Engineer and resides in Colorado. He is also a Certified Personal trainer, receiving his accreditation through the National Academy of Sports Medicine (NASM-CPT), with a focus on endurance running.

Running Log

Welcome to the WattsRunning Training Log! This is a basic running lot to get you started. If you're going to track more than the basic time, mileage and comments, I encourage you to use one of the many online tracking websites such as Garmin, Endomondo, Strava, etc. There are many other logs, spreadsheets and tracking websites on the internet — you simply have to find one that you like. Since it is a basis log, we'll cover the various fields and I'll show you an example of how to fill it in. Feel free to copy this sample or download them from WattsRunning at no charge.

At the very least, note the *distance, time, pace* and *comments*. The comments field will be crucial in constructing your training plan, so the more detail you have, the better information you'll have to create your plan.

Week	Day	Distance	Time	Pace (Avg)	HR (Avg)	HR (Max)	Type	Route	Comments
1	SUN	4 miles	:35:24	8:51	125	141	Fartleks	Track	Felt sluggish, weather was nice
	MON		: :						
	TUE	X-train	:30:00						Lap swimming
	WED		: :						
	THU	2 miles	:22:40	11:20	140	156	Hills	Apex Park	Felt great!
	FRI	11 miles	1:35:20	8:40	147	159	Progression run	River Run	Very cool weather, but felt good.
	SAT		: :						
2	SUN		: :						
	MON								

*For best results, use with the **WattsRunning Training Plan Builder** and **Training Plan Schedules**. For "Race Day," see the **WattsRunning Racing Log**.*

Running Log

Month _____ Year _____

Week	Day	Distance	Time	Pace (Avg)	HR (Avg)	HR (Max)	Type	Route	Comments
1	SUN		: :						
	MON		: :						
	TUE		: :						
	WED		: :						
	THU		: :						
	FRI		: :						
	SAT		: :						
2	SUN		: :						
	MON		: :						
	TUES		: :						
	WED		: :						
	THU		: :						
	FRI		: :						
	SAT		: :						
3	SUN		: :						
	MON		: :						
	TUE		: :						
	WED		: :						
	THU		: :						
	FRI		: :						
	SAT		: :						
4	SUN		: :						
	MON		: :						
	TUE		: :						
	WED		: :						
	THU		: :						
	FRI		: :						
	SAT		: :						
TOTALS									

Racing Log

Welcome to the WattsRunning Racing Log! Similar to the Running Log, this log is formatted for your race day achievements. Be sure to log your overall and division placements so you can you see your improvements! Feel free to copy this sample or download them from WattsRunning at no charge.

Date	Race Name	Distance	Time	Pace (Avg)	Pace (Max)	HR (Avg)	HR (Max)	Overall Place	Division Place	Comments
11/25	Turkey Day 5k	3.1 miles	:25:13	8:07	7:22	144	160	15/221	2/11	2nd in my age group!
12/7	Santa Claus 10k	6.2 miles	:53:37	8:38	7:44	142	153	35/412	16/23	Didn't place but had fun anyway
12/15	Snowman Stomper	10	1:27:08	8:43	8:12	130	145	67/888	14/109	Avg HR lower each time!
			: :							
			: :							
			: :							
			: :							
			: :							

Racing Log

Year _____

Date	Race Name	Distance	Time	Pace (Avg)	Pace (Max)	HR (Avg)	HR (Max)	Overall Place	Division Place	Comments
			: :							
			: :							
			: :							
			: :							
			: :							
			: :							
			: :							
			: :							
			: :							
			: :							
			: :							
			: :							
			: :							
			: :							
			: :							
			: :							
			: :							
			: :							
			: :							
			: :							
TOTALS										

www.ingramcontent.com/pod-product-compliance
Lightning Source LLC
Chambersburg PA
CBHW061959090426
42811CB00006B/990